Respiratory Care
of the Newborn

Contributors

Marlis E. Amato, B.S.R.T., R.R.T.
Chapters 8–10
Director of Clinical Education, Respiratory Therapy Programs,
Onondaga Community College, Syracuse, New York

Kathleen M. Beney, M.S., R.R.T.
Chapter 16
Research Associate, Department of Critical Care and Emergency
Medicine, SUNY Health Science Center, Syracuse, New York

Michael Boroch, M.B.A., R.R.T.
Chapter 17
President, Health Network Associates, Houston, Texas

Daniel V. Cleveland, B.S.R.T., R.R.T.
Chapters 11, 12
Director, Respiratory Therapy Department,
St. Mary's Health Care Services,
Rochester, New York

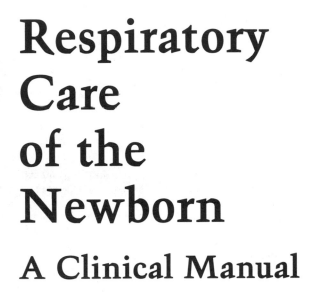

Respiratory Care of the Newborn

A Clinical Manual

Claire A. Aloan, M.S.E., R.R.T.

Program Director, Respiratory Therapy Programs,

Onondaga Community College, Syracuse, New York

With Four Additional Contributors

J.B. Lippincott Company

Philadelphia   London   Mexico City   New York

St. Louis   São Paulo   Sydney

Acquisitions Editor: Lisa A. Biello
Sponsoring Editor: Sanford J. Robinson
Manuscript Editor: Leslie E. Hoeltzel
Indexer: Angela Holt
Art Director: Tracy Baldwin
Design Coordinator: Don Shenkle
Designer: Arlene Putterman
Production Supervisor: Kathleen P. Dunn
Production Coordinator: Carol A. Florence
Compositor: TAPSCO, Inc.
Printer/Binder: R. R. Donnelley & Sons Company

6

Library of Congress Cataloging-in-Publication Data

Respiratory care of the newborn.

Includes bibliographies and index.
1. Respiratory organs—Diseases. 2. Infants
(Newborn)—Diseases. 3. Respiratory therapy for
newborn infants. I. Aloan, Claire. [DNLM:
1. Respiratory Tract Diseases—in infancy & childhood. 2. Respiratory Tract Diseases—therapy.
WS 280 R4332]
RJ434.R47 1986   618.92'2   86-7270
ISBN 0-397-50666-X

The author and publisher have exerted every effort to
ensure that drug selection and dosage set forth in this
text are in accord with current recommendations and
practice at the time of publication. However, in view of
ongoing research, changes in government regulations,
and the constant flow of information relating to drug
therapy and drug reactions, the reader is urged to check
the package insert for each drug for any change in
indications and dosage and for added warnings and
precautions. This is particularly important when the
recommended agent is a new or infrequently employed
drug.

Preface

Over the past decade and more, the art and science of respiratory care for the newborn has expanded rapidly. From initial attempts to modify adult treatments and equipment for the tiniest newborns, we have progressed to the present-day proliferation of equipment intended solely for infants and small children. Our ability to support very premature infants, and our ability to do so without replacing an acute problem with a chronic one, has increased markedly. Respiratory therapists are increasingly involved in the care of newborns in nurseries of all sizes and intensities. The development of Level III nurseries, with their increasing sophistication in treating and monitoring the sick newborn, requires more knowledge of perinatal medicine in general and respiratory care in particular on the part of all care personnel, including both therapists and nurses. On the other hand, the nursery in the small, community-based hospital must be able to stabilize these infants and keep them going until the transport team from the Level III facility arrives to take over. In between, many hospitals have found that they can manage infants who are not terribly sick but who require some degree of "intensive care" provided that they have a respiratory care staff that can support their needs.

Respiratory Care of the Newborn: A Clinical Manual is intended to be used both as a textbook for students of respiratory care who are learning to care for the compromised newborn and as a reference book for those currently involved in respiratory care of the newborn, both therapist and nurse. It is not intended to serve as a procedures manual, but rather as a *clinical* text and reference. The major content of the book is directly related to the evaluation and management of the newborn with respiratory disease, or with some other disorder that compromises the respiratory system. Because the best patient care seems to flow from the team approach, in which physicians, nurses, and therapists work in close association, each lending special expertise to the management of the newborn, this book also touches on several subjects of peripheral interest to the respiratory therapist but of primary concern to other members of the team (and, of course, to the patient!), such as prenatal and perinatal assessment, hematology, and special problems of the newborn, including bilirubin excretion and intracranial hemorrhage. *Respiratory Care of the Newborn* begins with a discussion of the development of the fetus and of the transition from fetal to neonatal life, which forms the basis for understanding the problems that may arise in the newborn period. Evaluation of the newborn is addressed from several aspects, including those that alert us to possible problems prenatally, physical assessment techniques so vital to the minute-to-minute care of the newborn, various types of laboratory and radiologic assessment, and noninvasive monitoring techniques such as transcutaneous monitors and oximetry. Disorders that appear commonly and not so commonly in the newborn are reviewed, including primary respiratory disease and cardiovascular disorders and congenital anomalies. Finally, techniques used to treat these various disorders are reviewed, including oxygen therapy, positive pressure, bronchial hygiene, airway care, and resuscitation, as well as the application of respiratory care to the patient well enough to be transferred to the home.

It is my hope that *Respiratory Care of the Newborn: A Clinical Manual* will help the members of the team to move forward in our mutual understanding of the various facets of respiratory care so vital to the lives of our very special patients, and thereby to increase our movement toward our goal of increasing the quality of life for all of them.

Claire A. Aloan, M.S.E., R.R.T.

Acknowledgments

Special thanks to those who have inspired and nurtured me both personally and professionally, and who have supported me without reserve:

> To Roger and my family, for your love and support.
>
> To Jack Lyda, who got me started and kept me going.
>
> To Marlis, Dan, Larry, Sherry, Betty, Linda, Jan, Kathy, Amy, Mary, Mary Jane, Keith, Paul, and all the rest of the OCC staff, past and present, for your dedication to the cause in spite of the obstacles.
>
> To Dr. Siddiqui and the nursery staff at the Holy Cross Hospital in Fort Lauderdale, Florida, who taught me what teamwork is all about.
>
> And to Lisa and Sanford, who knew all along I'd make it.

Contents

I·
From
Fetus
to
Neonate

1·
Gestational
Development

Development of the pulmonary system

The lung develops as a bud off the anterior portion of the foregut at approximately 3 weeks of gestation and continues to develop by both single budding and irregular branching. Cartilage appears at the 4th week, with distinct rings in the trachea by the 7th week. By week 6, the embryo has a tracheobronchial tree with 18 segmental bronchi. Pulmonary arteries and veins develop along with the branching airways. By week 16, the conducting airways of the tracheobronchial tree are present in miniature form, but respiratory bronchioles have not yet developed. By the 24th week, respiratory bronchioles, alveolar ducts, alveoli, pulmonary vessels, and lymphatic vessels have begun to develop. The alveoli are still rudimentary. By the 26th week, formation of the alveolar–capillary unit is sufficient to allow extrauterine life, although many capillaries still are not in contact with air spaces. By weeks 27 to 28, there are more alveolar sacs and more capillaries in contact with them, allowing for better gas exchange potential. The connective tissue spaces between terminal gas-exchange units remain quite large, making the lung compliance low and allowing for accumulation of fluid and air (interstitial emphysema). The large interstitial space also widens the distance for diffusion of gases from alveoli to capillaries, thus impeding gas exchange. From this point forward, new alveolar growth is rapid. By weeks 34 to 36, the alveoli are mature in form. Alveoli continue to develop after birth in both number and size. Alveolar growth in numbers has usually been completed by the age of 8 years, while alveoli increase in size until adulthood. The growth and the development of the pulmonary structures are summarized in Table 1-1.

PHASES OF LUNG DEVELOPMENT

Reid has described four phases of lung development, which is an ongoing process from the beginning of fetal development through adulthood. These phases are the glandular phase, the canalicular phase, the alveolar phase prenatally, and the postnatal phase. The glandular period extends from conception to about 16 weeks of gestation. During this period, development of the tracheobronchial tree is the major event. The canalicular phase is from 16 to 24 weeks, during which respiratory bronchioles develop, along with other components of the gas-exchange unit (alveolar ducts, alveoli, and pulmonary capillaries). Cartilage and glands also develop during this period. The alveolar phase begins at 24 weeks and lasts until term. As the name implies, the major event during this period is the formation of alveolar sacs. Postnatally, alveoli grow in both number and size.

Surfactant development

Pulmonary surfactants are a mixture of phospholipids and proteins and are responsible for altering the surface tension at the alveolar level. These surfactants are secreted by Type II alveolar cells (also called Type II pneumocytes). The major surfactant is phosphatidyl choline, commonly called lecithin. Without an adequate supply of surfactant, alveoli tend to collapse on expiration (atelectasis), making the lungs very stiff and noncompliant. The occurrence of noncompliant lungs caused by immature surfactant production in the newborn is called hyaline membrane disease (HMD) or respiratory distress

Table 1-1
Sequential development of the pulmonary system

Gestational age	Development
24 days	Primitive lung bud appears
26–28 days	Lung bud divides into beginnings of two major (main-stem) bronchi
By 6 weeks	Segmental bronchi are formed
By 12 weeks	Major lobes are differentiated
16 weeks	Respiratory bronchioles are differentiated
24 weeks	Alveolar sacs are formed
25–26 weeks	Alveolar–capillary surface is capable of sustaining extrauterine life
28–29 weeks	Terminal sacs are lined with mature Type II cells from which surfactant is released
30–33 weeks	New alveolar units appear rapidly
34–36 units	Mature alveolar structures are evident

syndrome (RDS). Two pulmonary surfactants, lecithin and sphingomyelin, produced by the fetus and secreted into the amniotic fluid have been found to change in concentration during gestation and to correlate well with the development of lung maturity.

SPHINGOMYELIN AND LECITHIN

Sphingomyelin is a pulmonary surfactant found in amniotic fluid in fairly constant amounts with advancing gestation. Beginning at about 18 weeks of gestation, sphingomyelin concentrations rise slowly to a peak at 30 weeks and then decline to term. Lecithin concentrations also rise from about 18 weeks but surge abruptly at approximately 34 weeks and reach a peak at 38 weeks. Lecithin may be produced by several metabolic pathways. The surge in production at 34 weeks represents synthesis of lecithin by a more mature and stable pathway, which coincides with fetal lung maturity (Fig. 1-1).

Assessment of lung maturity

The production of these two types of surfactants and their secretion into amniotic fluid can be detected by chemical analysis of amniotic fluid obtained from amniocentesis. The relationship or ratio of lecithin concentration to sphingomyelin concentration (L/S ratio) is calculated and used as an estimate of fetal lung maturity.[1] L/S ratios of greater than 2.0 predict mature lungs and are rarely associated with respiratory distress. If the L/S ratio is less than 1.0, severe lung immaturity is present and respiratory distress syndrome is likely. If the L/S ratio is between 1.0 and 2.0, respiratory distress syndrome may or may not develop. The incidence and the severity of respiratory distress correlate with L/S ratio and with factors such as low birth weight and birth asphyxia.

The shake test is another procedure that attempts to determine lung maturity.[3] Samples of amniotic fluid are mixed with alcohol and shaken, forming bubbles at the surface. The samples are then allowed to stand, and the stability of the bubbles is observed. A complete ring of bubbles at the surface after 15 minutes indicates that the L/S ratio is 2.0 or greater, predictive of fetal lung maturity. If bubbles are absent, pulmonary immaturity is likely. The absence of bubbles is not as

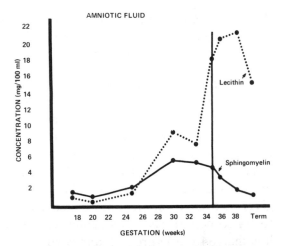

AMNIOTIC FLUID

Fig. 1-1. Lecithin and sphingomyelin levels in amniotic fluid during gestational development. (Avery GB: Neonatology: Pathophysiology and Management of the Newborn, 2nd ed, p 109. Philadelphia, JB Lippincott, 1981)

specific as a low L/S ratio. Because this test is simple to perform, it may be used as a screening test. A positive test, determined by the presence of stable bubbles, indicates maturity and should not require further testing. In the absence of bubbles, an L/S ratio should probably be performed.

Under certain conditions, the L/S ratio may not correlate well with gestational age, although it will still be predictive of pulmonary maturity. Some conditions may accelerate the maturation of the lungs, whereas others may delay maturation. Thus an L/S ratio of 2.0 or greater, which would usually indicate a gestational age greater than 34 weeks, may occur in a fetus who is less than 34 weeks but who has accelerated lung maturation. This accounts somewhat for the occurrence of relatively mild or no respiratory distress in some infants of low gestational age. Conditions that may be associated with accelerated maturation of the lungs include toxemia, maternal hypertension, severe diabetes, maternal infection, prolonged rupture of the membranes, and placental insufficiency. Conditions associated with delayed maturation of the lungs include mild diabetes, fetal Rh disease, and smaller identical twins.

Other variables may affect the accuracy of the L/S ratio measurement: If there is maternal bleeding into the amniotic fluid, for example, the L/S ratio will tend to read falsely low. Meconium in the amniotic fluid may also affect results, with both false-negative and false-positive results possible.

Acceleration of lung maturation

The maturation of the lungs, through the induction of surfactant production, has been shown to be accelerated by the administration of corticosteroids.[2] This fact has allowed the administration of corticosteroids to the mother before delivery if the fetus is known to have immature lungs. Betamethasone and dexamethasone have been used and should be given at least 48 hours, but not more than 7 days, before delivery to be effective. Additionally, only gestational ages of less than 34 weeks are affected by this therapy, with the most significant results occurring between 30 and 32 weeks of gestation. The use of these drugs does not entirely prevent the development of RDS, but both the incidence and the severity of RDS may be reduced.

Fetal circulation

The placenta is the nutrient, gas exchange, and waste removal organ for the fetus. It provides direct contact between the circulation of the mother and the circulation of the fetus while keeping the two blood supplies separate. Segments called cotyledons that contain fetal vessels, chorionic villi, and an intervillous space comprise the placenta. The chorionic villi are fingerlike projections of tissue that invade the uterine wall at the site of implantation of the placenta. These villi contain the fetal capillaries. The spaces formed in the uterine wall by the villi are surrounded by maternal blood. These blood-filled areas are the intervillous spaces and are the site of exchange of nutrient, gaseous, and waste substances between the maternal and fetal blood. The surface area for exchange provided by this system increases throughout pregnancy to meet the needs of the growing fetus.

Maternal blood is supplied to the placenta by the uterine arteries, and oxygenated blood from these arteries surrounds the villi. Fetal blood enters the placenta through two umbilical arteries in the umbilical cord, and these vessels branch and terminate in capillaries within each villus. After exchange has taken place, fetal blood returns to the fetus through a single umbilical vein, and maternal blood drains back into the venous system.

As a gas-exchange organ, the placenta acts to allow diffusion of oxygen from the maternal arterial blood into the fetal circulation and to allow diffusion of carbon dioxide from the fetus into the maternal circulation, and subsequently to be returned to the lungs by way of the maternal venous system. Fetal blood that has supplied fetal tissues, thus losing oxygen and gaining carbon dioxide, enters the placenta by way of the umbilical arteries. Once it has exchanged with the maternal circulation, fetal blood leaves the placenta by way of the umbilical vein, now richer in oxygen and poorer in carbon dioxide. Thus, in the fetus, the umbilical vein carries the highest oxygen concentration. Average oxygen saturation in the umbilical vein is about 80%, equivalent to a P_{O_2} of about 29 mm Hg. Some of the blood in the umbilical vein supplies the fetal liver, with the remaining blood being diverted through the ductus venosus into the inferior vena cava. The inferior vena cava already contains some blood that is returning from the lower part of the body after having supplied the tissues there, and it is thus low in oxygen. The mixing of oxygenated blood from the umbilical vein and deoxygenated blood from the tissues results in an oxygen saturation of about 67% in the inferior vena cava. This blood then returns by way of the inferior vena cava to the heart, where it enters the right atrium. At this point, there is some mixing with deoxygenated blood from the superior vena cava, which drains the upper part of the body, resulting in a slight drop in oxygen saturation to about 62%. Most of the blood from the inferior vena cava, however, is diverted directly from the right atrium into the left atrium through an opening called the foramen ovale. The left atrium also receives some blood from the pulmonary veins. This blood now proceeds from the left atrium to the left ventricle and is ejected into the ascending aorta, where it supplies the coronary arteries and the vessels of the head and the upper extremities of the left side of the body. Thus, blood that is relatively rich in oxygen supplies the brain and heart of the fetus, the organs that use the most oxygen.

Blood returning to the heart from the superior vena cava enters the right atrium, flows into the right ventricle, and is ejected into the pulmonary artery. This blood is relatively low

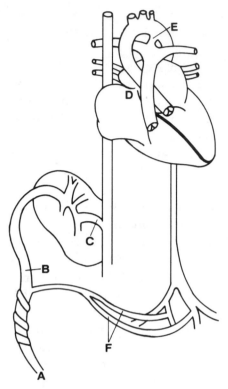

Fig. 1-2. Fetal circulation. (A) Placenta, (B) umbilical vein, (C) ductus venosus, (D) foramen ovale, (E) ductus arteriosus, (F) umbilical arteries.

in oxygen, with a saturation of about 52%. Once it has entered the pulmonary artery, most of the blood is diverted into the descending aorta through the ductus arteriosus. This blood supplies the lower part of the body and the umbilical arteries. Only about 10% of the blood ejected from the right ventricle passes into the pulmonary circulation; there is, of course, no reason to provide a large supply of blood to the pulmonary system because the fetal lung is filled with fluid and does not play a role in gas exchange. The pulmonary vascular resistance in the fetus is high because of several factors: The pulmonary vessels are kinked and tortuous, and the fluid filling the alveoli exerts pressure against them; and the very low P_{O_2} leads to hypoxic vasoconstriction of these vessels.

In summary, there are several unique features of the fetal circulation (Fig. 1-2). The *placenta* serves as the organ of gas exchange. The *umbilical vein* serves to return oxygenated blood from the placenta to the fetus. The *ductus venosus* diverts some of this blood into the inferior vena cava. Blood returning to the right atrium through the inferior vena cava is selectively diverted to the left atrium through an opening called the *foramen ovale*, which allows blood relatively rich in oxygen to be supplied to the brain and heart. Blood entering the right heart from the superior vena cava, which is low in oxygen, enters the pulmonary artery, where most of the blood is diverted to the descending aorta through the *ductus arteriosus*, a vessel that connects the pulmonary artery and the descending aorta. Blood from the descending aorta supplies the lower part of the body and also supplies the *umbilical arteries*, which will return blood to the placenta to pick up oxygen and remove carbon dioxide.

Objectives

Having completed this chapter, the reader should be able to do the following:

1. Describe the sequence of events that occurs in the normal development of the pulmonary system.
2. Discuss the four phases of lung development as described by Reid.
3. Explain the significance of pulmonary surfactants and their relationship to gestational age.
4. Discuss the use of the L/S ratio and the shake test to predict fetal maturity and lung function.
5. Explain the intrinsic and extrinsic factors that may influence fetal lung maturation.
6. Describe the anatomy and function of the placenta.
7. Describe the fetal circulation.
8. List the factors that contribute to elevated pulmonary vascular resistance in the fetus.
9. Define the following terms:

glandular phase	chorionic villi
canalicular phase	intervillous space
alveolar phase	umbilical artery
surfactant	umbilical vein
L/S ratio	ductus venosus
shake test	ductus arteriosus
placenta	foramen ovale
cotyledon	

References

1. Gluck L, Kulovich MV, Borer RC Jr: Estimates of fetal lung maturity. In Nesbitt REL (ed): Clinics in Perinatology, vol 1. Philadelphia, WB Saunders, March 1974
2. Liggins GC, Howie RN: A controlled trial of antepartum glucocorticoid treatment for prevention of the respiratory distress syndrome in premature infants. Pediatrics 50:515, 1972
3. Platzker A, Tooley W et al: Prediction of the idiopathic respiratory distress syndrome by a rapid new test for pulmonary surfactant in amniotic fluid. Clin Res 20:283, 1972
4. Reid L: The embryology of the lung. In DeReuck AVS, Porter R (eds): Ciba Foundation Symposium: Development of the Lung. Boston, Little, Brown and Company, 1967

Bibliography

Dancis J: Fetomaternal interaction. In Avery GB (ed): Neonatology: Pathophysiology and Management of the Newborn, 2nd ed. Philadelphia, JB Lippincott, 1981
Gluck L: Fetal lung development. In The Surfactant System and the Neonatal Lung, Mead Johnson Symposium on Perinatal and Developmental Medicine no. 14, 1978
Murray JF: The Normal Lung: The Basis for Diagnosis and Treatment of Pulmonary Disease. Philadelphia, WB Saunders, 1976
Richmond B, Galgoczy M: Development of the cardiorespiratory system. In Lough MD, Williams TJ, Rawson JE (eds): Newborn Respiratory Care. Chicago, Year Book Medical Publishers, 1979

2·
Fetal–
Neonatal
Transition

Initiation of respiration

It is now known that intrauterine breathing movements occur commonly in the human fetus. Little is currently understood about the significance of these movements, or about what factors may stimulate or depress them. Perhaps they occur naturally as a prelude to extrauterine breathing. The factors that stimulate the infant to initiate respiration at birth are better known, although the relative roles of various factors are unclear. Stimulation to breathe is probably caused by several factors, both chemical and sensory in nature.

During the normal birth process, placental circulation is impaired; because the placenta provides for gas exchange, transient fetal asphyxia (hypoxia, hypercapnia, and respiratory acidosis) results. These chemical stimulae, through their effects on chemoreceptors, provide a strong stimulus to breathe. Prolonged asphyxia, however, resulting in metabolic acidosis as well as in the previous chemical changes, tends to depress rather than to stimulate respiration.

Sensory stimuli may also play an important role in the initiation of respiration. The fetus is enveloped in a warm, wet atmosphere *in utero*. The sudden departure from this environment into the relatively cool, dry air of the delivery room stimulates nerve endings in the skin and causes subsequent transmission of impulses to the respiratory center in the brain. In addition, handling of the newborn infant provides tactile stimuli, which may also contribute to the first efforts at breathing.

The lung *in utero* is normally filled with fluid. After the infant is delivered, the fluid must be replaced with air as the lungs replace the placenta as the organ of gas exchange. Several factors assist in this transition. During normal vaginal delivery, the thoracic cage is greatly compressed as the fetus passes through the birth canal. This "squeezing" of the chest cage helps to eject some of the fluid from the lungs. After birth, the chest cage recoils, which may passively introduce some air into the lungs. As the newborn infant receives stimuli from the chemical and sensory changes associated with birth, he initiates nerve impulses to the muscles of respiration, resulting in an expansion of thoracic volume and a decrease in intrathoracic pressure. Thus a pressure gradient is established, allowing air to flow into the lungs. To overcome the surface tension of the alveoli and the viscosity of the remaining lung fluid, the newborn infant must often generate negative intra-thoracic pressures of 60 to 80 cm H_2O. The volume of the first breath varies from infant to infant, averaging about 40 ml. Not all of this air is exhaled after the first inspiration, with approximately 20 to 30 ml remaining in the lungs as the infant begins to establish his functional residual capac-ity (FRC).

Subsequent breaths will require lower transpulmonary pressures, as more and more alveoli remain inflated after each breath. The opening of alveoli occurs serially, so that each alveolus becomes fully inflated before the next one opens. A normal FRC is usually established within the first few hours after birth. This sequence of events, of course, represents the normal course of events and requires the presence of surfactant in sufficient quantities to prevent alveolar collapse at the end of expiration. In infants who are born prematurely or who for other reasons have insufficient surfactant, the alveoli collapse and the infant cannot establish a normal FRC. This means that the effort to inflate the lungs with each succeeding breath does not decrease and accounts for the respiratory distress seen in these infants.

As previously mentioned, it is necessary not only to move air into the lungs but also to move fluid out. There are three primary mechanisms through which this occurs. As much as one third of the total lung fluid may be squeezed out during passage through the birth canal. Infants born by cesarean sec-tion do not experience this "squeezing" and may be more likely to have difficulty in clearing lung fluid, resulting in the transient tachypnea syndrome; however, many infants born by cesarean section do not develop this problem because they apparently clear lung fluid adequately through the remaining two mechanisms: absorption into the pulmonary capillaries and clearance by the pulmonary lymphatic system. Because of the very negative pressures created in the pleural space dur-ing the first breaths, a pressure gradient is established from the alveoli to the interstitial space, favoring movement of fluid out of the alveoli. In addition, the opening of the alveoli stretches the alveolar walls and enlarges the normal alveolar wall openings or pores, allowing fluid easier exit from the alveoli into the interstitial space. The large increase in pulmonary blood flow that occurs after birth also helps to remove fluid from the lungs. In the normal term infant, fluid removal to the interstitial space is complete within several breaths, although it may take several hours to remove excess fluid from the interstitial space by means of the capillaries and lymphatics.

Transition to neonatal circulation

The unique aspects of the fetal circulation have previously been described. After birth, several events occur that cause the circulation to change from the fetal to the neonatal (or "adult") circulatory pathway. As with the initiation of respiration and removal of lung fluid, these changes occur very rapidly following delivery and are not sequential.

CLOSURE OF THE FORAMEN OVALE

Once the infant has been delivered, the umbilical cord is clamped, thus removing the infant from the placental circulation. This results in less blood flow returning to the right atrium and thus decreases the pressure on the right side of the heart. In addition, the placenta is a low-pressure circuit. Loss of this low-pressure outlet for aortic blood flow results in an increased pressure on the left side of the heart. Following birth, pulmonary vascular resistance falls, pulmonary perfusion increases greatly, and a much greater volume of blood is returned to the left atrium through the pulmonary veins, further increasing the pressure on the left side of the heart. This difference in pressure between the right and left sides results in functional closure of the foramen ovale, which is essentially a flap valve. When the pressure on the left is greater than the pressure on the right, the flap closes. If these pressures are reversed, the flap opens. Functional closure of the foramen occurs almost immediately after birth. Anatomic closure does not occur for weeks or months after birth, and the foramen ovale may remain patent throughout adult life. Should the pressures on the right side of the heart be elevated, the foramen may reopen and allow for shunting of blood from the right side of the heart to the left side without passing through the pulmonary circulation.

PULMONARY VASCULAR RESISTANCE

The major event that alters pressure on the right side of the heart is pulmonary vascular resistance, or resistance to outflow from the right side of the heart. Normally, pulmonary vascular resistance falls abruptly at birth for several reasons. As the fluid is removed from the alveoli, there is less pressure on the pulmonary vessels. As the alveoli expand, they exert traction on the pulmonary vessels, helping to straighten them. As the infant begins to breathe, oxygen tensions rise and the hypoxic vasoconstriction of pulmonary vessels seen in the fetus is reversed. Carbon dioxide tensions fall, also helping to reverse vasoconstriction. Thus we can see that a number of factors may contribute to an elevated pulmonary vascular resistance in the newborn: failure to remove lung fluid adequately; failure to inflate the lungs adequately; hypoxia; and hypercapnia. If pulmonary vascular resistance does not fall, the infant is likely to continue to use fetal circulatory pathways rather than perfusing the pulmonary capillary bed. This makes it very difficult to oxygenate the infant because there is little blood coming in contact with air spaces.

DUCTUS ARTERIOSUS

Constriction and closure of the ductus arteriosus occur for several reasons. The decrease in pulmonary vascular resistance allows a much greater portion of the blood ejected from the right ventricle to enter the pulmonary circulation, thus decreasing the blood flow through the ductus. Unlike the foramen ovale, the ductus arteriosus does not close functionally immediately at birth. During the first few hours of life, the ductus remains open and ductal blood flow, although greatly reduced, continues. The direction of flow will usually be from the aorta (left side) to the pulmonary artery (right side) since, as previously discussed, the pressures on the left or systemic side of the circulation become much greater than the pressures on the right or pulmonary side immediately after birth. Over the next several hours, the ductus will begin to constrict, primarily in response to elevated oxygen tensions. This is the opposite response from the pulmonary circulation: Hypoxia causes vasoconstriction in the pulmonary vascular bed, whereas elevated oxygen causes vasoconstriction of the ductus arteriosus. Conversely, hypoxia will result in failure of the ductus to constrict. Anatomic closure of the ductus arteriosus is usually complete by 3 weeks of age. Following complete constriction, the ductus arteriosus becomes a ligament (the ligamentum arteriosum).

The premature infant may have some difficulty in constriction and closure of the ductus arteriosus because his capacity to respond to elevated oxygen tensions is not well developed. This is probably related to the levels of prostaglandins in the ductus of the premature infant. Prostaglandins E1 and E2 are responsible for keeping the ductus open during fetal life. In the premature infant, they may continue to do so. The enzyme complex responsible for the formation of prostaglandins is called prostaglandin synthetase. Prostaglandin synthetase inhibitors, by decreasing the activity of this enzyme complex, can help to decrease the levels of prostaglandins and thus promote constriction of the ductus arteriosus. Indomethacin is a prostaglandin synthetase inhibitor commonly used with good success in infants with patent ductus arterious.

DUCTUS VENOSUS

The ductus venosus closes anatomically within 3 to 7 days after birth. There is very little blood flow after closure of the umbilical circulation. The mechanism of closure of this vessel is unknown.

Fetal hemoglobin

Fetal hemoglobin differs from adult hemoglobin in its affinity for oxygen. The relationship between oxygen and hemoglobin is represented by the oxyhemoglobin dissociation curve (Fig. 2-1), which relates partial pressure of oxygen to the percentage of hemoglobin saturation. In other words, for any given oxygen partial pressure (P_{O_2}), a hemoglobin saturation can be predicted. Fetal hemoglobin has a greater affinity for oxygen

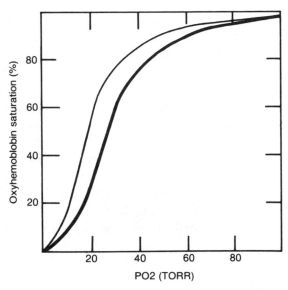

Fig. 2-1. The oxygen dissociation curves for normal adult blood and, to the left, the dissociation curve for fetal blood, demonstrating an increase in the affinity of fetal hemoglobin for oxygen and a decrease in the release of oxygen.

than does adult hemoglobin, which means that at any given P_{O_2}, fetal hemoglobin will have a higher percentage of saturation with oxygen than will adult hemoglobin. This is often expressed as a shift of the curve to the left. Another way of expressing this relationship is the P_{50}, which is the partial pressure of oxygen at which the hemoglobin will be 50% saturated. The P_{50} of adult blood is normally 27 mm Hg. Fetal blood has a P_{50} that is 6 to 8 mm Hg lower than that of the normal adult. This means that fetal hemoglobin binds oxygen more readily and releases it less readily.

The major reason for the difference in oxygen affinity of adult and fetal hemoglobin is related to an organic phosphate, 2,3-diphosphoglycerate (2,3-DPG), which, when bound to hemoglobin, reduces the affinity of hemoglobin for oxygen. In other words, it shifts the curve to the right or increases the P50. Fetal hemoglobin cannot bind 2,3-DPG as well as can adult hemoglobin, and thus has more affinity for oxygen.

In the newborn, the ability to bind and release oxygen will thus be related both to the level of fetal hemoglobin present and to the amount of 2,3-DPG in the blood. The level of

2,3-DPG rises throughout gestation and is similar at term to that of adults. It then falls for the first several days after birth, rising again to values exceeding those at birth by the end of the first week of life. Fetal hemoglobin is high in the term newborn and diminishes gradually over the first year of life, causing the oxyhemoglobin dissociation curve to shift gradually to the right. The P_{50} value is usually increased to the adult level by 6 months of age. This shift differs for premature infants, who have lower 2,3-DPG values and higher fetal hemoglobin levels. The shift in the curve (rise in P_{50}) for premature infants is much more gradual than that for term infants, which means that for any given P_{O_2} level, the premature infant will usually have less oxygen available for release at the tissue level.

Objectives

Having completed this chapter, the reader should be able to do the following:

1. Describe the chemical and sensory factors that stimulate respiration at birth.
2. Discuss the factors that contribute to the removal of fetal lung liquid.
3. Describe the establishment of functional residual capacity in the newborn.
4. Discuss the pressure gradients involved in initial respiratory efforts.
5. Describe the changes that occur in the circulatory system at birth.
6. Discuss the factors that influence the transition from fetal to neonatal circulation at birth.
7. List the factors that contribute to a decrease in pulmonary vascular resistance and closure of the ductus arteriosus at birth.
8. Describe the role of prostaglandins and oxygen tensions in circulatory transition.
9. Compare fetal and adult hemoglobin function.
10. Discuss the significance of the presence of fetal hemoglobin.
11. Define the following terms:
    P50   oxyhemoglobin dissocia-
    2,3-DPG   tion curve
                                             prostaglandin synthetase

Bibliography

Avery ME, Fletcher BD: The Lung and Its Disorders in the Newborn Infant. Philadelphia, WB Saunders, 1974

Escobedo MB: Fetal and neonatal cardiopulmonary physiology. In Schreiner RL, Kisling JA (eds): Practical Neonatal Respiratory Care. New York, Raven Press, 1982

Nelson NM: The onset of respiration. In Avery GB (ed): Neonatology: Pathophysiology and Management of the Newborn, 2nd ed. Philadelphia, JB Lippincott, 1981

Sanderson RG: Anatomy, embryology, and physiology. In Sanderson R, Kurth CL (eds): The Cardiac Patient: A Comprehensive Approach, 2nd ed. Philadelphia, WB Saunders, 1983

II·
Evaluation
of the
Newborn

3.
Prenatal and Perinatal History

The high-risk mother

Many factors lead to the categorization of a high-risk pregnancy, including maternal age and parity, history of previous births, use of drugs, tobacco, and alcohol, maternal disease, and anatomic problems of the mother.

MATERNAL AGE AND PARITY

Neonatal morbidity and mortality are affected by maternal age, with infants of both young and older women being at increased risk. The highest risk occurs if the mother is younger than 16 years of age or older than 40. The upper age limit is reduced if it is a first pregnancy. The term *gravida* is used to refer to pregnancy. A woman who is pregnant for the first time is referred to as a *primigravida.* The term *para* refers to completion of pregnancy resulting in a potentially viable infant. Thus a woman who delivers for the first time is a *primipara* or *primiparous*, sometimes abbreviated as *primip.* This term is used regardless of the outcome of the pregnancy, so that whether the birth results in a live or stillborn infant or whether one or more than one infant is delivered, the woman who delivers for the first time is a primipara. A woman who has delivered more than once is referred to as *multiparous.* Grand multiparity (*e.g.*, more than five previous pregnancies) is also associated with increased risk to the fetus.

HISTORY OF PREVIOUS BIRTHS

If a mother has had difficulty with previous pregnancies, she will be considered high risk. Some of these previous problems include cesarean section, miscarriage, premature or postmature birth, fetal or neonatal death, infant of high birth weight, and infant requiring either intrauterine or neonatal exchange transfusion.

TOXEMIA OF PREGNANCY AND UTEROPLACENTAL INSUFFICIENCY

Many maternal diseases are also associated with increased risk to the fetus. The most common of these are toxemia of pregnancy and other hypertensive disorders, diabetes mellitus, and maternal infection. Toxemia is characterized by hypertension, edema, and proteinuria in the third trimester of pregnancy. Toxemia that leads to convulsions is referred to as *eclampsia.* The term *pre-eclampsia* is used interchangeably with toxemia. Maternal hypertension that occurs in toxemia may lead to decreased placental blood flow, resulting in uteroplacental insufficiency (UPI). Other causes of hypertension, such as renal disease, essential hypertension, or diabetes, may also result in UPI. In addition, UPI may occur in postmaturity, cyanotic maternal heart disease, and chronic hypoxia associated with maternal pulmonary disease. It is more likely to occur in elderly primigravidas and should be suspected when third trimester bleeding or oligohydramnios (deficient amount of amniotic fluid) occurs. The decrease in intervillous blood flow associated with maternal vascular disease results in a limitation of gas and nutrient exchange across the placenta, which may produce no growth of the fetus (intrauterine growth retardation), intrauterine fetal death, chronic intrauterine asphyxia, or the passage of meconium into the amniotic fluid, with the subsequent possibility of meconium aspiration into the lungs of the fetus.[15] If UPI is suspected, assessment of placental function will be performed, using urinary estriol levels and evaluation of fetal heart rate patterns during fetal movement or during induced contractions. In addition, fetal lung maturity should be assessed, usually by determining the L/S ratio of amniotic fluid. Delivery of the immature fetus is avoided whenever possible, but if UPI appears to be severe, as indicated by both falling estriol levels and abnormal fetal heart rate responses, intervention may be necessary even with fetal immaturity because the fetal prognosis is very poor under these circumstances.

MATERNAL DIABETES MELLITUS

Maternal diabetes mellitus (DM) is also associated with increased fetal risk. Some of the more common problems occurring in infants of diabetic mothers (IDMs) include prematurity, stillbirth, congenital anomalies such as congenital heart disease, and birth injury due to very large (macrosomic) infants. In addition, maternal diabetes predisposes to the development of toxemia and hypertension, with the consequent possibility of UPI. The classic IDM is described as a fat, plethoric, large infant, but maternal diabetes may also result in diminished fetal growth owing to placental insufficiency. White has classified diabetes in pregnancy, and this classification helps to predict fetal outcome.[18] Class A diabetes in pregnancy is characterized by mild diabetes that is controlled by diet alone. Class A diabetics tend to have large infants but do not usually have infants with other problems. Classes B through F are insulin-dependent diabetics, with classification dependent on age of onset, duration of diabetes before current pregnancy, and presence of vascular disease. Class B diabetics tend to have had recent onset of diabetes, short duration of diabetes, and no vascular involvement, whereas Class F diabetics have had juvenile onset of diabetes, long duration of diabetes, vascular disease, and kidney involvement. Class B mothers tend to have classic large IDMs, whereas Classes C through F are more likely to deliver infants who are of normal size or small for gestational age. It should also be remembered that maternal DM influences maturation of the fetal lungs. Less severe classes of diabetes are associated with delayed maturation of the lungs, whereas chronic intrauterine stress associated with severe DM may accelerate lung maturation.[10] This means that many of the infants seen in the nursery born to diabetic mothers are large yet premature, with lungs that are even less mature than gestational age would predict. Thus respiratory distress syndrome is likely to occur in these infants and is an important cause of perinatal morbidity and mortality in the IDM. In addition, IDMs tend to have increased susceptibility to infection, partly because of their prematurity but possibly related to the increased incidence of urinary tract infections in the diabetic mother. They are also likely to manifest hypoglycemia, hypocalcemia, and hyperbilirubinemia in the neonatal period.[7]

ALCOHOL, DRUGS, AND TOBACCO

The maternal use of alcohol, drugs, and tobacco is also associated with increased risk to the fetus. Smoking more than one pack per day of cigarettes is associated with an increased risk of low birth weight with its concomitant problems. Acute alcohol consumption before delivery, although it may cause withdrawal symptoms such as tremors and seizures in the newborn, does not result in fetal abnormality. Chronic alcohol consumption during pregnancy is much more ominous, often resulting in the fetal alcohol syndrome, which includes low birth weight, fetal wasting, and various developmental disorders, such as abnormal brain development and cardiac anomalies.[5] Other drugs consumed by the mother may affect the fetus. Those that most commonly affect respiration are the sedative drugs, including those given during labor, which may result in depression of respiration in the newborn. Maternal narcotic addiction may result in withdrawal symptoms in the infant, including tremors, dyspnea, cyanosis, convulsions, and death and may also cause intrauterine growth retardation.[9]

MATERNAL INFECTIONS

Maternal infections may also result in increased risk of abnormal fetal outcome. Although many infectious processes may compromise the fetus, the most notable examples include rubella, toxoplasmosis, herpes, cytomegalovirus, and syphilis.

Rubella infection is associated with a wide range of outcomes, including intrauterine death and severe multiple organ-system disease. Most commonly, though, rubella infection results in no obvious neonatal disease, although most of these symptom-free neonates will develop later evidence of infection. Common disorders seen in infants born with effects of rubella infection include cardiac defects, cataracts, and deafness. Rubella infection is also associated with intrauterine growth retardation. The most serious outcomes are usually associated with infection early in pregnancy.[14]

Toxoplasmosis is caused by a protozoa that may be acquired from consumption of contaminated raw or undercooked meat or from oral contact with contaminated cat feces or soil. Maternal infection is difficult to diagnose because it rarely causes symptoms more specific than swelling of lymph glands. Congenital infection may result in various fetal outcomes, including inflammation of the eye, anemia, convulsions, jaundice, splenomegaly and hepatomegaly, hydrocephalus, and pneumonia. Varying degrees of sight loss, including blindness, and of retarded psychomotor development are not uncommon.[1]

Cytomegalovirus infection, like toxoplasmosis, is difficult to recognize in the adult. Infection of the fetus may result in a broad spectrum of neonatal disorders, including bleeding disorders, CNS disorders that may cause apnea or seizures, hyperbilirubinemia, and pneumonia. Intrauterine growth retardation may also occur.[16]

Herpes simplex virus occurs in two strains, called types 1 and 2. Type 2 is sexually transmitted and infects the genitalia. The infant usually acquires herpes infection during birth by contact with infected genital secretions or by vertical transmission from the mother to the fetus following rupture of the membranes. Recognition of maternal disease is often difficult because the infection does not always result in noticeable symptoms. Disease in the neonate falls into one of two classes: disseminated or localized.[13] Disseminated disease affects almost every organ system, including the lungs, and is associated with a high mortality rate. Localized disease most commonly affects the CNS, eyes, and skin and is much less likely to cause death. Since infection is rarely acquired in the presence of intact membranes, cesarean section is recommended in the presence of active genital infection to avoid perinatal infection of the newborn.

Maternal syphilis, a sexually transmitted disease caused by the spirochetal bacteria *Treponema pallidum*, is relatively easy to detect using antibody testing of maternal blood. Unfortunately, clinical manifestations of this disease are often overlooked, and many women (specifically, those most likely to harbor this infection) do not avail themselves of prenatal care and thus of the opportunity for blood testing for syphilis. Clinical features of congenital syphilis include intrauterine death, prematurity, hepatitis, hyperbilirubinemia, hepatosplenomegaly, CNS abnormalities, skin lesions, bone disorders, and, occasionally, pneumonia.[16]

ANATOMIC ABNORMALITIES

Maternal anatomic abnormalities such as small bony pelvis, uterine malformations, and incompetent cervix may increase fetal risk. The risk of birth trauma is increased if the bony pelvis is small, and cesarean section delivery may be necessary. Uterine malformations and incompetent cervix may increase the risk of premature delivery of the infant.

Other risk factors

Several other factors may increase fetal risk, including multiple gestation, problems with the placenta, premature rupture of the membranes, and postmaturity.

MULTIPLE GESTATION

Perinatal mortality is increased among twins, with identical twins having higher risk than fraternal twins. The most common event affecting multiple gestation pregnancies is prematurity. In addition, problems of the placenta and cord occur more frequently, as does intrauterine growth retardation. In some twin births, one placenta is considerably smaller than the other, and the twin supported by this placenta is markedly smaller. This occurrence is referred to as discordant twins. Abnormal fetal presentation, particularly breech, is also more common in twins.

Another problem that sometimes occurs in multiple gestation pregnancies is the twin transfusion syndrome, also called the intrauterine parabiotic syndrome, in which the circulations of the fetuses are connected. This allows for transfer of blood from one fetus to the other, resulting in one twin with polycythemia and one with anemia. The polycythemic twin may have congestive heart failure caused by volume overload and is also more susceptible to increased bilirubin levels because there are more red cells available for hemolysis. The anemic twin may be in shock owing to acute and dramatic blood loss to the other twin.

PLACENTAL PROBLEMS

Problems that affect the placenta include abnormal implantation, referred to as placenta previa, and abnormal separation, called abruptio placentae or placental abruption. Normally, the placenta is implanted in the upper wall of the uterus; in placenta previa, it is implanted in the lower wall. Three types of placenta previa occur: In total placenta previa, the placenta completely covers the cervical opening of the uterus; in partial placenta previa, the cervix is partially occluded by the placenta; and in low implantation, the cervix is not occluded at all, although the placenta is implanted very close to the cervical orifice. The major problems resulting from placenta previa are an increased incidence of premature labor and early separation of the placenta, reducing fetal–maternal gas exchange and resulting in fetal asphyxia. Maternal or fetal hemorrhage may also occur. Placenta previa is usually identified by ultrasound examination.

Abruptio placentae involves premature separation of a normally implanted placenta. When the placenta separates at its margin, referred to as marginal abruption, bleeding occurs along the uterine wall and ultimately presents as vaginal bleeding. This is the most common type of abruption. Bleeding may also occur in the central portion of the placenta, but this does not usually result in vaginal bleeding and is thus more difficult to recognize. Both types of abruption increase the incidence of fetal asphyxia and premature delivery, as well as fetal hemorrhage and shock.

PREMATURE RUPTURE OF MEMBRANES

Premature rupture of membranes (PROM) increases the likelihood of fetal infection, especially pneumonia. Generally, rupture is considered premature if it occurs more than 24 hours before delivery of the infant. Early rupture with prolonged labor further increases the risk of fetal infection. PROM is more likely to occur in premature infants than in full-term infants. At this point the relative risks of infection versus premature delivery must be considered. If the risk of infection appears high, as judged by maternal fever or infected amniotic fluid, acceleration of fetal lung maturity with steroids followed by delivery of the fetus may be indicated.

POSTMATURITY

An infant delivered after the 42nd week of gestation is defined as postmature. Placental function begins to decline after term, and these infants are often small for gestational age with signs of wasting. Physical signs of postmaturity include dry, cracked skin, long nails, excessive scalp hair, and loose skin, owing to loss of subcutaneous fat. Postmature infants also may have meconium staining of the skin, nails, and umbilical cord. This decline in placental function, in addition to diminished fetal growth, also predisposes the postmature infant to intrauterine asphyxia and death. These infants do not tolerate the stress of labor well, since labor interferes with an already malfunctioning placental circulation. Assessment of the postmature fetus may involve amniocentesis, urinary estriol testing, and stress testing to determine placental function. Meconium staining of fluid, oligohydramniosis, poor response to stress testing, and falling estriols may all indicate that placental function is impaired and that delivery, either by induction of labor or by cesarean section, is indicated.

Consequences of increased fetal risk

The major consequences to the fetus who is determined to be at risk because of any of these factors include prematurity, intrauterine growth retardation, and asphyxia.

PREMATURITY

Prematurity is defined as delivery before the end of the 37th week of gestation. Although most premature infants are of low birth weight, not all low-birth-weight infants are premature. Thus, classification of prematurity by gestational age rather than by birth weight is appropriate. Premature infants have the highest infant mortality rate, which is inversely proportional to gestational age (*i.e.*, the lower the gestational age, the higher the mortality). The major problem of prematurity is, as has previously been described, with the respiratory system. The surface area for gas exchange develops rapidly during the last weeks of gestation, as does the mature form of pulmonary surfactant. Both of these are necessary for adequate extrauterine respiratory function. Impaired gas exchange caused by inadequate surfactant is referred to as hyaline membrane disease or respiratory distress syndrome and is discussed in Chapter 8. In addition to respiratory problems, premature infants have difficulty absorbing nutrients from the digestive tract, poor defenses against infection, problems with thermoregulation because of increased rate of heat loss, poor tissue perfusion owing to immature capillary development, and an increased incidence of hemorrhage, particularly into the ventricles of the brain. The most common disorders occurring in the premature infant are thus hyaline membrane disease (HMD), intraventricular hemorrhage (IVH), asphyxia, and infection.

INTRAUTERINE GROWTH RETARDATION

Intrauterine growth retardation (IUGR) is also known as small for gestational age or small-for-dates. These terms do not imply anything about the maturity of the infant, nor do they tell the cause of the diminished growth rate of the fetus. The type of growth retardation that occurs depends on when during the pregnancy factors causing diminished growth occur. If the insult occurs early in pregnancy, when fetal growth occurs primarily due to formation of new cells, growth retardation will manifest as hypoplasia, with fewer new cells formed and small underweight organs. Later in pregnancy, fetal growth occurs primarily due to increase in size rather than number of cells. Growth retardation then causes underweight organs with a normal number of cells that are reduced in size, referred to as hypotrophic IUGR. The growth of the brain tends to be spared if the insult occurs late in pregnancy. These infants often appear to have an oversized head, although they actually have normal heads and undergrown bodies. They often have loose, dry skin, little subcutaneous fat, and sparse scalp hair and appear more active than expected for their birth weight. The most common causes of this type of IUGR are disorders that interfere with placental blood flow, such as toxemia, maternal hypertension, and maternal renal disease. Infants with hypoplastic IUGR, on the other hand, have uniform reduction of head and body size, with all measurements of fetal growth (head circumference, body weight, and body length) falling below the tenth percentile. This is usually a result of insults beginning early in pregnancy or occurring throughout pregnancy, such as chronic maternal malnutrition or intrauterine infection. These infants appear small but proportionate, with skin that may be slightly thickened. They are usually quite active and often have major congenital malformations.

Growth-retarded infants may have several problems in the newborn period. They often are chronically hypoxic *in utero;* they thus have difficulty withstanding the stress of labor and often develop asphyxia. Intrauterine hypoxia also predisposes these infants to meconium aspiration, which is apparently due to hypoxic stimulation of meconium release by the fetus and reflex gasping respirations *in utero.* Hypoglycemia also occurs frequently, and these infants have more difficulty than appropriately sized infants in the conservation of body heat. Cerebral edema also occurs more commonly owing to chronic intrauterine asphyxia and to birth asphyxia.

Most infants with IUGR are term infants who are small for gestational age. These infants have a higher mortality than do appropriately grown term infants, but not as high as low-birth-weight preterm infants, who have the highest mortality rates. Mortality rates are also affected by the type of IUGR (hypoplastic or hypotrophic) and by associated congenital defects.

ASPHYXIA

Fetal asphyxia is most commonly associated with impaired maternal blood flow to the placenta, and it results in hypoxia, hypercarbia, and both metabolic and respiratory acidosis. Heart rate monitoring and fetal scalp blood sampling are helpful in the assessment of fetal asphyxia. The passage of meconium-stained amniotic fluid also suggests fetal asphyxia, and meconium aspiration may occur. Hypoxemia associated with asphyxia may result in several types of brain injury, including cerebral edema and necrosis, intraventricular hemorrhage, and subarachnoid hemorrhage.

A list of conditions commonly associated with prematurity, IUGR, and asphyxia follows.

Prematurity

Abruptio placentae	Placenta previa
Diabetes	PROM
Incompetent cervix	Toxemia
Multiple gestation	

IUGR

Advanced diabetes	Intrauterine infection
Alcohol consumption	Malnutrition
Cigarette smoking	Multiple gestation
Chronic renal disease	Single umbilical artery
Essential hypertension	Toxemia

Asphyxia

Abnormal fetal presentation	Placenta previa
Abruptio placentae	Postmaturity
Cord prolapse	Prematurity
Hypertension	Pulmonary disease
Meconium staining	Prolonged labor
Multiple gestation	Single umbilical artery
	Toxemia

Fetal assessment

When a fetus is determined to be at risk, several methods of assessment may be useful, including ultrasound imaging of the fetus, measurement of maternal urinary estriol levels, amniocentesis, nonstress testing, and stress or oxytocin challenge testing.

ULTRASOUND IMAGING

Ultrasound imaging involves transmission of high-frequency sound waves from a scanner in contact with the maternal abdominal wall. The sound waves are reflected back from the various organs and tissues, creating a visual image that can be converted to a permanent photographic record. In addition to still photographic images, a "moving picture" can be generated, called real-time imaging, which allows the observation of fetal movement and the assessment of fetal heart and respiratory activity.[8] Ultrasound is helpful in the evaluation of multiple gestation, fetal position, and location of the placenta. It may also be used to evaluate fetal growth *in utero* and fetal maturity by assessment of head and thoracic diameter.[4]

URINARY ESTRIOL

Estriol is a steroid that is transferred across the placenta and excreted in maternal urine. Estriol levels normally increase throughout pregnancy with advancing gestational age, especially in the third trimester. The patterns of excretion are evaluated and compared with normal patterns for the estimated gestational age of the fetus. If the estriol levels are normal or consistently elevated, placental function is assumed to be normal. A falling estriol level is a poor prognostic sign, often preceding fetal death. A chronically low estriol level may indicate chronic uteroplacental insufficiency or an inaccurate estimation of gestational age. If the estriol level is falling or chronically low, further testing is usually indicated.[11]

AMNIOCENTESIS

Amniocentesis involves the withdrawal of a sample of amniotic fluid through the maternal abdominal wall. Assessment of amniotic fluid for fetal lung maturity through measurement of the L/S ratio has been discussed in Chapter 1. Additionally, amniotic fluid may be examined for bilirubin concentration, creatinine levels, and cellular abnormalities. Bilirubin is a by-product of the breakdown of red blood cells. In maternal–fetal Rh incompatibility (fetal erythroblastosis), an excessive rate of hemolysis occurs and increased amounts of bilirubin are present in the amniotic fluid. Bilirubin concentrations measured in amniotic fluid can be compared against normal values and the severity of disease estimated.[3] Severe disease may require intrauterine transfusion of the fetus or interruption of the pregnancy. Milder disease can be followed with repeated amniocentesis for bilirubin levels.

Creatinine levels in amniotic fluid increase throughout pregnancy with advancing gestational age. In uncomplicated pregnancies, creatinine levels may be used to assess fetal maturity. Unfortunately, creatinine levels are not reliable in many high-risk situations, such as toxemia, diabetes, and Rh disease.[17]

The amniotic fluid also contains cells shed from the developing fetus. These cells can be examined to determine the presence of genetically transmitted disorders, such as Down's syndrome. In addition, the sex of the fetus can be determined from cellular examination, which may be of consequence in sex-linked inherited disorders such as hemophilia.

NONSTRESS TESTING

Nonstress testing is based on the association of changes in fetal heart rate with fetal movement. Fetal heart rate is recorded externally through the maternal abdominal wall. A normal pattern involves acceleration of the fetal heart rate during fetal movement. If this does not occur, the pattern is abnormal. Nonstress testing is a very useful screening test because it does not involve administration of any drugs and is harmless to the mother and fetus. If a normal pattern is recorded, there is probably no need for further testing. In the presence of an abnormal pattern, stress testing may be needed.[6]

STRESS TESTING

Stress testing, also called oxytocin challenge testing, is used to assess the ability of the placenta to remain functional during uterine contractions, and thus the ability of the fetus to withstand labor. As with the nonstress test, fetal heart rate is recorded externally. In addition, uterine contractions are recorded externally through a pressure-sensitive device strapped to the abdominal wall. After measurement of fetal heart rate in the resting state, oxytocin is administered. Oxytocin (Pitocin, Syntocinon) stimulates contraction of the uterus and is administered in increasing dosages until uterine contractions occur. The fetal heart rate is monitored during this process. A negative (normal) test occurs if the fetal heart rate is stable. A positive (abnormal) test occurs if the fetal heart rate decelerates after the onset of uterine contractions (late deceleration pattern); this pattern is associated with uteroplacental insufficiency and may indicate fetal jeopardy.[15] Stress testing is not usually performed in placenta previa, vaginal bleeding, or in any woman at high risk for premature labor.

Labor and delivery

Labor begins with the onset of contractions and ends with the delivery of the placenta. If is usually divided into three stages.

In the first stage of labor, contractions are widely spaced. The uterine wall begins to differentiate into a thick upper segment and a thin lower segment; the upper segment supplies most of the force of contraction, thus helping to apply the force necessary for descent of the fetus into the birth canal. Cervical effacement (thinning of the cervical wall and incorporation into the uterine wall) occurs and the cervix dilates. As dilation progresses to completion, the second stage of labor begins. Fetal descent occurs primarily during this stage, owing to uterine contractions and increased abdominal pressure caused by voluntary contraction of abdominal muscles by the mother. The face and shoulders of the fetus rotate to accommodate the dimensions of the birth canal. In a normal vaginal delivery, the head presents first with the face down, then the shoulders, and, rapidly, the rest of the body. The cord is cut and the infant begins extrauterine life. The third stage of labor involves separation of the placenta from the uterine wall and continued contractions until the placenta is delivered.

DYSTOCIA

Dystocia refers to difficult labor, or prolongation of labor. The first stage of labor may last for many hours, but the second stage should not last for more than an hour or two. It is normally longer in primiparas. If labor is abnormally prolonged, early placental separation is more likely, thus reducing the surface area for gas exchange to the fetus and predisposing the fetus to asphyxia. In addition, compression of the cord is more likely, which also reduces gas exchange and contributes to the development of asphyxia.

CORD PROLAPSE

Prolapse of the umbilical cord occurs when the cord advances through the cervical opening and is compressed between fetal and maternal parts. Visible prolapse occurs when the cord can be seen in advance of the fetus through the cervical opening, and occult prolapse occurs when cord compression is evident but the cord cannot be visualized. Some compression of the cord occurs commonly during labor and delivery and is usually harmless; however, if cord compression is prolonged, gas exchange to the fetus is compromised and severe asphyxia is likely. Fetal heart rate monitoring reveals a pattern of variable decelerations (*i.e.*, decelerations not related to uterine contractions) during cord compression, and is thus a useful monitoring procedure in cord prolapse. Cord prolapse is more likely to occur in abnormal fetal presentations, such as breech or transverse lie, in multiple gestation, and in premature rupture of the membranes.

FETAL PRESENTATION

The normal presentation of the fetus is head first, called the vertex presentation. This occurs in almost all deliveries. Several abnormal presentations may occur, all of which present an increased risk to the fetus. The most common abnormal presentation is breech, which has several variations. Frank breech occurs when the buttocks present first; complete breech involves presentation of both the buttocks and the lower extremities; and footling breech or incomplete breech involves presentation of the lower extremities first. Breech deliveries carry a much higher mortality than vertex deliveries owing to the increased risk of trauma and asphyxia. Trauma most commonly occurs to the head owing to sustained pressure from contractions and may result in intracranial bleeding with consequent permanent brain damage or death. Compression of a prolapsed cord is much more common in breech presentation and may result in fetal asphyxia. In addition, breech is more common in the presence of placenta previa, which may further increase the risk of asphyxia. Face and shoulder presentations may also occur, which may prolong labor, since fetal passage through the birth canal is difficult in this position. A shoulder presentation occurs when the fetus is in a transverse position rather than a vertical position. Fetal passage is impaired and labor prolonged. If the position of the fetus cannot be corrected, cesarean section is performed.

MEMBRANES

Rupture of membranes may occur spontaneously during labor or may be artificially performed by the obstetrician. Membranes may also rupture well before the onset of labor, leading, as has been discussed, to increased risk of fetal infection. When the membranes rupture, amniotic fluid should be examined.

Foul-smelling, discolored amniotic fluid may be indicative of an infectious process, whereas meconium passage into the amniotic fluid may cause discoloration of the fluid or obvious observation of meconium itself in the fluid.

FETAL MONITORING

Fetuses who have been identified as high risk will be monitored during labor and delivery. There are, however, a significant number of fetuses who have not been identified as high risk who nevertheless tolerate the stress of labor poorly. Thus fetal monitoring has become popular for most deliveries, regardless of previous assignment of fetal risk. The most common method used to monitor the fetus during labor is fetal heart rate monitoring. Before rupture of the membranes, external monitoring must be used. This procedure is the same as that for stress testing during pregnancy. After rupture of the membranes, direct fetal monitoring can be employed, which involves placement of a monitoring electrode directly on the fetal presenting part (usually the scalp) to record fetal heart rate, and placement of a pressure monitoring device directly into the uterus to record uterine contractions. This method is more accurate than external monitoring. The three most significant patterns observed during fetal heart rate monitoring are early deceleration, late deceleration, and variable deceleration (Fig. 3-1).[12]

Early deceleration means that the fetal heart rate decreases at the same time that uterine contractions occur and returns to normal (120 to 160/min) between contractions. This is thought to be due to stimulation of the vagus nerve following compression of the head and does not seem to have any clinical significance or to be associated with any increase in abnormal fetal outcomes.

Late deceleration means that the fetal heart rate decreases after the onset of contraction and returns to normal after the contraction has ended. Thus the deceleration lags behind the uterine contractions. This is believed to be due to impaired maternal blood flow to the placenta and is associated with uteroplacental insufficiency. It is often associated with fetal asphyxia and low Apgar scores. Administration of oxygen to the mother may help to correct this, as well as attention to maternal hemodynamic status.

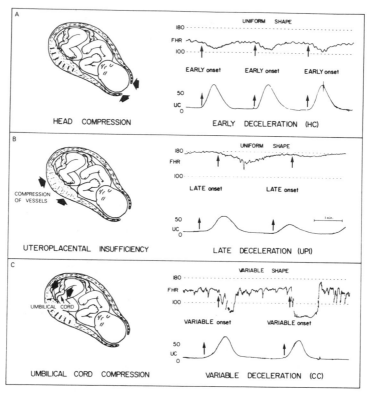

Fig. 3-1. Fetal heart rate patterns. (Avery GB: Neonatology: Pathophysiology and Management of the Newborn, 2nd ed, p 123. Philadelphia, JB Lippincott, 1981)

Variable deceleration means that there is no relationship between uterine contractions and decreases in fetal heart rate. This is the most common deceleration pattern and is believed to be caused by compression of the umbilical cord by fetal parts. Most fetuses can tolerate short periods of cord compression, but longer periods usually result in asphyxia. Changes in maternal position often help to alleviate this problem.

Another method of monitoring fetal status during labor is the sampling and analysis of fetal capillary blood.[2] A blood sample is drawn from the presenting fetal part (usually the scalp) and the pH of the blood measured. Normally, fetal blood pH falls somewhat during labor owing to the transient effects of contractions on maternal–fetal gas exchange. The pH at the beginning of labor is usually about 7.35, falling to 7.25 as the second stage of labor progresses. If the pH falls below 7.20, fetal distress is likely. There are two reasons for the fall in pH: Interference with placental blood flow inhibits the removal of carbon dioxide from the fetus, resulting in increased blood carbon dioxide levels and decreased pH (respiratory acidosis). This probably accounts for the normal drop in pH seen during routine deliveries. If, however, interference with blood flow is prolonged, oxygen levels supplied to the fetus will drop to dangerously low levels. The fetus will no longer be able to carry out metabolism through normal aerobic pathways and will revert to secondary pathways operative in the absence of oxygen (anaerobic metabolism). One of the end products of the anaerobic pathway is lactic acid, which builds up in the fetal blood, producing lactic acidosis, and accounts for the severe drops in pH seen in fetal asphyxia. Fetal scalp blood sampling and analysis are usually reserved for those cases in which the fetus has demonstrated an abnormal response to labor, such as a late deceleration pattern, or in which the fetus is known to be at high risk of asphyxia for various reasons previously discussed.

Objectives

Having completed this chapter, the reader should be able to do the following:

1. Discuss the effects of maternal age on pregnancy risk.
2. Describe the features of toxemia of pregnancy.
3. List conditions related to uteroplacental insufficiency.
4. Describe the possible results of uteroplacental insufficiency.
5. Explain the possible effects of maternal diabetes on fetal development in general and on lung maturation in particular.
6. Discuss the effects of maternal alcohol, drug, and tobacco use on pregnancy outcomes.
7. Describe the possible effects of maternal infection with rubella, toxoplasmosis, herpes, cytomegalovirus, and syphilis on the fetus.
8. List anatomic abnormalities that may increase fetal risk.
9. Describe the risks associated with multiple gestation pregnancies.

10. List problems associated with placental function that may influence fetal outcomes.
11. Describe the risks associated with premature rupture of fetal membranes.
12. Discuss the possible effects of postmaturity.
13. List the major consequences of high-risk pregnancy.
14. Describe the major problems associated with prematurity.
15. Discuss the types of intrauterine growth retardation and the problems that this development may cause.
16. List the features and common complications of fetal asphyxia.
17. Describe the use of ultrasound imaging, urinary estriol levels, and amniocentesis in the assessment of the fetus.
18. Differentiate between stress and nonstress testing and identify abnormal results of each type of test.
19. Describe the normal labor process.
20. Discuss the significance of dysstocia, cord prolapse, and abnormal fetal presentation to the fetus.
21. Explain the ways in which the fetus may be monitored during labor and delivery.
22. List the types of fetal heart rate patterns that may occur and discuss the significance of each pattern.
23. Define the following terms:

gravida
primigravida
primiparous
multiparous
toxemia
pre-eclampsia
eclampsia
uteroplacental insuffi-
    ciency
oligohydramnios
IUGR
IDM
macrosomic
fetal alcohol syndrome
discordant twins
twin transfusion syn-
    drome
placenta previa
abruptio placentae
PROM
postmaturity

prematurity
IVH
fetal asphyxia
ultrasound
estriol
amniocentesis
nonstress testing
stress testing
oxytocin challenge test
first, second, and third
    stages of labor
effacement
dystocia
vertex presentation
breech presentation
frank, complete, and
    footling breech pre-
    sentation
prolapsed cord
transverse lie
early, late, and variable
    deceleration

References

1. Alford CA, Stagno S, Reynolds DW: Congenital toxo-plasmosis: Clinical, laboratory and therapeutic consid-erations, with special reference to subclinical disease. Bull NY Acad Med 50:160, 1974
2. Beard RW, Morris ED, Clayton SG: pH of fetal capillary blood as an indicator of the condition of the fetus. J Obstet Gynaecol Br Commonw 74:812, 1967
3. Bowman JM, Pollack JM: Amniotic fluid spectrophotom-etry and early delivery in the management of erythro-blastosis fetalis. Pediatrics 35:815, 1965
4. Campbell S: The assessment of fetal development by di-agnostic ultrasound. Clin Perinatol 1:273, 1974
5. Clarren SK, Smith DW: The fetal alcohol syndrome. N Engl J Med 298:1063, 1978
6. Evertson L, Paul RH: Antepartum fetal heart rate testing: The nonstress test. Am J Obstet Gynecol 132:895, 1978
7. Fletcher AB: The infant of the diabetic mother. In Avery GB (ed): Neonatology: Pathophysiology and Management of the Newborn, 2nd ed. Philadelphia, JB Lippincott, 1981
8. Fox HE, Hohler CW: Fetal evaluation by real-time im-aging. Clin Obstct Gynecol 20:339, 1977
9. Giacoia GP, Yaffe SJ: Drugs and the perinatal patient. In Avery GB (ed): Neonatology: Pathophysiology and Man-agcment of the Newborn, 2nd ed. Philadelphia, JB Lip-pincott, 1981
10. Gluck L, Kulovich MV: Lecithin/sphingomyelin ratios in amniotic fluid in normal and abnormal pregnancy. Am J Obstet Gynecol 115:539, 1973
11. Greene JW, Beargie RA: The use of urinary estriol excre-tion studies in the assessment of the high-risk pregnancy. Pediatr Clin North Am 17:43, 1970
12. Hon EH: An Atlas of Fetal Heart Rate Patterns. New Haven, Harty Press, 1968
13. Nahmias AJ, Visintine AM: Herpes simplex. In Reming-ton JS, Klein JO (eds): Infectious Diseases of the Fetus and Newborn Infant. Philadelphia, WB Saunders, 1976
14. Peckham GS: Clinical and laboratory study of children exposed in utero to maternal rubella. Arch Dis Child 47: 571, 1972
15. Quilligan EJ, Nochimson DJ, Freeman RK: Management of the high-risk pregnancy. In Avery GB (ed): Neonatol-ogy: Pathophysiology and Management of the Newborn, 2nd ed. Philadelphia, JB Lippincott, 1981

16. Reynolds DW, Stagno S, Alford CA: Chronic congenital and perinatal infections. In Avery GB (ed): Neonatology: Pathophysiology and Management of the Newborn, 2nd ed. Philadelphia, JB Lippincott, 1981
17. Roopnarinesingh S: Amniotic fluid creatinine in normal and abnormal pregnancies. Obstet Gynaecol Br 77:785, 1970
18. White P: Pregnancy and diabetes. In Marble A et al (eds): Joslin's Diabetes Mellitus, 11th ed. Philadelphia, Lea & Febiger, 1971

Bibliography

Hon EH, Koh KS: Management of labor and delivery. In Avery GB (ed): Neonatology: Pathophysiology and Management of the Newborn, 2nd ed. Philadelphia, JB Lippincott, 1981
Korones SB: High-risk Newborn Infants, 3rd ed. St Louis, CV Mosby, 1981
Lubchenco LO: The High Risk Infant. Philadelphia, WB Saunders, 1976
Quilligan EJ, Nochimson DJ, Freeman RK: Management of the high-risk pregnancy. In Avery GB (ed): Neonatology: Pathophysiology and Management of the Newborn, 2nd ed. Philadelphia, JB Lippincott, 1981

4·
Physical Examination

The Apgar scoring system

Evaluation of the newborn begins as soon as the infant is delivered. While standard care procedures following delivery are being performed, including bulb suction of the upper airway, drying and warming of the infant, and cutting and clamping of the cord, a preliminary assessment is done. The most important observation is the infant's heart rate. Additionally, the infant's respiratory effort, skin color, and response to handling and stimulation are evaluated. These parameters are incorporated into a standardized evaluation system developed by Dr. Virginia Apgar in the 1950s, commonly referred to as the *Apgar score*, which allows rapid evaluation of a depressed infant and of the severity of the depression.[1] The infant is scored in five categories at 1 minute and 5 minutes after delivery. (These scores are traditionally recorded in the infant's chart as "Apgars 8 and 10," for example, meaning that the infant had a score of 8 at 1 minute and 10 at 5 minutes.) The maximum score in each category is 2 points. Thus the total Apgar score ranges from 0 (no points in any category) to 10 (2 points in each of five categories). The five parameters scored in this system include heart rate, respiratory effort, muscle tone, reflex irritability, and skin color. Scoring in each category is described in Table 4-1.

The following system may be helpful in remembering the five categories of the Apgar system:

A: *"Appearance"* (skin color)
P: *"Pulse"* (heart rate)
G: *"Grimace"* (reflex irritability)
A: *"Activity"* (muscle tone)
R: *"Respiration"* (respiratory effort)

The 1-minute score is especially useful in identifying the infant who needs immediate intervention. An Apgar score of 2 or less indicates a severely depressed infant who requires immediate resuscitation, including ventilatory assistance. If the score is between 3 and 6, the infant may need some assistance, usually requiring stimulation and oxygen. Infants with scores of 7 or more are considered normal and require only routine observation and care.

The 5-minute score is useful in assessing the infant's recovery from depression and in assessing the effectiveness of any previous interventions. If the infant remains depressed at 5 minutes, with a score less than 6, major depression is present and the infant should be under special care. These infants are at high risk of developing major complications of the newborn period, including respiratory distress, aspiration syndromes, and hypoglycemia. They will usually need intravenous fluids and oxygen, and many will require ventilatory assistance.

Estimation of gestational age

Soon after admittance to the nursery, the infant's gestational age is assessed. One common system used for estimating gestational age is that developed by Dubowitz and co-workers in the early 1970s, commonly referred to as the *Dubowitz score*.[3] This system involves the scoring of 10 external characteristics and 11 neuromuscular signs and is one of the most accurate systems available. It has some disadvantages in that no score can be obtained and thus no gestational age estimated unless all external and neuromuscular criteria have been evaluated. The Dubowitz score also does not provide the examiner with a picture of irregularities in the infant's development because

Table 4-1
Apgar scoring system criteria

Category	0 Points	1 Point	2 Points
Heart rate	Absent	Under 100	Over 100
Respiratory effort	Absent	Irregular, weak, or gasping	Crying infant, vigorous breathing
Muscle tone	Flaccid, limp	Some flexion of extremities	Active flexion of extremities, good motion, resistance to extension
Reflex irritability	Unresponsive	Frown or grimace when stimulated	Active movement, crying, cough, or sneeze
Skin color	Totally cyanotic, or pale or gray	Acrocyanosis (cyanotic hands and feet with pink body)	Completely pink

the system does not include a notation of what gestational age is normally associated with which particular developmental sign.

Various investigators and hospitals have modified the systems used for estimation of gestational age, but all are based on evaluation of one or more of the external and neurologic criteria that have been defined for gestational age, and which are summarized in Table 4-2.[3,5,6]

EXTERNAL CRITERIA

Vernix. The amount of vernix covering the infant decreases with advancing gestational age, so that the preterm infant is covered with vernix, the term infant has very little vernix, usually only in the body creases, and the post-term infant has no vernix at all.

Skin. The skin becomes thicker and less transparent with increasing gestational age, so that the preterm infant's skin is thin (almost transparent), the term infant's skin is pale with few visible vessels, and the post-term infant's skin may be thick and soft and begin peeling and cracking after birth. The skin in the early preterm infant appears dark red in color, gradually fading to pink, then to pale pink over the entire body, becoming generally pale with pink ears, lips, palms, and soles by term.

Nails. Nails are present and cover the nail bed in any viable infant. Post-term infants may have especially long fingernails.

Sole (plantar) creases. Creases develop on the soles of the feet during gestation beginning with the ball of the foot and proceeding toward the heel. An infant of about 32 weeks' gestation will have one or two anterior creases. By 37 weeks, the creases should be present over about two thirds of the sole, and by 40 weeks the entire sole is covered. The post-term infant has deeper creases.

Breast tissue and areola. The areola develops at about 34 weeks, with a palpable nodule of breast tissue present after the 36th week.

Table 4-2
Criteria for assessment of gestational age

Criteria	Changes as gestation advances
External criteria	
Vernix	Decreases
Skin thickness	Increases
Skin transparency	Decreases
Skin color	Changes from dark red to pale with pink extremities during gestation
Plantar creases	Increase
Breast tissue	Increases
Pinna	Increased incurving
Ear cartilage	Increases
Lanugo	Decreases
Genitalia (female)	Clitoris becomes less prominent, and labia majora increase in size to cover clitoris
Genitalia (male)	Testes descend into scrotal sacs, rugae appear late in gestation
Neurologic criteria	
Posture	Initial hypotonia changes to frog-leg position, then to flexion of all extremities, with recoil of extremities following extension at term
Popliteal angle	Decreases as muscle tone increases
Ankle dorsiflexion	Angle diminishes toward zero as joint becomes more flexible
Square window	Wrist angle same as ankle dorsiflexion
Heel to ear	Changes from little or no flexion of knee with heel very close to ear, to increasing flexion
Scarf sign	Increased resistance to placing infant's hand around neck to opposite shoulder
Head lag	Head initially lags behind trunk as supine infant is pulled erect by arms; becomes more in line with trunk as gestation advances
Ventral suspension	Infant suspended in prone position will be hypotonic initially, then begin flexion of extremities and lift head even with and eventually above back with extremities fully flexed

Ears. Before 33 weeks gestation, the pinna (external ear) is flat with very little incurving of the edge. At 33 or 34 weeks' gestation, the upper pinna begins incurving, and by 38 weeks the upper two thirds of the pinna is completely curved. This curving extends to the lobe by 39 or 40 weeks. Additionally, ear cartilage development proceeds throughout gestation. Before 32 weeks' gestation, there is little cartilage and the ears are soft, easily folded, and remain folded. By 36 weeks, they recoil from folding, and by term they are firm and erect and recoil instantly.

Hair. Preterm infants tend to have very fine hair that mats. In term infants, the hairs tends to lie flat in single strands. A receding hairline may be present in post-term infants.

Lanugo. Early in gestation, fine body hair (lanugo) is present over the entire body. As gestation progresses it disappears first from the face, then the trunk and extremities. By term, it is usually inconspicuous or present only in small amounts on the upper back.

Genitalia. The clitoris is prominent in the female at 30 to 32 weeks. The labia majora are widely separated and the labia minora protruding. As gestation proceeds, the labia majora increase in size until they completely cover the clitoris by term. In the male, the testes gradually descend toward the scrotum during gestation. At 30 weeks, they can be palpated in the inguinal canal. By 37 weeks they are located high in the scrotal sacs and by 40 weeks should be completely descended. Rugae (folds or wrinkles) begin to appear at about 36 weeks and cover the entire scrotum by 40 weeks.

NEUROLOGIC SIGNS

Posture and extremities. Before 30 weeks' gestation, the infant will tend to be hypotonic with arms and legs extended. By 34 weeks, flexion of the legs occurs, resulting in the "frog-leg" position, but the arms remain extended. By 36 to 38 weeks, both arms and legs should be flexed, but the infant will not recoil the extremities if they are extended. By 38 to

40 weeks, the infant should recoil the extremities after extension.

Flexion angles. The popliteal angle is measured by placing the infant's knee to his chest and attempting to extend the leg. As muscle tone develops during gestation, the angle formed when the leg is extended as far as possible becomes smaller and smaller. Ankle and wrist angles are signs of joint flexibility and diminish toward zero as term approaches. The test for wrist flexion is often referred to as "square window" and involves flexing the hand onto the forearm and measuring the angle formed at the wrist. Ankle dorsiflexion is measured by flexing the foot onto the anterior leg and measuring the angle formed at the ankle. Premature infants tend to have less flexible joints than do term infants.

Muscle tone. Heel to ear, scarf sign, head lag, and ventral suspension are signs evaluated in the Dubowitz scoring system that are related to muscle tone. The heel to ear test involves placing the infant's foot as near to the head as possible and observing how close it comes and also the degree of flexion of the knee. The very preterm infant will have little or no flexion and the examiner will be able to place the heel very close to the ear. The knee becomes increasingly flexed as gestation proceeds. The scarf sign involves trying to put the infant's hand around his neck and around the opposite shoulder. Resistance to this maneuver increases with advancing gestational age. Head lag involves grasping the hands or arms of a supine infant and pulling him slowly up into a sitting position. The position of the head in relation to the trunk is observed. Before 34 weeks' gestation, the head always tends to lag behind the trunk. After this, the infant begins to have control of his head and by 38 weeks is able to keep his head and body in the same plane as he is pulled up. Ventral suspension involves suspending the infant in the prone position by placing one or both hands under his chest. The degree of extension of the back and flexion of the extremities is then observed. Until about 36 weeks of gestation, the infant will appear hypotonic, with back slightly rounded and arms and legs hanging straight. After this, he will begin to show flexion of extremities and to lift his head even with his back. By term he should have his head lifted above his back and extremities fully flexed.

Once gestational age has been estimated, a comparison can be made between the growth of the infant being evaluated and appropriate growth for the estimated gestational age. The most common method of comparing normal and actual growth is the Colorado intrauterine growth curves. These curves plot gestational age against birth weight, length, and head circumference. An example of a Colorado growth curve for birth weight and gestational age is shown in Figure 4-1. These curves are based on data obtained for infants born in Colorado from 1948 to 1961.[7] Infants who score between the 10th and 90th percentiles on the Colorado curve are considered appropriate for gestational age; those scoring below the 10th percentile are small for gestational age, or intrauterine growth retarded (IUGR); and those scoring above the 90th percentile are large for gestational age. As previously discussed, identification of each of these groups is important in determining which infants are at high risk, and what those particular risks might be.

Vital signs

RESPIRATION

The normal respiratory rate for a newborn varies between 35 and 60 breaths per minute. Fluctuation of the respiratory rate is normal, and respirations are not necessarily regular, particularly in the preterm infant. Periodic breathing is defined as respiration interrupted by short periods of apnea, lasting up to 10 seconds, which is not associated with any other abnormalities such as cyanosis or bradycardia. This breathing pattern occurs commonly in preterm infants, is not considered pathologic, and does not require treatment. There is very little chest wall movement in the newborn, with most of the respiratory excursion caused by movement of the diaphragm. Thus the abdomen rises and falls quite obviously with each inspiration and expiration.

HEART

Heart rate in the newborn is generally determined by auscultation. The normal heart rate fluctuates between 120 and 160

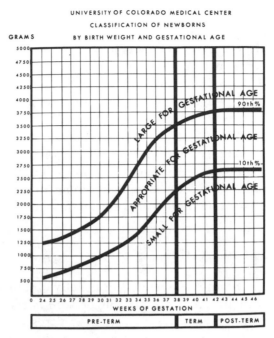

UNIVERSITY OF COLORADO MEDICAL CENTER

CLASSIFICATION OF NEWBORNS

BY BIRTH WEIGHT AND GESTATIONAL AGE

Fig. 4-1. Colorado intrauterine growth chart. (Avery GB: Neonatology: Pathophysiology and Management of the Newborn, 2nd ed, p 206. Philadelphia, JB Lippincott, 1981)

beats per minute; it may be slightly higher in the preterm infant. Transient increases may occur when the infant is agitated. Persistent tachycardia is usually associated with congenital heart defects, particularly if they result in congestive heart failure, or with shock. Bradycardia is usually secondary to significant apnea. In addition to heart rate, palpation of the apical impulse is important in evaluating cardiac status. The apical impulse is used to locate the position of the heart and is normally felt at the fifth intercostal space in the midclavicular line. This may also be visible as a localized pulsation. Several abnormalities may result in a shift of the apical impulse from its normal position: For instance, pneumothorax will result in a shift of the apical impulse away from the affected side.

BLOOD PRESSURE

Blood pressure is usually measured with a Doppler apparatus and a blood pressure cuff. The blood pressure cuff must be appropriate for the size of the infant in order to obtain accurate measurements. Usually a cuff of 1 inch width or less is used, although larger infants may require a larger cuff. Blood pressures are often obtained from the leg with the cuff around the thigh, in addition to being obtained from the arm. In low-birth-weight infants, blood pressure averages 50/30 mm Hg. Infants with birth weights above 2000 g have an average blood pressure of 60/35 mm Hg, whereas infants above 3000 g have an average blood pressure of 65/40 mm Hg. Evaluation of peripheral pulses (brachial, radial, femoral) is also valuable in the indirect assessment of blood pressure. Weak peripheral pulses commonly indicate a hypotensive state.

TEMPERATURE

An infant's temperature is usually obtained from the rectum, skin, or axilla. Rectal temperature is the best assessment of core temperature. Skin temperatures are good because they provide constant measurement and do not interfere with the care of the baby. In addition, the metabolic response of the infant to cold temperatures is sensed and mediated by the skin receptors. Axillary temperature is usually somewhat lower than rectal temperature but may be falsely high; it is recommended only for routine monitoring in the absence of any problems with thermoregulation. In general, continuous monitoring of skin temperature is recommended for infants who require close thermal monitoring and regulation. Skin temperature is usually maintained at about 36.5° Celsius to minimize oxygen consumption, which increases with both elevated and depressed body temperatures.

Signs of respiratory distress

Five signs commonly appear in the infant with respiratory distress to varying degrees: tachypnea, cyanosis, nasal flaring, expiratory grunting, and retractions. Additionally, periods of apnea and bradycardia may occur.[4] None of these signs is specific for any particular disease or type of disease. Many of these signs occur in both respiratory and cardiac disorders, and some may be associated with disorders of other body systems.

Tachypnea in the newborn is defined as a respiratory rate in excess of 60 breaths per minute, although a rate in excess of 50 breaths per minute should increase one's index of suspicion for respiratory or cardiac difficulty. Because of the normal fluctuations in respiratory rate and pattern in the newborn, tachypnea should be ascertained by several counts of respiratory rate rather than by an isolated one.

Cyanosis, or blue discoloration, may be localized or generalized, with the latter indicating a more serious problem. A well-lighted environment is essential to the evaluation of cyanosis. Central cyanosis, which involves the mucous membranes, indicates that there is an excessive amount of unsaturated hemoglobin present (in excess of 5 g %). Peripheral cyanosis (acrocyanosis, or cyanosis of the hands and feet) is common in newborns and is not necessarily a sign of difficulty. Because of the presence of fetal hemoglobin in the newborn, with its increased affinity for oxygen, cyanosis occurs at a lower partial pressure of oxygen in newborns than in adults. The presence of central cyanosis usually indicates an arterial oxygen tension of less than 40 mm Hg. This is an ominous situation because even a slight drop in the oxygen partial pressure at this point will result in a sharp decline in hemoglobin saturation and thus in oxygen-carrying capacity of the blood. Further, because cyanosis is related to the amount of unsaturated hemoglobin present, the anemic infant is unlikely to demonstrate cyanosis at all even though he may be extremely hypoxemic. Thus cyanosis is a very serious sign if present; its absence does not, however, preclude difficulty.

Nasal flaring involves flaring of the nostrils (alae nasi) during inspiration and is believed to be a sign of air hunger. Presumably the more pressure that must be generated to move air, the higher is the degree of flaring. Flaring may be present intermittently and may be barely discernible or very obvious.

Expiratory grunting is typical of the infant with hyaline membrane disease, although it may be seen in other disorders. It is believed to be an attempt on the part of the neonate to maintain positive pressure on expiration and prevent alveolar collapse. Grunting involves exhalation against a partially closed glottis (partial Valsalva maneuver) and may vary from mild (audible only with a stethoscope) to severe (audible with the naked ear).

Retractions involve indrawing of the chest wall either between the ribs (intercostal), above the clavicles (supraclavicular), or below the rib margins (subcostal). They may also occur at the top (suprasternal) or the bottom (xyphoid) margins of the sternum. Retractions may occur in any age group but are much more common in the newborn because of the very compliant nature of the chest cage. As the infant develops difficulty moving air and generates more pressure in an attempt to move more air, the wall of the chest cage is pulled in. Initially, with moderate distress, slight subcostal and intercostal retractions occur. As distress increases, retractions become more widespread and obvious, and eventually the retractions at the sternal level (xyphoid retractions) may mimic the appearance of pectus excavatum. As the infant forcefully contracts the diaphragm in an attempt to move more air, the abdomen protrudes. The high negative pressures generated in the chest cage with this diaphragmatic contraction result in the entire anterior chest wall and sternum moving inward, producing a characteristic "see-saw" or paradoxical type of respiratory pattern.

Apnea in the newborn is defined as periods of absence of respiration for at least 20 seconds, or periods of absence of respiration that are accompanied by bradycardia (generally defined as a heart rate less than 100/min) or cyanosis, or both. Apnea, which will be discussed in detail later, is associated with many types of disorders, among which are prematurity, sepsis, cardiorespiratory disease, and central nervous system disorders.

Auscultation of the chest

Auscultation of the newborn chest is much less valuable than in any other age group and requires an experienced listener. The newborn chest is very small, and localization of findings with a stethoscope is extremely difficult. Breath sounds are easily referred from one area of the chest to another. Nevertheless, an experienced neonatal care provider can augment the physical examination of the infant with auscultation.

Three basic types of breath sounds can be distinguished: diminished breath sounds, rales, and rhonchi. Diminished breath sounds in one area of the lung are difficult to appreciate because sounds from unaffected areas may be transmitted to the affected area; however, a difference in air entry between the two lungs may be appreciated and may be helpful in the detection of pneumothorax, atelectasis, or lobar emphysema. A general decrease in air entry may also be noticed in diseases that result in loss of lung volume, notably hyaline membrane disease. Rales, which are also called crackles, are described as short, interrupted, nonmusical sounds heard most readily during inspiration. Rales are associated most often with hyaline membrane disease, pulmonary edema, and pneumonia. Rhonchi are described as changes in pitch of the breath sounds and probably result from a narrowing of the airways by secretions, swelling, foreign matter, or spasm of bronchial smooth muscle. Rhonchi in infants are usually low pitched (sometimes referred to as coarse rhonchi) and are associated with secretions or foreign (aspirated) matter. Very high-pitched rhonchi are referred to as wheezes and are unusual in the newborn period. Infants who subsequently develop bronchopulmonary dysplasia after treatment for hyaline membrane disease may develop wheezing.

Objectives

Having completed this chapter, the reader should be able to do the following:

1. Describe the Apgar scoring system.
2. Interpret Apgar scores and suggest appropriate treatment.
3. Describe the criteria used in the assessment of gestational age and the assessment of appropriateness of intrauterine growth.
4. Describe the normal respiratory rate and pattern of a newborn.
5. State normal heart rate for the newborn.
6. List the most common causes of newborn tachycardia and bradycardia.
7. Describe the use of the apical impulse in the evaluation of the newborn.

8. Recognize normal blood pressure ranges for the newborn.
9. Describe temperature assessment in the newborn.
10. List and describe the most common signs of respiratory distress in the newborn.
11. Describe normal breath sounds in the newborn.
12. Discuss the difficulties associated with auscultation of the newborn.
13. Recognize the significance of abnormalities in breath sounds.
14. Define the following terms:

acrocyanosis	ventral suspension
Dubowitz score	periodic breathing
Colorado intrauterine growth curve	tachypnea of the newborn
square window	"see-saw" respirations
heel to ear sign	apnea of the newborn
scarf sign	rales
head lag	rhonchi

References

1. Apgar V: A proposal for a new method of evaluation of the newborn infant. Anesth Analg 32:260, 1953
2. Battaglia FC, Lubchenco LO: A practical classification of newborn infants by weight and gestational age. J Pediatr 71:159, 1967
3. Dubowitz LMS, Dubowitz V, Goldberg C: Clinical assessment of gestational age in the newborn infant. J Pediatr 77:1, 1970
4. Guthrie RD, Hodson WA: Clinical diagnosis of pulmonary insufficiency: history and physical. In Thibeault DW, Gregory GA (eds): Neonatal Pulmonary Care. Menlo Park, CA, Addison–Wesley, 1979
5. Korones SB: Significance of the relationship of birth weight to gestational age. In High-Risk Newborn Infants, 3rd ed. St. Louis, CV Mosby, 1981
6. Lubchenco LO: Assessment of weight and gestational age. In Avery GB (ed): Neonatology: Pathophysiology and Management of the Newborn, 2nd ed. Philadelphia, JB Lippincott, 1981
7. Lubchenco LO, Hansman C, Boyd E: Intrauterine growth in length and head circumference as estimated from live births at gestational ages from 26 to 42 weeks. Pediatrics 37:403, 1966

5·
Laboratory
and
Radiologic
Assessment

Blood gases

The assessment of respiratory and acid–base status of the newborn, as in other age groups, is greatly enhanced by the performance of blood gas studies. Some special procedures are used in the newborn, however, so that competence in obtaining and analyzing samples in older patients does not necessarily imply competence in handling of samples from the newborn.

Three basic types of samples are obtained for blood gas analysis in the newborn: arterial samples from an arterial line; arterial samples from single puncture of a peripheral artery; and arterialized capillary samples. In addition, samples from the umbilical vein are occasionally used in emergencies, although they are not valid for oxygen tension values.

ARTERIAL LINES

The most common site at which an arterial line is placed in the newborn is the umbilical artery. Placement of an umbilical artery line allows for frequent sampling without disturbance of the infant, provides a valid measurement of all traditional blood gas measurements, including P_{O_2}, P_{CO_2}, and pH, and allows continuous blood pressure measurement. Arterial lines may also be placed in a peripheral artery if the umbilical artery is not accessible or becomes nonfunctional. Peripheral arteries that have been used include the radial, ulnar, temporal, and posterior tibial arteries. Arterial lines are most commonly placed by catheterization of the artery, although occasionally cutdown may be required.

Umbilical artery lines are inserted through the umbilicus into one of the two umbilical arteries. After insertion, the position of the catheter should be checked by x-ray study. The tip of the catheter may be placed either at the L3–L4 position (called the low position) or above the diaphragm (high position) depending on physician preference. The length of the catheter required to reach either point may be determined from a graph that relates the shoulder-to-umbilicus measurement to various catheter locations (Fig. 5-1).[1] The catheter is secured in place with either suture or umbilical tape attached to both the umbilical stump and the line and then is taped to the abdominal wall.

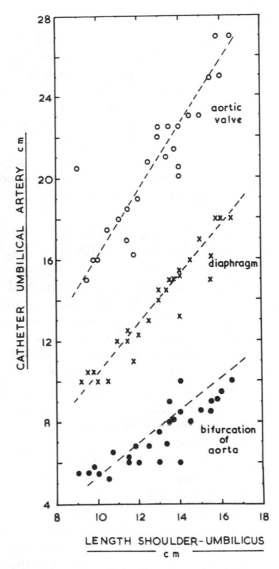

Fig. 5-1. The relationship between umbilical artery catheter insertion lengths and shoulder–umbilicus measurements (Dunn PM: Localization of the umbilical catheter by postmortem measurement. Arch Dis Child 41:69, 1966)

Although several risks are associated with the use of umbilical artery catheters, properly trained personnel should be able to avoid most of them. Infection may be avoided by maintaining strict attention to sterile technique during catheter insertion and during aspiration of blood from the catheter.

An obstructed arterial line should never be flushed because thromboembolism may occur. If the line is obstructed (blood cannot be withdrawn) or if there is any other sign of malfunction, such as diminished perfusion to the extremities, the catheter should be withdrawn and, if necessary, replaced. Hemorrhagic complications may be avoided by paying careful attention to blood withdrawal procedures, and by withdrawing the catheter only part way when it is to be removed and waiting for vasospasm to occur before removing it completely from the artery. Proper technique for infusing solutions, including the use of filters, will help to avoid the possibility of air embolism.

When obtaining blood from an arterial line for arterial blood gas studies, the following technique should be followed:

1. Using a sterile syringe, withdraw fluid from the umbilical artery line until blood is obtained and fills the line. Cap this syringe to maintain sterility and set it aside. This fluid and blood will be returned to the infant to minimize blood loss from sampling procedures.
2. Using another sterile syringe that has been heparinized, withdraw the blood sample to be analyzed. The amount of blood needed will vary with the type of equipment used for analysis of blood gases, but it is usually not more than 0.5 ml.
3. Reinfuse the fluid previously withdrawn. After attaching this syringe to the infusion port, aspirate to remove air from the sampling port, and then tap the syringe to make air bubbles rise to the top, so that they will not be infused through the line. Then infuse the fluid slowly, watching the line for any air bubbles that may remain. If a bubble is noted, reaspirate the line, tap the syringe again, and attempt to reinfuse.
4. Flush the line so that it is clear of blood, and be sure that all connections are tight.
5. Prepare the sample for analysis by rolling the syringe to mix the blood and the heparin, by labeling the syringe, and by immersing the syringe in ice water unless analysis is performed immediately.
6. Keep an accurate record of all blood samples withdrawn. Infants who require frequent sampling may require trans-

fusion, and an accurate record of blood withdrawn is very helpful.

PERIPHERAL ARTERY PUNCTURE

Samples may be obtained for blood gas analysis from one of several peripheral arteries, including the radial, brachial, temporal, and posterior tibial arteries. The femoral artery is never used for blood sampling in the newborn. The radial artery is preferred because there are no veins or nerves immediately adjacent to the artery and there is good collateral circulation to the hand through the ulnar artery. The puncture site may be determined by palpation of the arterial pulse. Transillumination of the infant's arm, by placing the transilluminator under the back of the wrist, will help to visualize the artery and may be useful if the artery is difficult to locate.

A heparinized tuberculin syringe is used, with care taken to eject all heparin from the deadspace of the syringe to avoid dilutional effects and decreases in *p*H from excess heparin. Puncture is usually accomplished with a 25- or 26-gauge needle. Alternatively, puncture may be accomplished with a 25-gauge scalp vein butterfly needle, and blood withdrawn from the infusion tubing with a heparinized syringe. The skin of the infant and the palpating finger of the sampler should be cleansed with alcohol or iodophor before puncture. When sampling from the radial artery, the nondominant hand should be used to stabilize the infant's arm. The needle should be inserted at a 30° to 45° angle into the direction of arterial blood flow. The bevel of the needle normally faces in the direction of blood flow ("up," in the case of the radial artery), although there is some controversy over whether this is necessary. The radial artery of a newborn is, of course, quite small, and it is possible to puncture completely through the artery. If blood is not obtained after initially advancing the needle, slowly withdraw while watching for blood to enter the needle hub.

Once a sample has been obtained, withdraw the needle from the artery and immediately apply pressure to the puncture site for 5 minutes. Any air bubbles present should be removed from the sample, and the sample prepared for analysis.

Complications from peripheral artery puncture, including hematoma formation, infection, and hemorrhage, are uncommon in the face of proper puncture procedures. The major problem associated with peripheral puncture is that it requires considerable disturbance of the infant. Many infants will cry, which makes the blood gas values quite different from what they might be in the resting state, and therefore of questionable value. If the puncture cannot be accomplished quickly and with minimal discomfort to the infant, it is probably not worthwhile.

ARTERIALIZED CAPILLARY SAMPLING

Peripheral artery puncture requires some skill and cannot be performed frequently on the extremely small vessels of the newborn. For these reasons, capillary blood obtained from the heel of the infant is sometimes used in place of arterial blood. The heel is warmed for several minutes before puncture is performed to "arterialize" the capillary blood. When properly performed, arterialized capillary samples ("heel sticks") may provide fairly accurate values for pH and P_{CO_2}. There is, of course, relatively little difference in the arterial and venous values for these measurements in any case. Unfortunately, the same cannot be said for P_{O_2}. The measurement of oxygen tension using capillary samples, however well "arterialized," is always risky. Most studies show that there is very poor correlation between capillary and arterial values when the actual arterial P_{O_2} is greater than 60 mm Hg,[3] meaning that an infant who has an acceptable range for capillary oxygen levels might well have an excessively high arterial oxygen level and thus be at risk for the development of retrolental fibroplasia. On the other hand, it is possible to have an acceptable capillary oxygen tension when the actual arterial oxygen tension is unacceptably low, allowing the infant to be exposed to dangerously low levels of oxygen and the possible consequences, including brain damage and pulmonary vasoconstriction. A falsely high capillary oxygen tension is usually the result of exposure of the blood to room air during sampling. Capillary samples are not recommended for assessing oxygenation status of the newborn, although they may be acceptable for monitoring acid–base and ventilatory status using pH and P_{CO_2}.

Arterialized capillary samples are obtained from the lateral heel surface of the infant. After warming of the heel with a warm water bath, a warm cloth, or a warming pack, the skin is cleansed with alcohol and punctured with a lancet to a depth of about 3 mm. A quick, stabbing motion should be used, not a slash. The first drop of blood is discarded. The tip of a heparinized capillary sampling tube is placed as close as possible to the puncture site and freely flowing blood collected in the tube. Every effort should be made to avoid exposing the blood to the atmosphere and to avoid introducing air bubbles into the tube. The foot should not be squeezed to increase blood flow because this may both damage the foot and alter blood gas values. If blood does not flow freely, another puncture should be performed.

Once the capillary tube has been filled, the blood may be aspirated from the tube into a heparinized tuberculin syringe and prepared for analysis. Alternatively, one end of the tube may be sealed, after which a small steel wire is inserted into the open end of the tube. A magnet is passed along the length of the tube to mix the blood and heparin. As with arterial samples, the capillary sample should be iced and analyzed as soon as possible. Pressure should be applied to the heel as needed to stop blood flow and a dry dressing applied to the site.

INTERPRETATION OF BLOOD GAS RESULTS

The standard measured values from a blood gas analysis include pH, P_{CO_2}, and P_{O_2}. In addition, bicarbonate level is measured (from its relationship to P_{CO_2} and pH) and reported. Oxygen saturation may be determined from its relationship to pH, P_{CO_2}, and P_{O_2} or may be directly measured separately from blood gases using an oximeter. Base excess, like bicarbonate, is calculated and represents the amount of acid or base added from metabolic (nonrespiratory) causes. A positive base excess means either an excess of base or a deficit of fixed acid, whereas a negative base excess, also called base deficit, means either a deficit of base or an excess of fixed acid.

The normal values for blood gases in the newborn are similar but not identical to those in the adult population. The pH is normally slightly acidotic (less than 7.4) at birth and rises to the normal or "neutral" value of 7.4 over the first 24 hours of life. The P_{CO_2} is normally quite high at birth (greater than 50 mm Hg), since the birth process interferes with placental blood flow, and the P_{O_2} is usually fairly low (less than 55 mm Hg) for the same reason. In the term infant, P_{O_2} usually rises above 60 mm Hg by the first hour of life. The premature infant may take much longer to reach this level. The P_{CO_2} usually falls to about 35 mm Hg by 1 hour and remains low. Bicarbonate values are slightly below the "normal" of 24 mEq/liter, so that the pH, which results from the relationship between bicarbonate and P_{CO_2}, remains in the normal range (7.35–7.45).

Four major classes of acid–base disturbance may be present in the newborn as well as in other age groups: respiratory acidosis, metabolic acidosis, respiratory alkalosis, and metabolic alkalosis. In addition, mixed disorders may occur (e.g., mixed respiratory and metabolic acidosis). After the initial disturbance, the body may attempt to compensate. The pH is determined by the relationship between bicarbonate and P_{CO_2}. If one rises or falls, the other may move in the same direction as a compensatory mechanism. As long as the relationship between the two values (or the ratio, as it is usually expressed) remains the same, the pH will not change. Thus, to compensate for a disturbance that results in an increase or decrease in one component (bicarbonate or CO_2), the body will attempt to move the other component in the same direction to maintain the ratio.

Respiratory acidosis

Respiratory acidosis occurs when the P_{CO_2} rises above the normal value (greater than 40 mm Hg). This will initially result in a decrease in the pH (acidosis). Over a period of hours or days, the kidneys may compensate for this disturbance by conserving bicarbonate and eliminating hydrogen ions, thus attempting to return the pH toward its normal value. If no compensation has occurred (bicarbonate value is normal), the disturbance is termed uncompensated respiratory acidosis. If compensation has occurred to the point where the pH has been returned to the normal range (7.35–7.45), the disturbance is termed fully compensated respiratory acidosis. If compensation has begun (bicarbonate is elevated) but is not complete (*p*H remains less than 7.35), it is termed partially compensated respiratory acidosis. The initial disturbance remains respiratory acidosis, regardless of compensation.

Respiratory acidosis always indicates that ventilation is not adequate to keep up with metabolic production of carbon dioxide. This may occur in many types of diseases that affect the cardiopulmonary, central nervous, or musculoskeletal system. The usual treatment for respiratory acidosis is to increase ventilation or to reverse the cause of inadequate ventilation if possible. In some cases, chronic respiratory acidosis may occur and may not require treatment.

Respiratory alkalosis

Respiratory alkalosis occurs when the P_{CO_2} falls below the normal range (less than 35 mm Hg). This will initially result in an increase in the *p*H (alkalosis). Respiratory alkalosis results from excessive ventilation. As in respiratory acidosis, the kidneys may gradually compensate by altering levels of bicarbonate and hydrogen ion to return the ratio toward normal and thus restore the *p*H to its normal range. Uncompensated, partially compensated, or fully compensated respiratory alkalosis may occur. The most common cause of respiratory alkalosis in the newborn is mechanical hyperventilation. This may be intentional (*e.g.*, in the treatment of persistent fetal circulation to reverse pulmonary vasoconstriction) or accidental, in which case ventilator settings should be adjusted to decrease minute ventilation. Additionally, an infant who is actively resisting peripheral artery puncture (crying) will usually show a transient respiratory alkalosis. Finally, the P_{CO_2} may fall below normal levels in an attempt to compensate for a very low bicarbonate concentration.

Metabolic acidosis

Metabolic acidosis occurs when the serum bicarbonate level is decreased. This will initially result in a decreased *p*H (acidosis). The respiratory system may compensate for this problem quite rapidly by decreasing the P_{CO_2}, thus restoring the relationship between bicarbonate and P_{CO_2} toward normal. As with respiratory disturbances, metabolic acidosis may be uncompensated, partially compensated, or fully compensated. It is rare to see an uncompensated disturbance unless the patient has poor pulmonary function and cannot increase ventilation and decrease CO_2 or is being mechanically ventilated with no ability to increase ventilation. Metabolic acidosis results from either an addition of fixed acids or a loss of base from the body. The most common cause of metabolic acidosis in the newborn is from the accumulation of lactic acid. Lactic acid is produced as a byproduct of metabolism that occurs in the absence of oxygen (anaerobic metabolism) and occurs any time the tissues are deprived of an adequate supply of oxygen. Inadequate tissue oxygenation may occur from various causes, including low blood oxygen levels, diminished or abnormal hemoglobin, diminished perfusion of tissues, and sepsis. Additionally, an increased rate of anaerobic glycolysis associated with hypothermia contributes to lactic acidosis. Treatment of metabolic acidosis involves identification of the primary disturbance and attention to the reversal of that disturbance. If, for instance, acidosis is due to hypoxia, oxygen administration or manipulation of ventilator settings is indicated. If acidosis is due to hypothermia, maintenance of a neutral thermal environment is indicated. Circulatory support may be needed if acidosis is due to poor perfusion, and transfusion may be needed if the oxygen-carrying capacity of the blood is too low to supply tissue oxygen needs. Bicarbonate therapy should be reserved for those cases in which severe or persistent metabolic acidosis occurs and should be administered with caution.

Metabolic alkalosis

Metabolic alkalosis occurs when the serum bicarbonate level is increased. This will initially result in an increased pH (alkalosis). Metabolic alkalosis may be caused by either a gain of base or a loss of acid. The compensation mechanism for this disturbance would be to retain CO_2 to offset the increase in bicarbonate and to maintain the normal ratio. This compensation mechanism is not adequate to reverse alkalosis, since retained CO_2 results in a strong stimulation to breathe. In other words, it is difficult to decrease ventilation to the point at which sufficient CO_2 is retained to compensate for metabolic alkalosis. This disturbance may occur when gastric acid is lost through vomiting or nasogastric suctioning, as a result of diuretic therapy, or iatrogenically secondary to the administration of excessive bicarbonate.

Oxygenation status

In addition to evaluating acid–base status, blood gases provide an indication of oxygenation. The P_{O_2} is only one aspect of oxygenation; adequate and functional hemoglobin must also be present for sufficient oxygen-carrying capacity. Normally, P_{O_2} is maintained at between 50 and 70 mm Hg in the newborn. Slightly lower values may be accepted when capillary samples are used, although it must be remembered that oxygen values of capillary samples are not accurate. Frequent monitoring of blood oxygen levels is extremely important in the infant receiving oxygen therapy because excessive oxygen levels may lead to serious complications, including retrolental fibroplasia and bronchopulmonary dysplasia.

Hematology

HEMOGLOBIN AND HEMATOCRIT

Normal hemoglobin levels in newborns vary according to sample site and age. Initially, hemoglobin values tend to be higher than adult values (16–19 g %) and fall to lower than adult values (11–13 g %) over the first several weeks of life. There may be some variation depending on whether a venous or capillary sample is analyzed. Similarly, the hematocrit values for newborns tend to be high (55–60%) and to decrease to 30% to 40% during the first weeks. Venous hemoglobin levels of less than 13 g % indicate anemia, whereas hemoglobin concentrations above 23 g % or hematocrit values above 70% indicate polycythemia. Some infants may be symptomatic at lower levels. Anemia may be due to hemolysis secondary to Rh incompatibility (erythroblastosis fetalis), ABO incompatibility, or infection; it may also occur secondary to blood loss either prenatally or postnatally. Polycythemia may occur from placental transfusion at birth, from transfusion of blood to the fetus from either the mother or a twin fetus, or from increased production of red blood cells by the stressed fetus (*e.g.,* after chronic intrauterine hypoxia).

THROMBOCYTES

Platelets (thrombocytes) are blood cells that are vitally important to the coagulation process. A platelet count of less than 100,000/mm^3 (thrombocytopenia) is considered abnormally low and may result from several problems. Thrombocytopenia is often associated with perinatal infection, particularly bacterial sepsis, and the TORCH infections (toxoplasmosis, rubella, cytomegalovirus, and herpes). Some drugs taken by the mother may cause decreased platelet counts, including thiazide diuretics that may be used to treat maternal preeclampsia. Symptoms of thrombocytopenia include petechiae and bruising (ecchymoses). The principal hazard of thrombocytopenia is hemorrhage, particularly into the central nervous system.

The syndrome known as disseminated intravascular coagulation (DIC) also results in a decreased platelet count. In this syndrome, some stimulus (such as infection) results in clotting in the bloodstream. Platelets and other clotting factors are rapidly "consumed" by this intravascular coagulation process. DIC syndrome is thus sometimes called "consumption coagulopathy" and may result in bleeding anywhere in the body. Paradoxically, heparin may help to treat this disease because it interrupts the ongoing coagulation and thus the consumption of platelets and clotting factors.

LEUKOCYTES

The white blood cell (leukocyte) count in the newborn has a wide normal range, with a low value of 9,000 and a high value of 30,000/mm^3. Initially, the most numerous white blood cell is the polymorphonuclear leukocyte (neutrophil), which averages 11,000/mm^3. The lymphocyte becomes the most prominent white blood cell during the first week of life and remains so throughout the early childhood years. Band (immature) forms of neutrophils range from 5% to 10% of the total white blood cell count. Elevated bands are associated with infection but may result from other causes. Neutropenia (neutrophil count of less than 7,800 in the first 60 hours of life or less than 1750 thereafter) is the most useful indicator of infection in the newborn.[2] In addition, abnormalities of neutrophil structure, such as toxic granulation, may be indications of infection. The most common cause of severe neutropenia in the newborn is overwhelming sepsis. Neutropenia may also occur as a primary deficiency not secondary to infection, such as that secondary to maternal neutropenia.

Chest radiograph

Chest films are invaluable in evaluating the initial cause of cardiorespiratory disturbance and in following the course of treatment. Alterations in specific diseases will be discussed in later chapters. It is essential, however, to have some understanding of the normal film before discussing alterations from the normal.

NORMAL CHEST FILM

The normal lung field can be described as "lucent" (Fig. 5-2), meaning that it appears well aerated, or black, on chest x-ray film but that the pulmonary vasculature can be distinguished from the hilum to the chest wall. The lung fields appear symmetrical and the rib interspaces equal. The overall configuration of the chest is that of a cone or triangle. The diaphragms are well rounded and the costophrenic angles clear. In the lateral film, the ribs appear to slope downward from back to front.

The heart is somewhat difficult to evaluate on the normal neonatal chest film because cardiovascular changes occur rapidly in the first hours and the thymus gland outline, which is prominent in the newborn chest, blends with the cardiac silhouette. The size of the heart is usually evaluated by comparing the transverse diameter of the heart to the transverse diameter of the lungs on an inspiratory film. The heart diameter should not exceed 60% of the lung field diameter. A poor inspiration or an expiratory film will make the heart appear larger.

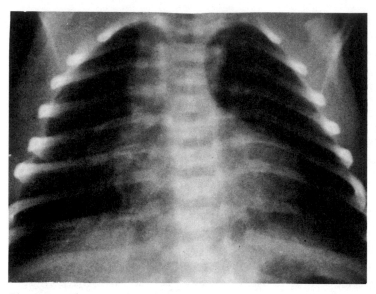

Fig. 5-2. The normal newborn chest film. (Avery GB: Neonatology: Pathophysiology and Management of the Newborn, 2nd ed, p 463. Philadelphia, JB Lippincott, 1981)

The mediastinum should be evaluated for midline position, since several conditions can alter its position. Increases in the volume of one hemithorax (*e.g.*, from pneumothorax) will cause the mediastinum to shift away from the affected side, whereas decreases will cause the mediastinum to shift toward the affected side.

ABNORMAL CHEST FILM

Major alterations in appearance of the chest film associated with cardiopulmonary disorders include hyperaeration, underaeration, infiltrates, granularity, "bubbly lungs," opaque lungs, vascular congestion, hazy lungs, air bronchograms, and extrapulmonary air.

Hyperaerated lungs appear hyperlucent, with depressed diaphragms. The anterior chest wall begins to protrude and the retrosternal air space increases. Rib interspaces may bulge. The upper ribs lose their downward slope and become more horizontal (Fig. 5-3).

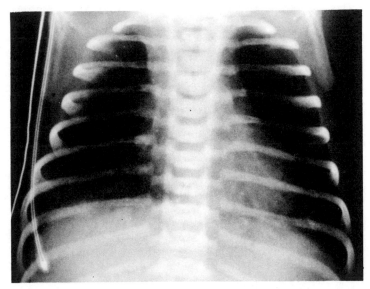

Fig. 5-3. Radiologic appearance of hyperaeration in the newborn chest film. (Avery GB: Neonatology: Pathophysiology and Management of the Newborn, 2nd ed, p 389. Philadelphia, JB Lippincott, 1981)

Underaerated lungs may appear less radiolucent (hazy) owing to crowding of lung tissue or may appear clear if the actual lung size is reduced. Diaphgrams appear elevated, and the anterior chest wall may appear to be depressed on the lateral view.

Granularity, also called reticulogranular appearance or ground-glass lungs, involves the appearance of small radiopaque (white) "dots" in the lung fields (Fig. 5-4). Granularity is usually associated with hyaline membrane disease, although it may occur in other disorders, including transient tachypnea and neonatal pneumonias (particularly Group B strep).

"Bubbly lungs" are of several types and have been described as Types I, II, and III bubbles.[4] The Type I bubble is small and spherical and occurs in hyaline membrane disease, caused by overdistended terminal airways. The Type II bubble is tortuous in appearance, usually occurs first in one lung near the hilus rather than bilaterally, and tends to radiate out from the hilar regions to the periphery. This pattern occurs in pulmonary interstitial emphysema (PIE) and is associated with

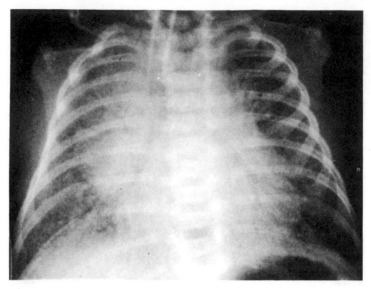

Fig. 5-4. Granularity, reticulogranular appearance, or ground-glass appearance on the chest film. (Avery GB: Neonatology: Pathophysiology and Management of the Newborn, 2nd ed, p 379. Philadelphia, JB Lippincott, 1981)

mechanical ventilation. The Type III bubble is associated with bronchopulmonary dysplasia and is oval or spherical in appearance. Types II and III bubbles are often difficult to differentiate. Both Types I and III bubbles, because they are within the pulmonary airspace, tend to be influenced by inspiration, expiration, and positive pressure. Type II bubbles, because they are extrapulmonary, do not diminish with expiration and may seriously compromise gas exchange. Figure 5-5 illustrates Type II bubbles as typically seen in a patient with PIE.

Opaque lungs are also referred to as "whiteout" on chest x-ray film. This pattern indicates that there is little, if any, residual volume in the lung; it is most commonly seen in severe hyaline membrane disease (Fig. 5-6).

Vascular congestion may produce various x-ray patterns, including prominent hilar and perihilar vessels, a reticular pattern of engorged veins and lymphatics, and a diffuse hazy pattern associated with interstitial fluid (edema).

Infiltrates may be localized or diffuse, producing varying degrees of fluffy densities within the lung fields. Well-localized

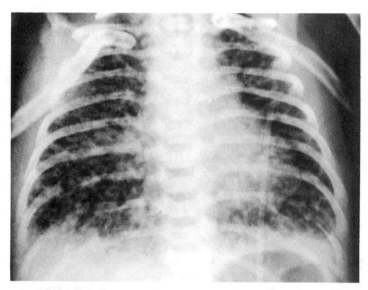

Fig. 5-5. An example of "bubbly lungs" on the chest radiograph, in this case type II bubbles associated with pulmonary interstitial emphysema. (Avery GB: Neonatology: Pathophysiology and Management of the Newborn, 2nd ed, p 385. Philadelphia, JB Lippincott, 1981)

Fig. 5-6. "White-out" of lung fields associated with severe hyaline membrane disease. (Avery GB: Neonatology: Pathophysiology and Management of the Newborn, 2nd ed, p 381. Philadelphia, JB Lippincott, 1981)

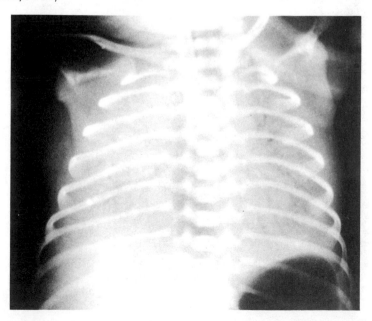

or lobar infiltrates are usually associated with bacterial pneumonia. Scattered "nodules" of infiltrate throughout the lung fields occur most commonly with aspiration syndromes. Diffuse infiltrates are common in bacterial pneumonias.

Hazy lungs may occur because of underaeration, which itself may occur for various reasons. The lungs appear less radiolucent but without obvious infiltrative (fluffy) densities. A diffuse hazy appearance may also occur in interstitial pulmonary edema.

Air bronchograms represent air-filled bronchi outlined against lung tissue that does not contain air, either because of alveolar collapse (atelectasis) or alveolar consolidation. They are commonly seen in hyaline membrane disease (Fig. 5-7).

Fig. 5-7. Air bronchograms, as seen in hyaline membrane disease. (Avery GB: Neonatology: Pathophysiology and Management of the Newborn, 2nd ed, p 378. Philadelphia, JB Lippincott, 1981)

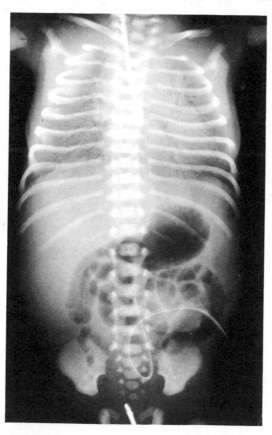

Extrapulmonary air may be in the form of pulmonary interstitial emphysema (previously described), pneumothorax, or pneumomediastinum. Mediastinal air classically collects centrally and elevates or surrounds the thymus gland. It is best seen on the lateral view, on which the elevated thymus produces the appearance of a sail ("sail sign"). Classic pneumothorax is easily identified, with a hyperlucent area along the chest wall and clear visualization of the free lung border (Fig. 5-8). Anterior pneumothoraces may be more difficult to visualize, producing only generalized hyperlucency as the air overlies the affected hemithorax and a sharpening of the mediastinal border. A cross-table view may be necessary to visualize this problem. Medial pneumothoraces may mimic pneumomediastinum, and a decubitus view may be helpful to allow the free air to move to the top of the chest cage and outline the edge of the lung.[5]

Fig. 5-8. Right tension pneumothorax, typified by widened rib interspaces, intercostal bulging, and shift of the mediastinum away from the affected side. Note also the outline of the collapsed lung on the affected side. (Avery GB: Neonatology: Pathophysiology and Management of the Newborn, 2nd ed, p 385. Philadelphia, JB Lippincott, 1981)

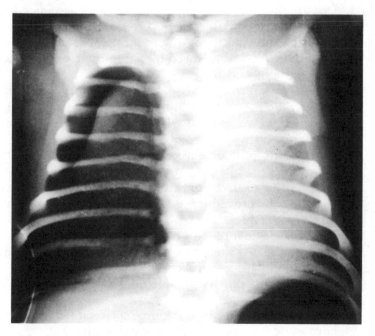

TUBE AND CATHETER POSITION

The x-ray film is also useful in evaluating the position of tubes and catheters, in particular the position of endotracheal tubes and umbilical artery and vein catheters. The endotracheal tube position should be evaluated for placement of the tip of the tube above the carina to ensure that endobronchial intubation does not occur, and should be rechecked periodically to assure that the tube has not migrated out of position. The carina is normally located at the level of the fourth thoracic vertebral body. The tip of the tube should be located above this level, at the second or third body. The umbilical artery catheter may be placed high in the descending aorta (between T4 and T11) or low in the abdominal aorta at approximately the level of L4. An umbilical vein catheter usually lies in the inferior vena cava just below the entrance into the right atrium or within the right atrium itself.

Objectives

Having completed this chapter, the reader should be able to do the following:

1. Discuss the advantages and disadvantages associated with the use of arterial lines.
2. Describe the placement of an umbilical artery catheter.
3. Explain the technique used for sampling from an arterial line in the newborn.
4. State the preferred site for peripheral artery puncture.
5. Explain the use of transillumination in arterial puncture.
6. Describe the technique used for peripheral artery puncture in the newborn.
7. Discuss the problems associated with peripheral artery puncture.
8. Discuss the accuracy of arterialized capillary samples.
9. Describe the procedure used for obtaining and preparing capillary samples.
10. Describe normal blood gases in the newborn period.
11. Discuss the features, causes, and treatment of the four major blood gas disturbances.
12. State the normal or acceptable ranges for oxygen tensions in the newborn period.
13. Compare hemoglobin and hematocrit values in the newborn period to those of the normal adult.

14. List possible causes of anemia and polycythemia in the newborn.
15. List possible causes and the major consequence of thrombocytopenia.
16. Discuss the use of the white blood cell count in evaluating the newborn.
17. Describe the features of the normal newborn chest film.
18. List and describe common radiographic abnormalities seen during the newborn period.
19. Describe the use of the radiograph in evaluating tube and catheter position.
20. Define the following terms:

"arterialized" capillary blood
base excess
base deficit
acidosis
alkalosis
compensation
uncompensated
partially compensated
respiratory acidosis
respiratory alkalosis
metabolic acidosis
metabolic alkalosis
anaerobic metabolism
lactic acidosis

anemia
polycythemia
erythroblastosis fetalis
thrombocytopenia
DIC
neutropenia
lucent
granularity
Types I, II, and II bubbles
PIE
"whitcout"
air bronchogram
"sail sign"

References

1. Dunn PM: Localization of the umbilical catheter by postmortem measurement. Arch Dis Child 41:169, 1966
2. Oski FA: Hematologic problems. In Avery GB (ed): Neonatology: Pathophysiology and Management of the Newborn, 2nd ed. Philadelphia, JB Lippincott, 1981
3. Schreiner RL et al: Techniques of obtaining arterial blood. In Schreiner RL, Kisling JA (eds): Practical Neonatal Respiratory Care. New York, Raven Press, 1982
4. Swischuk LE: Bubbles in hyaline membrane disease (differentiation of three types). Radiology 122:417, 1977
5. Swischuk LE: Radiology of pulmonary insufficiency. In Thibeault DW, Gregory GA (eds): Neonatal Pulmonary Care. Menlo Park, CA, Addison–Wesley Publishing, 1979

6·
Noninvasive
Monitoring

Apnea monitoring

One of the biggest problems in the monitoring of the neonate is the successful detection of respiration, and, more importantly, its absence (apnea). New noninvasive methods of measurement of oxygen and carbon dioxide tensions may eliminate the need to solve this problem because the ultimate concern in apnea monitoring is the degree of interference with oxygenation and the removal of carbon dioxide. Current methods of monitoring for apneic episodes include the use of transcutaneous oxygen and carbon dioxide monitors, which will be discussed below, and the direct assessment of respiratory movement.

All currently used methods of direct monitoring of respiration rely on detection of respiratory motion. The most common of these methods involves the use of impedance pneumography. The chest leads used to obtain the electrocardiographic tracing are also used for this type of apnea monitoring. A very small high-frequency electric current is passed between the electrodes. The electrical impedance that the current encounters is affected by the distance between the chest leads, which changes with respiratory motion, and by the type of tissue (alveoli relatively full of air or relatively empty) between the leads. The periodic changes in electrical impedance that would then occur with respiration produce an oscillating waveform that can be displayed and from which an average respiratory rate can be calculated. Unfortunately, monitors cannot always distinguish between artifactual patient motion and true respiratory motion. Additionally, apnea caused by upper airway obstruction may not be detected because chest cage movement continues. Other types of monitors have been developed that do not rely on the passage of an electrical current but are still designed to detect respiratory motion. The most common example of this is a monitoring system in which a mattress placed beneath the patient senses changes in position associated with respiration.

Two other methods of assessing respiration in the neonate show promise, although the technology for making these techniques accurate in the newborn is still under development. A temperature sensing device (thermistor) placed adjacent to the nares can be used to sense the temperature change associated with gas flow and thus to sense respiration. Unfortunately, securing this device to a neonate has not proved successful. End-tidal carbon dioxide monitoring can also be used to assess the presence of respiration, but the very small volumes of the neonate do not lend themselves well to some of the current measurement methods. In addition, end-tidal carbon dioxide is directly related to alveolar carbon dioxide and therefore to arterial carbon dioxide, which allows the monitoring of adequacy of ventilation as well as its presence or absence. Unfortunately, the small tidal volumes and relatively large mechanical dead space of a newborn make this a difficult technology to apply to the neonate. This is a promising area of respiratory monitoring.

Most systems designed to detect apnea have an adjustable delay time, after which an alarm will sound. This time delay should be adjusted individually to the infant; it is usually set at 15 or 20 seconds. A major problem occurs when the infant makes some ineffective respiratory movement, or any other type of movement that the monitor senses, during the apneic spell. The monitor will interpret this as a breath and "reset" the time delay. In effect, this means that the infant can have extremely long periods of apnea without an alarm sounding. Some sophisticated types of monitors have been designed to deal with this and other problems associated with apnea monitoring, such as the sensing of cardiac motion as respiration. Many institutions now use transcutaneous oxygen sensors or oxygen saturation monitors (oximeters) in conjunction with or in place of apnea alarm systems to avoid problems with apnea detection, since significant apneic periods are almost always associated with decreases in blood oxygen tensions and saturations.

Transcutaneous monitoring

Transcutaneous monitoring is based on the principle that gases diffuse through the skin and can be measured. The technology used to measure gas tensions is the same as that used to measure gas tensions in an arterial blood sample: A modified Clark electrode is used to measure oxygen tension and a modified Stow–Sevringhaus electrode to measure carbon dioxide. The electrodes are bathed in electrolyte solution and covered with a thin membrane, which allows gas diffusion. The major advantage associated with the use of transcutaneous monitoring is that it measures continuously, rather than relying on intermittent blood gas sampling. Transcutaneous monitors are designed to supplement the use of arterial sampling, providing a continuous assessment of the infant's oxygenation and ventilation status between samples. They are not designed to replace arterial blood gas monitoring.

Both oxygen (Fig. 6-1) and carbon dioxide (Fig. 6-2) electrodes incorporate heating elements and thermistors to measure and control the temperature of the electrode, in addition to the gas-measuring components of the electrode. The oxygen and carbon dioxide electrodes may be separate or may be incorporated into one sensing device. The electrode is secured to the skin surface with an airtight seal to eliminate contamination by room air gases. The skin surface beneath the electrode is then heated, which increases blood flow beneath the sensor, allowing for "arterialization" of the capillary blood in that area. This means that the gas tensions will more closely approximate arterial tensions. The function of the transcutaneous monitor is thus intimately related to the perfusion of the site: If perfusion is adequate, then gas tensions measured

Fig. 6-1. Schematic drawing of the electrode used to measure transcutaneous oxygen tension. (Redrawn from Novametrix Medical Systems: A User's Guide to Transcutaneous Gas Monitoring. Wallingford, CT, Novametrix Medical Systems, 1981)

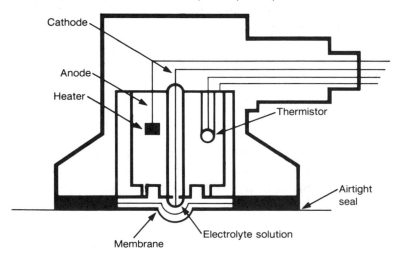

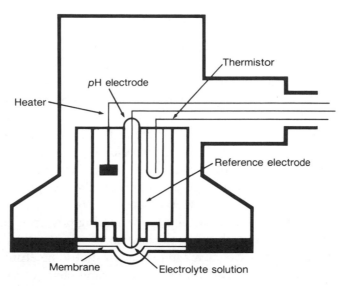

Fig. 6-2. Schematic drawing of the electrode used to measure trans-cutaneous carbon dioxide tension. (Redrawn from Novametrix Medical Systems: A User's Guide to Transcutaneous Gas Monitoring. Wallingford, CT, Novametrix Medical Systems, 1981)

transcutaneously will be linearly related to arterial gas tensions; if perfusion is poor, then transcutaneous oxygen tensions will be much lower than actual arterial tensions, and transcutaneous carbon dioxide tensions will be much higher.

Confusion often arises when interpreting transcutaneous values. The most important consideration is the difference between the terms "match" and "correlate" or "follow." The transcutaneous values are not necessarily the same as the arterial values, nor should they be expected to be the same ("match"), although oxygen values are often very close in neonates. Assuming adequate perfusion, though, they should correlate with, or follow, the arterial gas tensions. In other words, although a blood gas measurement may reveal an arterial oxygen tension that is 10 mm Hg higher than the transcutaneous oxygen value (Tc_{O_2}), the patient may subsequently be followed with transcutaneous monitoring, realizing that the arterial value is really higher than whatever value the Tc_{O_2} is. If the Tc_{O_2} value increases by 20 mm Hg, then it can be assumed that the Pa_{O_2} also increased by 20 mm Hg (always assuming that perfusion of the monitored site remains adequate).

MONITORING PERFUSION

Because the assurance of adequate perfusion is essential to the proper interpretation of transcutaneous measurements, these monitors incorporate a method of assessing perfusion of the monitoring site. The assessment is based on the principle that the amount of power required to maintain a given temperature at the electrode site is directly related to the perfusion of that site. If perfusion increases, it will take more electrical power to the heater to keep the site warm. Conversely, if perfusion decreases, it will take less power to keep the site warm. All transcutaneous monitors incorporate some system for monitoring changes in heating power. If the transcutaneous value changes, the heating power should always be evaluated, since changes in perfusion should be eliminated as a source of the problem before assuming changes in oxygenation or ventilation. Occasionally, an electrode is placed at a site at which blood supply has been periodically interrupted owing to movement of the infant. This is particularly likely to occur if the electrode is placed over a bony area. Movement of the infant may then cause the transcutaneous values to rise and fall, which could easily be interpreted as changes in the infant's cardiopulmonary status. Observing the relative heating power during these changes in transcutaneous readings would tell the operator that the values were changing because of intermittent interruption of site perfusion. The best treatment for this problem is to move the electrode!

MONITORING TRANSCUTANEOUS OXYGEN

To obtain correlation between transcutaneous and arterial oxygen tensions, the infant's skin surface must be heated to between 43° and 45°C. As a rule, infants weighing less than 1500 g require a temperature of 43°C, infants greater than 1500 g require a temperature of 44°C, and pediatric and adult patients require temperatures of 44° to 45°C. Heating of the skin surface serves three functions:

1. Vasodilation of cutaneous blood vessels, resulting in "arterialization" of capillary blood.
2. Increased blood temperature, resulting in a shift of the oxyhemoglobin dissociation curve to the right and an increase in the release of oxygen from hemoglobin.

3. Changes in the lipid structure of the outermost skin layer (stratum corneum), allowing oxygen to diffuse through the skin more readily.

Heating of the skin also increases the amount of oxygen consumed by tissue metabolism, which is at least partially offset by the shift in the oxyhemoglobin dissociation curve to the right.

If peripheral perfusion is good, then the transcutaneous oxygen value should correlate well with the arterial value. In the neonate, because of the very thin stratum corneum, arterial and transcutaneous values for oxygen may be very close.

CALIBRATION OF OXYGEN MONITORS

Transcutaneous oxygen monitors require a two-point calibration. The most accurate calibrations are performed with two gas mixtures of known oxygen concentrations. In clinical use, most oxygen monitors are calibrated to zero, using a "zero solution" that removes all oxygen from the sensor, and to room air oxygen values, which are calculated based on barometric pressure and F_{IO_2}. The zero solution contains sodium sulfite, which contains no oxygen. It is placed on the center of the electrode membrane. Oxygen tension should begin to fall as all oxygen is consumed and no further oxygen is allowed to reach the electrode. Once the reading has stabilized, the monitor is adjusted to read zero. For the high-point calibration, the sensor is exposed to room air. Barometric pressure and relative humidity should be taken into account when calculating the P_{O_2} of room air at a given location. The digital readout is then adjusted to the calculated room air value.

Electrodes should always be calibrated at the temperature at which they will be used and should be recalibrated if it is necessary to adjust the temperature. The calibration of the electrode to room air is usually checked each time the monitoring site is changed. Complete recalibration (two-point) is usually required only if the membrane is changed, or as recommended by the manufacturer of the particular monitor. The electrode *must not* be exposed to elevated oxygen concentrations during the room air calibration procedure (*e.g.*, remove the sensor from the isolette, which has been accumulating oxygen from the oxygen hood!).

MONITORING TRANSCUTANEOUS CARBON DIOXIDE

The optimal temperature for monitoring CO_2 in both infants and adults is 44°C. Heating is not strictly necessary to obtain good correlation, but the response time would be very slow without it. The increase in temperature results in three events:

1. As with oxygen monitoring, the structure of the stratum corneum is changed, resulting in increased diffusion of CO_2 through the skin.
2. Heating decreases the solubility of CO_2 in blood, thus allowing more CO_2 to escape through the skin.
3. Heating increases local metabolism and increases CO_2 production.

Because of the effects of heating, CO_2 values measured transcutaneously tend to be about 1.2 to 2 times greater than actual arterial CO_2 values; however, the correlation between transcutaneous and arterial values is excellent as long as perfusion is adequate. Many practitioners have difficulty with the display of "elevated" CO_2 values, and most monitors have been "recalibrated" to read closer to actual arterial values. This may decrease the correlation between transcutaneous and arterial values, although probably not significantly.

CALIBRATION OF CARBON DIOXIDE MONITORS

Like oxygen monitors, CO_2 monitors require a two-point calibration. Unfortunately, the amount of CO_2 in room air is negligible, and therefore room air values cannot be used. Calibration of CO_2 monitors thus requires the use of two gas mixtures with known concentrations of CO_2, usually 5% CO_2 for the low-point calibration and 10% CO_2 for the high point. Partial pressures for calibration must be calculated based on actual barometric pressure for accuracy. Calibration should be performed at monitoring temperature and is usually required every 4 to 6 hours.

APPLYING ELECTRODES TO THE SKIN

Site selection is important in transcutaneous monitoring. A site with good capillary blood flow, little fat deposit, and no bony prominences is best. Flat surfaces should be used to allow for a good airtight seal using double-sided adhesive rings on the electrode (Fig. 6-3). In the neonate, the common application sites include the upper chest, abdomen, and inner thigh, although almost every area of the infant's body that meets the requirements of a flat surface without bony prominences has been used. Transcutaneous monitors are also used in pediatric and adult patients, the upper chest and inner aspect of the arm being common sites. In the newborn, a major consideration in site selection may be the need for preductal or postductal values, which will be significantly different if a major right-to-left shunt through the ductus arteriosus is present (Fig. 6-3). Preductal values give a better approximation of the oxygen tension reaching the retinal vessels of the newborn, which is the most important consideration in preventing retrolental fibroplasia.

After the site has been selected, the skin surface is prepared. Normally, cleaning with an alcohol swab is sufficient.

Fig. 6-3. Transcutaneous oxygen electrode in place on the right upper chest (preductal area) of an infant receiving oxygen therapy. (Avery GB: Neonatology: Pathophysiology and Management of the Newborn, 2nd ed, p 419. Philadelphia, JB Lippincott, 1981)

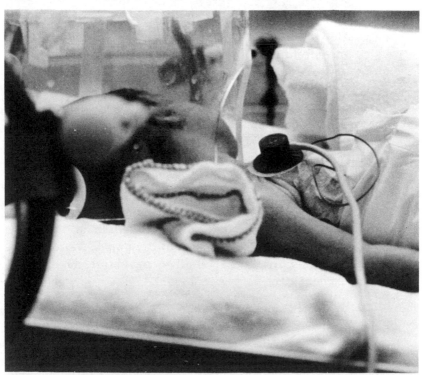

If the skin is oily, soap and water may be needed. In adults, shaving of the site is often necessary, and some of the upper skin layer may be removed using adhesive tape. A drop of contact solution or distilled water is placed on the membrane and the electrode applied to the skin site using a double-sided adhesive ring. The ring is pressed tightly to the skin surface. Often a cotton ball is used to press the adhesive ring to the skin to keep the applicant's fingers from adhering to the adhesive. An airtight seal at the skin surface is essential to accurate monitoring.

Once the electrode has been sealed to the skin, it must be allowed to stabilize. While the site is being warmed, the values that the monitor provides are meaningless. Oxygen values will fall rapidly as all oxygen under the sensor is consumed, and then begin to rise slowly as the site is warmed. Carbon dioxide values will rise slowly and steadily. Stabilization of values usually takes from 10 to 20 minutes. Prolonged stabilization times usually indicate poor site perfusion, and another site should be selected. Once the values have stabilized, the relative heating power should be zeroed, so that any changes in heating power, reflecting changes in perfusion, can be noted.

The monitoring site must be changed periodically to avoid burning the skin. Initially, the monitoring site should be evaluated after 1 hour and the time between site changes extended based on individual patient response. Most patients will require site changes every 3 or 4 hours; some may tolerate longer periods; and some may require more frequent changes to avoid burning. A red spot at the monitoring site is normal owing to the vasodilation effects of heating. Blistering, of course, is not normal and indicates that the site must be changed more frequently. The red spots may persist for some time but will eventually fade and do not leave any scars.

If the airtight seal is not maintained, the readings on the monitor will reflect room air values: Oxygen values will rise abruptly, and carbon dioxide values will fall. Erratic readings may occur in the presence of intermittent air leaks. If any of these situations arises, the adhesive ring should be checked and replaced if necessary.

CONTRAINDICATIONS AND PROBLEMS

Occasionally, transcutaneous monitors cannot be applied or will not produce accurate values. Excessive skin edema and deep hypothermia are contraindications to monitoring. Extremely sensitive skin, often present in very premature infants, may not tolerate the application of heat or adhesive rings. Some drugs may cause inaccurate values, particularly those that affect perfusion (tolazoline, dopamine). With proper selection of site, good calibration procedure, and careful attention to factors such as air leaks, perfusion state, and site changes, few problems should be encountered with the use of transcutaneous oxygen values.

In summary, transcutaneous monitoring has proved to be a valuable addition to the management of the newborn with cardiorespiratory disease. Most experience has been with oxygen monitoring because carbon dioxide monitors are relatively new in clinical use. The number of blood gases necessary can be reduced dramatically, decreasing the risk associated with peripheral punctures and decreasing the blood loss from sampling. In addition, the effect of various interventions, from simple nursing procedures involving the handling of the infant to complex manipulations of ventilator settings, can be evaluated almost immediately. Once a correlation has been established between arterial and transcutaneous oxygen values, heel sticks may be used to ascertain acid–base status. Most importantly, transcutaneous monitors allow a "real time" indication of the infant's status, rather than the intermittent "spot check" of arterial blood gas sampling.

Oximetry

One of the most recent advances in noninvasive monitoring of the newborn is the use of oximetry, or the measurement of blood oxygen saturation. An oximeter measures oxygen saturation by passing a light source through a perfused area to a photosensor. The amount of light reflected to the sensor depends on the amount of saturated hemoglobin present in the blood. The sensor can be attached to any patient, requires no heating or site preparation and no calibration solutions or gases, and provides a rapid assessment of oxygenation status. Current oximeter design allows for continuous monitoring of saturation as well as for intermittent "spot checks." Monitors include alarms for detecting decreases in saturation; they may also be used to check pulse rate. Pulse oximeters have been shown to be accurate to within 2% when compared to measurements made with standard laboratory instrumentation.

Fetal hemoglobin does not affect the accuracy of measurements, although abnormal hemoglobin forms such as methemoglobin may affect readings. Continuous monitoring of arterial oxygen saturation appears to be a promising tool for the care of the newborn with cardiorespiratory dysfunction.

Objectives

Having completed this chapter, the reader should be able to do the following:

1. Describe the methods used for direct monitoring of respiration in the newborn.
2. Discuss the problems associated with direct respiratory monitoring techniques.
3. List other methods that may be used to assess respiration in the newborn.
4. Explain why transcutaneous monitoring may be useful in detecting apneic episodes.
5. Describe the relationship between perfusion state and transcutaneous gas tensions.
6. Differentiate between the terms "match" and "correlate" and relate these terms to the interpretation of transcutaneous values.
7. Explain how perfusion status is monitored during transcutaneous monitoring.
8. State the temperatures used for transcutaneous monitoring.
9. Explain the effects of heating the monitoring site during transcutaneous oxygen and carbon dioxide monitoring.
10. Describe the procedure used for calibration of both oxygen and carbon dioxide monitors.
11. Explain the procedures used for application of monitoring electrodes to the skin.
12. Discuss the significance of placement of oxygen monitors in the newborn.
13. Discuss the importance of site selection, airtight sealing, stabilization, and site changes in transcutaneous monitoring.
14. Describe the contraindications and problems associated with transcutaneous monitoring techniques.
15. Discuss the use of oximetry in newborn monitoring.

16. Define the following terms:
    impedance pneumography   zero solution
    thermistor   preductal
    correlation   oximetry
    stratum corneum

Bibliography

Emrico J: Transcutaneous oxygen monitoring in neonates. Respir Care 24:601, 1979

Indyk L: Monitoring. In Goldsmith JP, Karotkin EH (eds): Assisted Ventilation of the Neonate. Philadelphia, WB Saunders, 1981

Jose JH, Schreiner RL: Neonatal apnea. In Schreiner RL, Kisling JA (eds): Practical Neonatal Respiratory Care. New York, Raven Press, 1982

Novametrix Medical Systems: A User's Guide to Transcutaneous Monitoring. Wallingford, CT, Medical Education Division, Novametrix Medical Systems, 1981

Tremper KK: Transcutaneous PO2 measurement. Can Anaesth Soc J 31:664, 1984

Yelderman M, New W: Evaluation of pulse oximetry. Anesthesiology 59:349, 1983

7.
Special Problems in the Newborn

Thermoregulation

Thermoregulation, or the maintenance of body temperature, poses special problems for the newborn, and particularly for the premature newborn. Because thermoregulation is important in determining oxygen consumption, and because the administration of many respiratory therapy procedures may influence heat loss or gain, those involved in respiratory care of the newborn need to pay special attention to this area.

REGULATORY MECHANISMS

The production, dissipation, and conservation of heat are all necessary and normal functions of the homeothermic organism, resulting in the maintenance of a constant core temperature over a wide variety of environmental temperature conditions. Heat is a normal byproduct of cellular metabolism. To prevent core temperature from rising, heat must be lost (dissipated) at the same rate at which it is produced. If the environmental temperature falls, then the organism must either conserve heat or increase heat production to maintain core temperature. If the environmental temperature rises, the organism must increase heat loss, usually through peripheral vasodilation and sweating mechanisms. This requires a thermoregulatory system with three major components: a sensory system for monitoring temperature (the skin); a central regulatory system to keep core temperature constant (probably located in the hypothalamus); and some method of regulating heat production and heat loss.

The newborn infant has the same homeothermic responses as the adult, although the range of environmental temperatures over which the newborn can maintain a constant temperature is narrower than that for adults.[13,55,56] The reasons for this narrower range include the relatively large surface area to weight ratio in the infant, resulting in an increased rate of heat gain or loss; relatively poor thermal insulation of the infant owing to minimal subcutaneous fat; and a small overall mass to hold heat.[29,53] In addition, shivering and sweating, which are major methods of heat gain and loss in the adult, are not well developed in the newborn.

The major receptors for monitoring temperature are located in the skin of the newborn, particularly in the trigeminal area of the face.[13,38] These sensors detect changes in environmental temperature and respond rapidly to increase heat retention or loss to maintain a constant internal temperature. This internal temperature is regulated through a central regulatory mechanism that is most likely located in the hypothalamus. The function of this central regulator may be altered by such factors as intracranial hemorrhage, birth trauma, asphyxia, and hypoglycemia, usually resulting in a decreased ability to respond to cold stress.[53]

In response to changes in environmental temperature, infants, like adults, must have ways of adjusting heat production (thermogenesis) and heat loss. The major mechanisms of heat loss are peripheral vasodilation and evaporative heat loss from sweat and insensible water. The ability to control peripheral blood flow through vasodilation of skin vessels is well developed even in very small infants and represents the most important method of dissipating heat in newborns.[13,28] Term infants have sweat glands, but this is not a very effective method of heat dissipation for them, and preterm infants have essentially no ability to sweat.[27]

THERMOGENESIS

It has been well demonstrated that increased heat production occurs even in very small premature infants, by both shivering and nonshivering thermogenesis.[52] Although shivering and other muscular activity that result in increased heat production do occur, they are much less effective than nonshivering thermogenesis. In general, visible shivering does not occur in newborns unless the environmental temperature is very low. The major mechanism of heat production in the newborn is through the metabolism of brown fat stores and is referred to as nonshivering thermogenesis.[30] This mechanism is impaired in the presence of hypoxemia; thus maintenance of oxygenation in the newborn is important to the maintenance of body temperature.[54]

Brown fat, the primary source of nonshivering thermogenesis, is stored in major deposits in the thorax and neck. Brown fat cells appear at 26 to 30 weeks of gestational age and disappear during the weeks following birth. Exposure to low environmental temperature rapidly depletes these stores. Brown fat is richly supplied with sympathetic innervation. In response to cold stress, these nerves release norepinephrine, which is thought to be the principal mediator of nonshivering thermogenesis.[31]

MECHANISMS OF HEAT LOSS

The four major mechanisms of heat loss in the newborn are conduction, convection, radiation, and evaporation. These mechanisms are summarized in Table 7-1.

Conduction refers to direct loss to a cooler surface in contact with the body. This is not usually a problem as long as care-providers avoid placing infants on cold surfaces without first covering the surface or wrapping the infant. In addition, mattresses should be made of material that is poorly conductive, so that cold temperatures of surfaces below the mattress will not be transmitted through the mattress to the infant.

Table 7-1
Mechanisms of heat loss

Mechanism	Definition	Prevention
Conduction	Direct heat loss to a cooler surface in contact with body surfaces	1. Avoid placing infant on cold, unprotected surface. 2. Use poorly conductive material for mattress.
Convection	Heat loss to cooler surrounding air	1. Heat environmental air. 2. Avoid drafts. 3. Heat inspired gas when infant is intubated.
Radiation	Loss of heat to cooler solid surfaces that are *not* in contact with body surfaces, such as the walls of the incubator	1. Avoid cooling of walls of incubator. 2. Keep room temperature high. 3. Use double-walled incubators or a heat shield within the incubator.
Evaporation	Loss of heat when a liquid such as body fluid becomes a gas (water vapor)	1. Increase the relative humidity of the environment. 2. Humidify inspired gas when infant is intubated.

Convection refers to loss of heat from a body surface to cooler surrounding air. The rate of convective heat loss depends on both the temperature of the air and the rate of airflow. Convective heat loss is minimized by maintaining surrounding air temperature and by avoiding drafts. In the intubated infant, heating the inspired gas will prevent heat loss across the respiratory tract.

Radiation involves the loss of heat to solid surfaces that are *not* in contact with the body. The rate of radiant heat loss depends on the temperature of the solid surfaces, usually the walls of the incubator. Radiant heat loss will be increased if the room is air conditioned or if the incubator is placed near a window and the incubator walls are cooled. Radiant heat loss can be minimized by keeping room temperature high, using double-walled incubators and heat shields around the infant inside the incubator, and by keeping incubators away from cold sources such as windows.

Evaporation is a heat-consuming process that results in heat loss when a liquid, including body fluids such as sweat and insensible water lost from the skin and respiratory tract, becomes a gas (evaporates or becomes water vapor). The rate of evaporation, and thus the rate of heat loss by this process, depends on the humidity of the surrounding air. If the humidity level is low, evaporation will occur at a faster rate and more heat will be lost. This is the major reason why a newborn infant should be dried immediately after delivery. In addition, bathing a newborn should be postponed until the infant is stable. Infants who are having difficulty conserving heat or those at high risk for such difficulty (particularly very small premature infants) may be supplied with increased humidity in their environment. Infants with an endotracheal tube in place must be supplied with adequately humidified gas to prevent both heat and fluid loss.

RESPONSE TO COLD STRESS

When an infant is exposed to cool environmental temperature, the first response will be to attempt to conserve body heat. This is achieved by constriction of cutaneous vessels, thus exposing less blood to the mechanisms of heat loss. Because the infant has a large ratio of body surface area to body weight, this method is not as effective as it is in the adult. If this is not sufficient, then the infant must generate heat by increased metabolism. The initiation of thermogenesis is through skin thermal sensors, which are activated when skin temperature drops below 35° to 36°C.[31] This occurs before core temperature drops, thus helping to maintain the constant internal temperature of the homeotherm, and can be diminished by increasing the environmental temperature and thus increasing the skin temperature.

CONSEQUENCES OF COLD STRESS

As previously discussed, the major mechanism for generating heat in the newborn is metabolism of brown fat. As with all metabolic processes, oxygen is consumed when brown fat metabolism is increased. This increase in oxygen consumption may result in hypoxemia. In addition, lack of adequate oxygen supply may result in metabolic acidosis caused by anaerobic metabolism (anaerobic glycolysis). Anaerobic glycolosis rapidly depletes body stores of glycogen, resulting in hypoglycemia. Infants who are classified as IUGR (see Chap. 3) already have reduced glycogen stores and are thus more susceptible to the development of hypoglycemia when cold-stressed. Additionally, infants who are hypoxemic before exposure to cold are more susceptible to these consequences; they are also less able to produce heat from nonshivering thermogenesis and are thus more susceptible to hypothermia. Infants who cannot compensate for cold stress and who become hypothermic (core temperature below normal) are likely to develop severe apnea.[3] Infants who are persistently hypoxemic may therefore require a higher environmental temperature to maintain body heat.

A further consequence of cold stress relates to the increased caloric demands of thermogenesis. Calories are consumed as heat is produced, resulting in an increased caloric requirement for the infant. If these calories are not replaced, the infant will experience difficulty with normal growth and weight gain.

In summary, cold stress may result in hypoxemia, metabolic acidosis, hypoglycemia, impaired weight gain, hypothermia, and apnea.

RESPONSE TO HEAT STRESS

Although exposure to cold air is a more common problem in the care of the newborn, overheating may occur if careful attention is not given to environmental temperature control. This is particularly true if heated gas is added to the infant's environment without monitoring the temperature of the gas. If the infant is overheated, peripheral vasodilation occurs in an attempt to increase heat loss. Increased evaporative loss may also occur from sweating and insensible sources. These heat-dissipating activities may cause increased oxygen consumption, resulting in hypoxemia. In addition, elevated temperatures have been associated with an increased incidence of apneic spells in the newborn.

NEUTRAL THERMAL ENVIRONMENT

Neutral thermal environment (NTE) refers to environmental conditions that allow the infant to maintain a normal internal temperature without increasing oxygen consumption. The temperature range required to maintain NTE is widest for full-term infants of normal birth weight; it becomes progressively narrower with decreasing birth weight or gestational age. Very premature infants who are small for gestational age have a very limited range of temperatures over which they can maintain normal core temperature, and thus require close control of their environment. These infants have very little body insulation and lose heat more easily than do larger, older infants. The temperature required to maintain NTE also depends on whether the infant is naked or clothed. Obviously, temperature maintenance will be more effective in the clothed infant, but critically ill infants often require minimal or no clothing in order for intensive care to be performed adequately.

Full-term infants who are clothed and covered with a light blanket in an open crib can maintain a normal body temperature with minimal oxygen consumption with a room temperature of 24° or 25°C. By contrast, a naked premature newborn weighing 1 kg, who is maintained in a double-walled incubator or with a heat shield in a single-walled incubator, with no drafts and with a relative humidity of 50%, will require an average NTE temperature of 35°C on the first day of life. NTE temperatures will be higher in a single-walled incubator without a heat shield and may be reduced if environmental humidity is increased. Average NTE temperatures for infants of several birth weights and ages are summarized in Table 7-2.

MAINTENANCE OF NTE

Temperature must be assessed to determine what temperature is required to maintain NTE. The three major methods of temperature assessment in the newborn are rectal, axillary, and skin temperatures. Rectal temperatures give the best estimation of core temperature; however, core temperature is a poor indicator of thermal balance in a cold environment, as the homeotherm will do everything possible to maintain this temperature. Once the core temperature begins to fall, the battle to maintain temperature in the face of cold stress may be nearly lost. Axillary temperatures are not particularly accurate. Brown fat deposits are located in the axillary region, and the increased metabolism of these deposits in the presence of cold stress may cause axillary temperatures to be falsely elevated. In addition, the measurement of temperature in the closed space of the axilla may also result in a falsely high temperature value. Since skin temperature sensors, particularly

Table 7-2
NTE temperatures

Birthweight	Age	Naked	Clothed
1 kg	0 days	35°C	32°C
	30 days	33°C	25°C
2 kg	0 days	34°C	28°C
	30 days	32°C	24°C
3 kg	0 days	32.5°C	27°C
	30 days	32°C	23°C

(Adapted from Hey EN: In Avery GB [ed]: Neonatology: Pathophysiology and Management of the Newborn, 2nd ed. Philadelphia, JB Lippincott, 1981)

All data are for infants in a draft-free environment with a relative humidity of about 50% and with a heat shield placed between the infant and the incubator walls.

over the face, are responsible for sensing the environmental temperature and mediating the infant's response, measurement of skin temperature provides the best method of temperature assessment. In addition, skin temperature can be monitored constantly, without interfering with care of the infant, which is preferable to intermittent monitoring of temperature at another site. Maintaining the abdominal skin temperature at approximately 36° to 36.5°C will avoid either overheating or underheating and the consequent problems, particularly increased oxygen consumption, of each.[57]

It is important to remember that the major skin temperature sensors of the infant are located on the face. If the rest of the body is well heated but the face is exposed to cold air, the infant will react as if cold-stressed. It is therefore necessary to heat the gas supply to an oxygen hood and to monitor the temperature of the hood, keeping it the same temperature as that of the incubator. In addition, the gas flow into the hood should be directed away from the infant's face to avoid convective heat loss.

Most of the time, temperature control for NTE in the newborn is achieved by servocontrol. This means that a temperature sensor is applied to the infant's skin, usually on the abdomen, and the environmental temperature automatically adjusts itself to maintain this temperature at a preset level, usually between 36° and 36.5°C. This may be achieved using either an incubator or an overhead (radiant) warmer. The sensor is usually attached to the skin of the exposed abdomen with adhesive tape. This may present a problem if the environmental humidity level is low and the evaporative heat loss is high. The skin under the adhesive tape will have low evaporative heat loss and a higher temperature than other areas. The incubator or warmer, however, sees only the temperature of the sensor and turns off and on in response to this temperature. If this temperature is falsely elevated, the infant will experience significant cold stress. This is particularly a problem with a very small premature infant, who has little ability to retain or produce heat and who is being cared for naked under a warmer. Increasing the relative humidity of the ambient air will decrease evaporative heat loss and help to eliminate this problem.[3]

RESPIRATORY CARE PROCEDURES AND THERMOREGULATION

It is obvious from the above discussion that respiratory care and thermoregulation in the newborn are closely related. Oxygenation and the maintenance of normal temperature are also very directly related. The hypoxemic infant has more difficulty maintaining a normal temperature when cold-stressed, and cold stress itself results in increased oxygen consumption and consequent hypoxemia. Thus careful attention to maintenance of adequate environmental temperature and adequate oxygenation is needed.

Oxygen hoods are a very common method of delivering oxygen to newborns. It is extremely important to heat the gas that supplies the hood and to monitor the temperature of the gas within the hood. The face is the major temperature sensing area of the newborn, and the temperature of the gas surrounding the face must be maintained at the same temperature as the NTE temperature of the incubator or radiant warmer. Underheating of hood gas may result in cold stress of the infant, whereas overheating may result in hyperthermia and its consequences. In addition, the gas supply to the hood should not be directed toward the infant's face.

Infants who are breathing through an endotracheal tube need inspired gas that is heated and humidified to avoid both humidity loss and heat loss from the respiratory tract. Supplying cool gas through an endotracheal tube or, for that matter, through a nasopharyngeal tube or nasal prongs may result in cold stress.

Finally, evaporative heat loss may be minimized by supplying humidified gas to the ambient environment, particularly for very small premature infants who are extremely susceptible to heat loss.

Bilirubin

FORMATION

Bilirubin is a substance formed from the catabolism of hemoglobin to its heme and globin portions. The heme portion is further broken down to form carbon monoxide (CO) and

biliverdin, which is converted by biliverdin reductase to bilirubin. About 75% of bilirubin is derived from the normal
destruction of circulating red blood cells. The life span of neonatal red blood cells is shorter than the average adult span of
120 days, so that production of bilirubin in the newborn is
increased over that of the adult. The remainder is derived from
heme catabolism from nonhemoglobin sources and from destruction of immature red blood cell precursors.[36]

CONJUGATION

The free bilirubin molecule formed in the spleen and liver is
a fat-soluble substance and is referred to as unconjugated or
indirect-reacting bilirubin. Because this unconjugated bilirubin is fat-soluble and not water-soluble, it cannot be excreted
in either bile or urine. Additionally, it has a high affinity for
both fatty tissue and brain tissue. This bilirubin is transported
bound to albumin in the plasma. In the liver, bilirubin is
conjugated to form a water-soluble complex, referred to as
conjugated or direct-reacting bilirubin. This water-soluble
complex is excreted through the biliary tract and into the gastrointestinal tract. If excess amounts are formed, it may also
be excreted through the kidneys in the urine.

The reactions that result in the conjugation of bilirubin
require protein carriers to accept the unconjugated bilirubin
when it enters the liver and an enzyme to catalyze the conjugation (glucuronyl transferase). A deficiency of either protein
carriers or the required enzyme, both of which may occur in
premature infants, will result in a decreased ability to form
conjugated bilirubin. In addition, oxygen and glucose are required, so that hypoxia and hypoglycemia, which occur commonly in sick newborns, will also decrease the ability to con-
jugate bilirubin.

EXCRETION AND ENTEROHEPATIC SHUNT

Once the conjugated bilirubin has entered the gastrointestinal
tract through the biliary system, it is either excreted in the
feces or converted back to unconjugated bilirubin by the enzyme beta-glucuronidase, which is found in increased amounts
in the fetal and newborn small intestine. This fat-soluble bil-

irubin is then absorbed through the intestinal walls into the portal (liver) circulation and into the bloodstream. An additional source of intestinal bilirubin is meconium, which normally contains bilirubin. If meconium passage is delayed (e.g., with intestinal obstruction or delayed feeding), more bilirubin will be absorbed across the intestinal walls. The reabsorption of unconjugated bilirubin through the intestines is referred to as the "enterohepatic shunt" and contributes significantly to the amount of bilirubin present in the newborn.[36]

JAUNDICE

An increase in serum bilirubin occurs in almost all newborns, for several reasons: because they have more circulating red cells per unit of body weight than do adults and because newborn red cells have a shorter life span. The rate of bilirubin production decreases postnatally but is still about twice as high as the normal adult rate at 2 weeks of age.[9] In addition, the enterohepatic shunt previously described results in more absorption of bilirubin in the neonate than in the adult, owing to an absence of bacterial flora and an increased activity of beta-glucuronidase in the newborn.[12] Research on newborn monkeys also suggests that ligandin, the predominant protein that binds bilirubin for conjugation in the liver, may be deficient in the first few days after birth, resulting in decreased uptake of bilirubin by the liver.[32] Glucuronyl transferase activity necessary for conjugation in the liver has also been demonstrated to be insufficient in monkeys. Activity of this enzyme increases postnatally, coinciding with the normal decrease in serum bilirubin levels. This enzyme is also decreased in activity in premature infants.[22] Finally, the ability of the newborn liver to excrete bilirubin is less than that of the adult, which may play a role if the bilirubin load is very high, as it might be in hemolytic disease of the newborn, causing an increase in conjugated bilirubin in the serum.

In about one half of newborns, the serum bilirubin is high enough to produce visible jaundice (clinical jaundice or icterus) within the first week of life. Serum bilirubin must be greater than 4 mg/100 ml for this to occur. In most instances, this is considered a normal event and is referred to as "physiologic jaundice." There are, however, many "nonphysiologic" causes for jaundice, and a distinction must be made between those cases that require further investigation and those which do not. Bilirubin levels generally peak in term infants between 3 and 4 days of age, and in preterm infants between 5 and 6 days of age, so that the appearance and rate of rise of bilirubin levels may be a helpful guide. Guidelines for the assumption of physiologic jaundice may include the following[36]:

1. The infant is otherwise well.
2. The jaundice first appears after 24 hours of age.
3. The jaundice lasts less than 1 week in the term infant, or less than 2 weeks in the preterm infant.
4. The total serum bilirubin is less than 13 mg/100 ml in the term infant, or less than 15 mg/100 ml in the preterm infant.
5. The level of conjugated serum bilirubin does not exceed 1.5 mg/100 ml.
6. The serum bilirubin concentration is not rising more than 5 mg/100 ml/day.

If any of these conditions are not met, an underlying cause for the jaundice should be sought, including factors known to influence bilirubin levels and underlying disease or abnormality in the infant.

CAUSES OF JAUNDICE

Many factors have been shown to influence serum bilirubin levels. Certain ethnic groups, including the Chinese, Japanese, Koreans, and American Indians, have higher average bilirubin values.[21,51] Some maternal drugs, including oxytocin, may alter bilirubin levels.[36] Early feedings tend to decrease bilirubin levels, probably because of a decrease in the enterohepatic shunt.[62] Delayed cord clamping may increase red cell and blood volume and thus cause an increase in bilirubin.[49] Infants of diabetic mothers and infants who have experienced asphyxia and hypoxia have an increased incidence and severity of jaundice.[18] Vitamin E, an antioxidant that prevents damage to red blood cell membranes and hemolysis and is often administered to preterm infants in an effort to prevent side-effects of oxygen therapy (retrolental fibroplasia and bronchopulmonary dysplasia), decreases serum bilirubin levels.[23] Finally, phenolic detergents that may be used as disinfectants have been associated with increased bilirubin, probably owing to inhibition of glucuronyl transferase, and should not be used.[16,65]

Diseases and disorders that may result in jaundice include those that increase the bilirubin load and those that decrease the ability of the liver to clear bilirubin. The bilirubin load is increased by hemolytic disease, most notably Rh and ABO incompatibility; by extravascular blood (hematomas, hemorrhage), which results in increased breakdown of the extravasated cells and increased bilirubin production; by polycythemia (*e.g.*, from twin-to-twin or maternofetal transfusion); and by an increase in the enterohepatic shunt (*e.g.*, secondary to intestinal obstruction). The ability of the liver to clear bilirubin may be influenced by inherited disorders, by biliary obstruction, and by infections, including bacterial sepsis, congenital syphilis, and the TORCH infections.

KERNICTERUS

Any of these disorders may result in hyperbilirubinemia and may lead to its most serious consequence, kernicterus. Kernicterus, or bilirubin encephalopathy, occurs when unconjugated bilirubin is deposited in brain cells, resulting in varying degrees of impaired perceptual, intellectual, or motor function or in deafness. As a general rule, kernicterus occurs when the serum bilirubin exceeds 20 mg/100 ml in term infants, 15 mg/100 ml in preterm infants, and 10 to 12 mg/100 ml in very small preterms (less than 1500 g), but many factors may alter the values. For bilirubin to be deposited in brain cells, it must be unbound. Normally, unconjugated bilirubin is carried in the blood bound to albumin. Bound bilirubin cannot leave the plasma and is therefore not a problem. In the term infant, bilirubin levels of higher than 20 mg/100 ml generally exceed the binding ability of the plasma. This is not a fixed number, however, and the bilirubin level varies greatly with many factors. Obviously, the albumin level itself is an important factor. In addition, binding capacity is decreased in the presence of acidosis and hypothermia. Some drugs and other substances can displace bilirubin from albumin. Fetal albumin has a decreased binding capacity compared to adult albumin, so that binding capacity increases with increasing gestational age and with increasing postdelivery age, up to about 5 months of age.

Lucey has described several factors that increase the likelihood of kernicterus in the low-birth-weight infant, including birth weight of less than 1500 g, hypothermia, asphyxia (either prenatally or postnatally), hypoalbuminemia, septicemia, meningitis, drugs that affect binding ability, and serum bilirubin of greater than 10 mg/100 ml.[35]

TREATMENT OF HYPERBILIRUBINEMIA

The two major methods used to treat hyperbilirubinemia are phototherapy and exchange transfusion. Phototherapy involves the use of blue light to decompose bilirubin by photooxidation, forming nontoxic byproducts that are water-soluble and can be excreted by the kidneys. Exchange transfusion is the classic treatment for neonatal jaundice and involves the actual removal of bilirubin by removing the infant's blood and replacing it with whole blood transfusions. In addition, administration of albumin before or during exchange transfusion may be helpful. Phenobarbitol can also be used because it accelerates normal excretion pathways through the liver; however, it is generally considered to be too slow to use to treat the jaundiced infant. Wennberg and colleagues have reported success with the use of this drug prenatally by administering it to mothers of fetuses with Rh disease, resulting in a slower rate of rise of bilirubin postnatally and in fewer infants requiring exchange transfusion.[61] The major considerations in the use of exchange transfusion or phototherapy are based on the actual serum bilirubin level, the birth weight of the infant, the rate of rise of bilirubin, and the presence of factors known to increase the risk of kernicterus, such as acidosis, hypoxia, hypothermia, and hypoalbuminemia. In general, all infants with a serum bilirubin level of 20 mg/100 ml or greater should be transfused, whereas infants with levels of less than 5 mg/100 ml require no treatment. Guidelines commonly used for the management of hyperbilirubinemia are presented in Figure 7-1.

EXCHANGE TRANSFUSION

Exchange transfusion involves the removal of twice the infant's calculated blood volume and the replacement of this volume, usually with whole blood. The two major indications

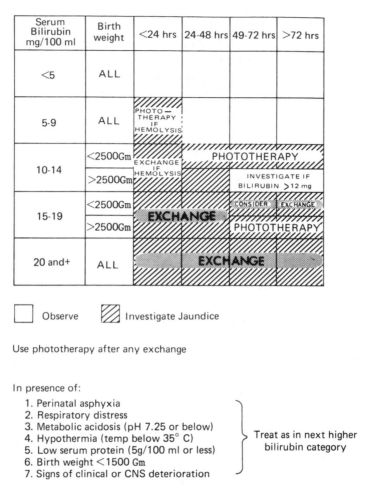

Serum Bilirubin mg/100 ml	Birth weight	<24 hrs	24-48 hrs	49-72 hrs	>72 hrs
<5	ALL				
5-9	ALL	PHOTO— THERAPY IF HEMOLYSIS			
10-14	<2500Gm	EXCHANGE IF HEMOLYSIS	PHOTOTHERAPY		
10-14	>2500Gm			INVESTIGATE IF BILIRUBIN >12 mg	
15-19	<2500Gm	EXCHANGE		CONSIDER EXCHANGE	
15-19	>2500Gm			PHOTOTHERAPY	
20 and+	ALL	EXCHANGE			

☐ Observe   ▨ Investigate Jaundice

Use phototherapy after any exchange

In presence of:
 1. Perinatal asphyxia
 2. Respiratory distress
 3. Metabolic acidosis (pH 7.25 or below)
 4. Hypothermia (temp below 35° C)   } Treat as in next higher
 5. Low serum protein (5g/100 ml or less)   bilirubin category
 6. Birth weight <1500 Gm
 7. Signs of clinical or CNS deterioration

Fig. 7-1. Guidelines for the management of hyperbilirubinemia. (Avery GB [ed]: Neonatology: Pathophysiology and Management of the Newborn, 2nd ed, p 511. Philadelphia, JB Lippincott, 1981)

for this procedure are to prevent or treat hyperbilirubinemia and to correct the anemia of severe erythroblastosis. The need for transfusion of the infant with hemolytic disease can be predicted by following the rate of rise of the bilirubin. These infants are at risk for developing hydrops fetalis, which is characterized by massive edema, pleural effusions, and ascites. Factors that predispose these infants to this disorder include severe anemia and decreased serum protein levels. In addition to treatment of hyperbilirubinemia and anemia, these infants should be treated for asphyxia, acidosis, hypoglycemia, and hypothermia, since any or all of these disorders may precipitate heart failure or cardiovascular collapse. Assisted ventilation with positive end expiratory pressure (PEEP) is frequently required to treat associated pulmonary edema.

PHOTOTHERAPY

Phototherapy involves the placement of the infant "under the lights" to prevent or treat moderate hyperbilirubinemia and to reduce the need for exchange transfusion. Blue light is more effective than white light, although less is known about its side-effects. Phototherapy results in the breakdown of bilirubin into more water-soluble products that can be excreted in bile, feces, and urine. It also enhances the excretion of unconjugated bilirubin itself. This technique has been used for more than 20 years without the occurrence of apparent serious side-effects such as an increased metabolic rate (increasing caloric requirements, oxygen consumption, and carbon dioxide production), hyperthermia, increased water loss through the skin and gastrointestinal system, premature aging of retinal cells, and "sunburn."[31,36] Eye shields are used to protect the eyes from potential damage, and a plastic shield (such as the "roof" of the incubator) should be placed between the lights and the infant to protect the skin. Fluid balance should be monitored closely and fluid replacement increased as needed.

Fluid balance

Although fluid balance is important to critically ill patients in all age groups, there are some special considerations in the newborn. The amount of body water and the distribution of body water vary with gestational age and change after birth. Fluid management must allow for this variation. Fluid overloading, particularly in the low-birth-weight infant in the first days postnatally, may be associated with congestive heart failure and PDA and with necrotizing enterocolitis.[4,5] Additionally, insensible water loss (IWL) is relatively greater in the low-birth-weight infant because of increased skin permeability, larger body surface area per unit of body weight, and high skin blood flow in relation to weight. The high respiratory rate in these infants may also account for some of this increased IWL.[41] Ambient temperature must be closely monitored because a temperature of as little as 1°C above the NTE temperature range has been shown to increase IWL through increased evaporative heat loss.[5] Use of radiant warmers and phototherapy, as previously described, also increase IWL.[42,63] Use of a heat shield, increasing the relative humidity of the environment, and humification of inspired gases may decrease IWL.[6,19,27]

Immunity and infection in the newborn

The immune response serves three major functions in the human body: defense against microorganisms, removal of worn-out cells to maintain homeostasis, and recognition and destruction of mutant cells.[7] In respiratory care, we are primarily concerned with the prevention and treatment of infection, and thus our major concern with the immune system lies in its ability or inability to protect the infant from pathogenic organisms. The newborn has an immune system that is both immature in its development and inexperienced in responding to pathogens.[8] Newborns are therefore increasingly susceptible to infections, and respiratory care providers need to be sensitive to prevention and recognition of infection.

IMMUNE MECHANISMS

The immune response has many components, including non-specific responses such as phagocytosis and the inflammatory response, and specific responses of the T cells (cell-mediated response) and B cells (humoral response) of the immune system. The newborn infant may have abnormalities or deficiencies of any or all parts of this system, which may affect both his ability to defend himself and our ability to recognize an infectious process.

The inflammatory response in newborns is not well developed. Fever in the older child or adult is most commonly present with infection, but the febrile response is not well developed in the neonate. Thus the presence or absence of elevated temperature is not a reliable indicator of infection in this population; however, instability or lability of temperature may be a warning sign. Increases in white blood cell count (leukocytosis) and increased erythrocyte sedimentation rate, used to monitor infection in older patients, are similarly poor indicators in the newborn. An increase in bands (non-segmented neutrophils) is more significant and helpful in the diagnosis of neonatal infection. In addition, bacterial infection may activate the clotting system, eventually leading to disseminated intravascular coagulation (DIC), and the monitoring of clotting factors and other components of the clotting system may be helpful in predicting infection.

Chemotaxis involves the movement of phagocytic cells toward a foreign stimulus such as an invading bacteria or virus. Chemotaxis is present in the newborn but is diminished when compared to the adult response.[39] Phagocytosis, which involves the ingestion of foreign particles by specific scavenger cells, may also be deficient. Various studies have shown that neonatal leukocytes may have abnormal phagocytic ability under varying conditions, although there is conflicting evidence as to whether this occurs in all newborns.[20,40]

To prepare virulent particles for phagocytosis, specific antibodies and the complement system are necessary. This process, called opsonization, is relatively deficient in the term newborn and more so in the preterm infant. Immunoglobulin M is probably important in the opsonization of many infectious agents, but this immunoglobulin does not cross the placenta. This may account for the relatively high incidence of gram-negative infections in the newborn population. The complement system plays a major role in the natural resistance to infection. Many components of this system have been found to be decreased in the newborn period.[8] In addition, the ability of newborn white blood cells to kill bacteria (bacteriocidal activity) may also be deficient, particularly in sick newborns.[64]

B cells are responsible for the synthesis of antibodies, including IgG, IgA, and IgM. These antibodies are the major defense against pyogenic pathogens such as *Haemophilus influenzae* and the meningococcus. In addition to reacting with antigens such as bacteria, antibodies are important in phagocytosis, chemotaxis, and the release of mediators of the inflammatory response. Levels of these substances are affected by transfer across the placenta and by maturation of the antibody-producing system of the body. Immunoglobulin G is actively transported across the placenta from the mother to the fetus, but other immunoglobulins are not. At birth, the infant has almost exclusively IgG, with little or no IgA or IgM. Immunoglobulin G is passively acquired from the mother, and the newborn cannot form sufficient quantities of this substance, which has a relatively short life. Thus IgG levels decline during the first few months after birth, resulting in a condition referred to as physiologic hypogammaglobulinemia. After birth, the infant begins to produce increasing amounts of IgM, which reaches adult levels by 1 year of age, and IgA, which reaches adult levels by 10 years of age.[8]

SYSTEMIC INFECTION

Although localized infections such as skin lesions, conjunctivitis, and gastroenteritis do occur in the newborn, systemic infections are far more serious and difficult to recognize and treat. Signs and symptoms are often very subtle and nonspecific. Because of the deficiencies in the newborn's immune response, he cannot localize infections very well, and systemic infection occurs commonly. The deficiencies of the immune system also predispose the infant to more serious infections such as those caused by gram-negative organisms. Respiratory care providers should be aware of the risk factors that increase the likelihood of infection and of the signs and symptoms that may indicate infection. A high index of suspicion may help to identify infections in their early stages, when treatment is more effective. In addition, care providers should be constantly vigilant in their attempts to avoid introducing or spreading infection in the nursery.

Systemic infections of the newborn include sepsis, meningitis, and pneumonitis, all of which present in the same general manner and may occur at the same time. The initial approach to these problems is essentially the same. Infants who are at high risk of developing systemic infections include those born after premature rupture of the membranes (PROM, or more than 24 hours between membrane rupture and delivery of the infant); infants who required resuscitation at birth; any premature infant; infants with meconium aspiration; and

infants born to mothers with fever, known infection, or am-
nionitis. Foul-smelling amniotic fluid following membrane
rupture may be an indication of infection.

Signs of systemic infection are nonspecific and may include respiratory distress, apneic spells, and cyanosis even
without obvious involvement of the pulmonary system. Other
signs include unstable temperature, jaundice, difficulty feeding, lethargy, vomiting, and irritability. The presence of any
of these signs in the high-risk infant indicates that diagnostic
procedures should be performed, including Gram stain and
culture and sensitivity testing of both blood and spinal fluid,
along with a chest radiograph. Sputum sampling may also be
helpful if pneumonitis is present. Complete blood count may
be supportive of a diagnosis of infection, particularly if the
white blood cell count is less than 5000/mm^3 or bands are
greater than 2000/mm^3. A declining platelet count or an ab-
solute decrease in platelets below 100,000/mm^3 also supports
a diagnosis of systemic infection.[11]

Once a systemic infection is suspected, cultures should
be drawn and antibiotic therapy begun immediately with
broad-spectrum antibiotics to cover both gram-positive and
gram-negative possibilities. Combinations of ampicillin and
kanamycin or ampicillin and gentamycin are commonly used.
Escherichia coli, Group B beta-hemolytic streptococcus, and
Staphylococcus aureus are some of the more common agents
that may be responsible for these infections.

PREVENTION OF INFECTION

Prevention of infection is extremely important in the newborn,
particularly the premature newborn with other disorders such
as respiratory distress syndrome. Handwashing is the single
most important and effective method of preventing the introduction and spread of infection, and should be performed before and after every contact with an infant in the intensive
care nursery. The initial washing should employ an iodophor
preparation and should last at least 2 minutes. The effectiveness of iodophors is primarily related to the length of time
they are applied. Vigorous scrubbing, although often used, is
probably unnecessary. Handwashing between contacts requires about 15 seconds.

Other activities that will help to prevent nosocomial infections include the use of cover gowns by all personnel or visitors in street clothing and by any person who holds an infant. Personnel with acute febrile illness, or any highly contagious infection, should stay away from the nursery. Strict attention to aseptic technique during invasive procedures such as endotracheal suctioning, arterial puncture, and heel stick is mandatory. Skin puncture sites must be thoroughly cleansed. Sterile technique should be used for cutdowns and catheterizations. Standard cleaning procedures for equipment should be followed and surveillance procedures established to ensure their success. In general, incubators and other "housing" devices should be changed weekly and thoroughly cleaned when changed. Sterile water should be discarded after 24 hours. Oxygen hoods and equipment used for humidification and ventilation should be changed daily.

Intracranial hemorrhage

Intracranial hemorrhage in the newborn is often related to asphyxia and hypoxia, and respiratory care providers need to be aware of the need to respond quickly to insults that may result in either of these sequelae. In addition, infants with intracranial disorders often present with various respiratory difficulties, and the respiratory practitioner should recognize these potential signs of difficulty.

EVALUATION OF NEUROLOGIC STATUS

Although a thorough neurologic evaluation is the province of the neonatologist, all personnel involved in the care of sick premature newborns should be aware of the potential indicators of neurologic dysfunction, including changes in level of alertness, diminished cranial nerve function, changes in motor function, and decreased sensory response, as well as the more obvious indicators such as apneic spells and seizures.

A decrease from the normal level of alertness of an infant may be one of the first signs of CNS disorder. One should be aware of what the normal alert state of the infant is in order to determine deviations from normal. Infants of less than 28 weeks' gestation are generally not alert, whereas a distinct change in the level of alertness occurs after this time.[50] Infants over 28 weeks' gestational age can be aroused from sleep and will remain awake for several minutes; they may also experience spontaneous periods of increased alertness. By 32 weeks, frequent alert states occur without stimulation, and the infant begins to exhibit roving eye movements. By 37 weeks, alertness is further increased, and vigorous crying often occurs during awake periods. Term infants have additional ability to engage in periods of attention to specific stimuli.

Cranial nerve function may be evaluated by checking vision, pupillary reaction, hearing, and sucking and swallowing ability. Infants under 28 weeks blink when exposed to bright light.[50] By 32 weeks, infants exhibit the "dazzle reflex" described by Peiper, consisting of closing their eyes to bright light for as long as the light persists.[60] By 37 weeks, infants will turn their eyes toward a soft light, and by term they will exhibit visual following, which is the major definitive sign of cerebral function in newborns.[50] Pupillary reaction to light is not consistently present until 32 weeks, although it may appear as early as 29 weeks.[48] Fixed and dilated pupils are associated with hypoxic or ischemic brain injury and with intraventricular hemorrhage in newborns.[60] Hearing deficit is very difficult to evaluate in the newborn. Infants of 28 weeks will usually exhibit a startle response to a loud noise, whereas infants of more advanced gestational age may respond more subtly with such responses as changes in activity or respiratory pattern or widening of the eyes.[50,60] The complex series of activities necessary for sucking and swallowing, which are mediated by several cranial nerves, are present by 28 weeks. Infants of this age tire easily with oral feeding, however, and it may place them in a dangerous position and should be avoided. By 32 to 34 weeks, feeding should present no problem. Depression of the central nervous system associated with many disorders may disturb the ability to suck.

Motor function is evaluated by observing tone and posture, motility, muscle power, deep tendon reflexes (biceps, knee and ankle jerks), plantar response, and primary neonatal reflexes such as the Moro reflex and palmar grasp. All of these must be evaluated in relationship to the normal response for the infant's gestational age; for example, a generalized decrease in tone is expected at 28 weeks but not at term. Infants of 32 weeks may normally have decreased upper extremity tone but not lower extremity tone. Generalized hypotonia occurs in CNS disturbance, including hypoxic–ischemic encephalopathy and intracranial hemorrhage, although hypertonia may also occur.[60] Additionally, transillumination to detect increased intracranial fluid, skull radiographs, the EEG, CT and radionuclide brain scans, and evaluation of the cerebrospinal fluid for red and white blood cells and protein may be helpful in evaluating neurologic status.

PERIODIC BREATHING AND APNEA

Periodic breathing and apneic spells both occur commonly in the premature newborn. While apneic spells may be associated with central nervous system disorders, other causes may need to be excluded.

The classic pattern of periodic breathing, seen in 25% to 50% of premature infants, involves a pattern of apnea for 5 to 10 seconds, followed by ventilation at a rate of 50 to 60 breaths per minute, with an overall respiratory rate between 30 and 40 per minute.[2] There are no changes in heart rate, color, or temperature during the periods of apnea and only minor and inconsistent variations in blood gas values.[14,46,47] The occurrence of this pattern of breathing is highly related to the level of maturity, with the least mature infants exhibiting the most pronounced pattern of periodic breathing. The incidence of this pattern declines dramatically after 36 weeks of gestational age.[60] Periodic breathing probably results from immature development of the system that regulates respiration centrally.

True apneic spells in the newborn are defined as apnea of more than 20 seconds duration or apnea associated with bradycardia and cyanosis. At least 25% of premature infants in some nurseries have been shown to exhibit apneic spells.[15] This probably represents an exaggeration of the normally poor control of respiration seen in the premature newborn, in response to some stress or insult. Thus apnea and periodic breathing can be seen as variations on a continuum of abnormal regulation of respiration.

The most common factor associated with frequent apnea is extreme prematurity. Hypoxemia, either secondary to pulmonary disease or precipitated by airway obstruction, is also commonly associated with apnea. Primary central nervous system disorders may predispose the infant to apnea, and apnea may be one manifestation of seizure disorder. Metabolic disorders that disturb CNS metabolism, such as hypoglycemia, hypocalcemia, acidosis, and severe hyperbilirubinemia, may also be associated with an increased incidence of apnea.[60]

Treatment of apnea involves prompt recognition through the use of monitors and alarms, treatment of the underlying disorder whenever possible, and CPAP or theophylline therapy, or both, when necessary.

SEIZURES

Seizures are another manifestation of central nervous system disorder. Unlike the older child, the newborn does not usually exhibit well-organized, generalized seizures, and premature newborns are even less "well organized" than term newborns. The presentation of seizure may be very subtle and the recognition very difficult. Because seizures are very often related to significant underlying disease, recognition of their occurrence is very important, and care providers should become familiar with the more common modes of presentation.

The most common type of seizure in the newborn, particularly in the very premature infant, presents in a manner that may be readily overlooked. Eye deviation or jerking, eyelid blinking or fluttering, drooling or sucking, tonic limb posturing, or apnea may all occur. "Rowing" or "swimming" movements of the upper extremities may also be present and, less commonly, "pedaling" movements of the lower extremities. Full-term infants with anoxic brain damage are more likely to exhibit multifocal clonic seizures, in which clonic movements (characterized by alternate contraction and relaxation of muscles) occur in one limb and then migrate to another body part, without any particular ordering of the involved areas. Focal clonic seizures may also occur, with well-localized clonic movements, although these do not necessarily indicate localized disease in the newborn. Premature infants with intraventricular hemorrhage are most likely to exhibit generalized tonic seizures (sustained muscle contraction), often associated with noisy, snoring respirations, various abnormalities of gaze or eye movement, or clonic movements of a limb. Finally, seizures may be myoclonic, with single or multiple jerks of flexion of upper or lower extremities, or both.[60]

Jitteriness is another sign associated with central nervous system disorder in newborns; it should not be confused with seizure. Jitteriness is rarely seen outside the newborn period and is a movement disorder characterized by tremors and occasional clonus. The major differences between jitteriness and seizure include lack of abnormal gaze or eye movement with jitteriness, no stimulus sensitivity with seizures but extreme stimulus sensitivity with jitteriness, dominance of tremor in jitteriness and clonic jerking in seizure, and response of tremor to flexion of extremity in jitteriness but not in seizures.[60]

ETIOLOGY OF SEIZURES

The most common causes of seizures in the newborn are related to complications of the perinatal period, including hypoxic or ischemic brain damage, cerebral contusion from obstetric trauma, and intracranial hemorrhage. Of these, hypoxic–ischemic encephalopathy is the most common, usually resulting from preinatal asphyxia. Cerebral trauma is most commonly associated with difficult delivery of a large, full-term infant, whereas intracranial hemorrhage may be associated with either birth trauma or hypoxia, or both. Other causes of seizures include metabolic disturbances, infection, developmental disorders (most commonly of the cerebral cortex), and maternal addiction to narcotics or barbiturates.

CAUSES OTHER THAN INTRACRANIAL HEMORRHAGE

The most common metabolic disturbance associated with seizures is hypoglycemia (blood glucose less than 20 mg/100 ml in premature infants, or less than 30 mg/100 ml in full-term infants). In addition to seizures, these infants usually are jittery, stuporous, and hypotonic and may exhibit apneic spells. Hypocalcemia (serum calcium less than 7 mg/100 ml) may occur within the first 2 to 3 days of life, often in association with hypoxic–ischemic brain injury following asphyxic insult. It is unclear whether seizure in this setting is secondary to hypocalcemia or anoxic brain injury. Hypocalcemia occurring later in the first week is more likely to be etiologic in seizure production. Infections related to seizures include bacterial meningitis and the TORCH group of infections. Maternal addiction to narcotics or barbiturates results in passive fetal addiction and the development of withdrawal symptoms in the first 2 or 3 days of life.[10,66] Seizures are infrequently associated with addiction, with jitteriness and irritability occurring much more commonly.

INTRACRANIAL HEMORRHAGE

Intracranial hemorrhage is a relatively common occurrence in premature newborns and is related primarily to asphyxia in this group. In term infants, hemorrhage is more likely to be associated with trauma. Four major types of hemorrhage occur: subdural hemorrhage secondary to trauma, periventricular–intraventricular hemorrhage secondary to asphyxia, subarachnoid hemorrhage related to both trauma and asphyxia, and cerebellar hemorrhage, which is probably secondary to asphyxia.

Subdural hemorrhage may result from tears in various vessels. The most serious consequences result when infratentorial hemorrhage occurs, causing rapid and lethal compression of the brain stem. The infant with such hemorrhage usually has severe disturbance from birth, with stupor or coma, eye deviation, unequal pupils with disturbed response to light, and rapid respiration, progressing to coma, fixed and dilated pupils, ataxic respirations, and respiratory arrest. Rupture of superficial cerebral veins may also occur, resulting in subdural hemorrhage with few clinically significant consequences.

Primary subarachnoid hemorrhage occurs when there is hemorrhage into the subarachnoid space that is not the result of extension of a subdural or intraventricular hemorrhage. This occurs commonly but is usually not of major clinical significance.

Periventricular–intraventricular hemorrhage, commonly referred to as intraventricular hemorrhage or IVH, classically involves hemorrhage into the subependymal germinal matrix, which then bursts through into the ventricular system. Some of these hemorrhages, however, remain subependymal. The lesion begins in the capillaries of the periventricular vascular network.[25] This disturbance is almost invariably associated with prematurity, with the highest risk associated with the lowest gestational age.[58] In two studies of premature infants of less than 32 weeks' gestation or less than 1500 g birth weight, 40% to 50% had documented IVH.[1,45] Two major consequences are associated with IVH: rapid deterioration, which is usually associated with massive hemorrhage (conversely, massive hemorrhage does not always result in rapid deterioration); and a much slower, more subtle progression, which Volpe and Koenigsburger have referred to as "saltatory deterioration," referring to its halting progression.[60] Rapid deterioration usually occurs within 24 to 48 hours after a major episode of asphyxia.[26] The infant's condition evolves rapidly from stupor and hypoventilation, proceeding to coma and respiratory arrest, with fixed pupils, eye deviation, flaccid quadriparesis, and occasional tonic seizures and decerebrate posturing. CT scan of the brain reveals major hemorrhage, and severe hydrocephalus or death usually ensues. By contrast, saltatory deterioration may go unnoticed, with some of the signs mentioned previously occurring at various times, and with most infants surviving, a few with hydrocephalus.[60]

PATHOGENESIS OF IVH

Prematurity predisposes the infant to IVH for several reasons. First, the subependymal germinal matrix is present in the preterm but not in the term infant. This matrix provides very poor support for the vessels passing through it. Second, vascular autoregulation is not good in premature infants, so that increases in vascular pressure with resuscitation and fluid infusion may result in vessel rupture.[33,59] Periventricular vessels in preemies are thin and fragile. Third, the anatomy of the periventricular vessels involves a sharp "U-turn" of the blood vessels, which predisposes to venous stasis, congestion, and thus to increased intravascular pressure and consequent rupture of vessels.[60] Asphyxia may increase the incidence of this occurrence by causing circulatory failure and increased venous congestion, by directly injuring the vascular endothelium, or by impairing vascular autoregulation.[34,44]

INTERCEREBELLAR HEMORRHAGE

More recently, intercerebellar hemorrhage (ICH) has been demonstrated to occur with relative frequency in small premature infants. In two studies of infants younger than 32 weeks and 1500-g birth weight, 15% to 25% had major ICH.[24,37] There was a strong association between ICH and IVH, and it is postulated that ICH may be an extension of IVH.[17] Clinically, ICH is associated with perinatal asphyxia or respiratory distress syndrome, or both. It usually results in rapid deterioration and death, with apnea, bradycardia, decreasing hematocrit, and blood in the CSF. The onset varies over the first weeks of life, with death occurring within 12 to 36 hours of onset, very much like severe IVH. The pathogenesis remains unclear, although some relationship to mask CPAP has been demonstrated.[43]

Objectives

Having completed this chapter, the reader should be able to do the following:

1. Define the following terms:

   thermoregulation
   thermogenesis
   nonshivering thermo-
      genesis
   neutral thermal environ-
      ment
   servocontrol
   bilirubin
   conjugated bilirubin
   unconjugated bilirubin
   direct-reacting bilirubin
   indirect-reacting biliru-
      bin
   icterus

   physiologic jaundice
   kernicterus
   phototherapy
   exchange transfusion
   insensible water loss
   leukocytosis
   chemotaxis
   phagocytosis
   opsonization
   intraventricular hemor-
      rhage

2. List the three major components of the thermoregulatory system.
3. Describe the normal thermoregulatory mechanisms in the newborn.
4. List the factors that may interfere with thermoregulation in the newborn.
5. Discuss the mechanisms of heat loss in the newborn, including methods of prevention of each.

6. Describe the response of the newborn to cold stress and to heat stress.
7. Discuss the potential consequences of both cold and heat stress.
8. Explain the concept of neutral thermal environment and discuss its importance in the newborn.
9. Describe temperature assessment and its relationship to maintenance of NTE in the newborn.
10. Explain the importance of heating and monitoring temperature when administering oxygen by hood.
11. Describe the problems related to low humidity of environmental gas.
12. Discuss the relationships between respiratory care procedures and thermoregulation.
13. Discuss the origin and conjugation of bilirubin.
14. Describe the factors that may interfere with excretion of conjugated bilirubin in the newborn.
15. Discuss the significance of the enterohepatic shunt.
16. List the reasons for increased bilirubin levels in the newborn.
17. Differentiate between "physiologic jaundice" and "non-physiologic jaundice" in the newborn.
18. List the causes of jaundice.
19. Discuss the factors that increase the risk of kernicterus.
20. Describe the methods used to treat hyperbilirubinemia.
21. Discuss the possible side-effects of phototherapy.
22. List the reasons why insensible water loss is higher in the low-birth-weight infant.
23. Discuss the importance of NTE maintenance in fluid balance.
24. List factors that can increase or decrease IWL.
25. Discuss the changes that occur in the newborn when infection is present, as compared to the changes in older patients.
26. Describe the features of the immune response that may be deficient in the newborn.
27. List the types of infants who are at high risk of developing infection after birth.
28. List the signs of systemic infection in the newborn.
29. Discuss the methods used to prevent infection.
30. Describe the ways in which neurologic status of an infant may be evaluated.
31. Differentiate between periodic breathing and apnea.
32. List factors associated with apnea.
33. Describe the types of seizures that occur in the newborn.

34. Differentiate between jitteriness and seizures.
35. List the major causes of seizures in the newborn.
36. Discuss the types of intracranial hemorrhage that occur, including their usual cause, clinical presentation, and consequences.
37. Describe the pathogenesis of IVH, and explain its relationship to prematurity.

References

1. Ahmann PA, Lazzara A, Dykes FD et al: Intraventricular hemorrhage: Incidence and outcome. Ann Neurol 4:186, 1978
2. Avery ME, Fletcher BD: The Lung and Its Disorders in the Newborn Infant, 3rd ed. Philadelphia, WB Saunders, 1974
3. Belgaumkar TK, Scott KE: Effects of low humidity on small premature infants in servo-control incubators. Biol Neonate 26:348, 1975
4. Bell EF, Warburton D, Stonestreet BS, Oh W: High-volume fluid intake predisposes premature infants to necrotizing enterocolitis. Lancet 2:90, 1979
5. Bell EF, Warburton D, Stonestreet BS, Oh W: Randomized trial comparing high and low volume maintenance fluid administration in low birth weight infants with reference to congestive heart failure secondary to patent ductus arteriousus. N Engl J Med 302:598, 1980
6. Bell EF, Weinstein MR, Oh W: Heat balance in premature infants: Comparative effects of convectively heated incubator and radiant warmer, with and without plastic heat shield. J Pediatr 96:460, 1980
7. Bellanti JA: Immunology II. Philadelphia, WB Saunders, 1978
8. Bellanti JA, Boner AL: Immunology of the fetus and newborn. In Avery GB (ed): Neonatology: Pathophysiology and Management of the Newborn, 2nd ed. Philadelphia, JB Lippincott, 1981
9. Bertoletti AL, Stevenson DK, Ostrander CR, Johnson JD: Pulmonary excretion of carbon monoxide in the human infant as an index of bilirubin production: I. Effects of gestational age and postnatal age and some common neonatal abnormalities. J Pediatr 94:952, 1979
10. Bleyer WA, Marshall RE: Barbiturate withdrawal syn-

drome in a passively addicted infant. JAMA 221:185, 1972

11. Borer RC, Wall PM, Rothfelder BS: Bacterial Infection in the Newborn. Ann Arbor, University of Michigan, 1977

12. Brodersen R, Herman LS: Intestinal reabsorption of unconjugated bilirubin: A possible contributing factor in neonatal jaundice. Lancet 1:1242, 1962

13. Bruck K: Temperature regulation in the newborn infant. Biol Neonate 3:65, 1961

14. Chernick V, Heldrich F, Avery ME: Periodic breathing of premature infants. J Pediatr 64:330, 1964

15. Daily WJR, Klaus M, Meyer HBP: Apnea in premature infants: Monitoring, incidence, heart rate changes, and an effect of environmental temperature. Pediatrics 43:510, 1969

16. Daum F, Cohen MI, McNamara H: Experimental toxicologic studies on a pheonol detergent associated with neonatal hyperbilirubinemia. J Pediatr 89:853, 1976

17. Donat JF, Okasaki H, Kleinberg F: Cerebellar hemorrhage in newborn infants. Am J Dis Child 133:441, 1979

18. Drew JH, Barrie J, Horacek I, Kitchen WH: Factors influencing jaundice in immigrant Greek infants. Arch Dis Child 53:49, 1978

19. Fanaroff AA, Wald M, Gruber HS, Klaus MH: Insensible water loss in low birth weight infants. Pediatrics 50:236, 1972

20. Froman ML, Stiehm ER: Impaired opsonic activity but normal phagocytosis in low birthweight infants. N Engl J Med 281:926, 1969

21. Gartner LM, Lee K-S: Jaundice and liver disease. In Behrman RE (ed): Neonatal Perinatal Medicine. St. Louis, CV Mosby, 1977

22. Gartner LM, Lee K-S, Vaisman S et al: Development of bilirubin transport and metabolism in the newborn rhesus monkey. J Pediatr 90:513, 1977

23. Gross SJ: Vitamin E and neonatal bilirubinemia. Pediatrics 64:321, 1979

24. Grunnett ML, Shields WD: Cerebellar hemorrhage in the premature infant. J Pediatr 88:605, 1976

25. Hambleton G, Wigglesworth JS: Origin of intraventricular hemorrhage in the preterm infant. Arch Dis Child 51:651, 1976

26. Harrison VC, Heese H de V, Klein M: Intracranial hemorrhage associated with hyaline membrane disease. Arch Dis Child 43:116, 1968

27. Hey EN, Katz G: Evaporative water loss in the new-born baby. J Physiol 200:605, 1969
28. Hey EN, Katz G: The range of thermal insulation in the tissues of the newborn baby. J Physiol 207:667, 1970
29. Hey EN, Katz G, O'Connell B: The total thermal insulation of the newborn baby. J Physiol 207:683, 1970
30. Hull D: Brown adipose tissue. Br Med Bull 22:92, 1966
31. Korones SB: High-Risk Newborn Infants: The Basis for Intensive Nursing Care, 3rd ed. St. Louis, CV Mosby, 1981
32. Levi AJ, Gatmaitan Z, Adias I: Deficiency of hepatic organic anion-binding protein, impaired organic anion uptake by liver and "physiologic jaundice" in newborn monkeys. N Engl J Med 283:1136, 1970
33. Lou HC, Lassen NA, Friis–Hansen B: Impaired autoregulation of cerebral blood flow in the distressed newborn. J Pediatr 94:118, 1979
34. Lou HC, Lassen NA, Tweed WA et al: Pressure passive cerebral blood flow and breakdown of the blood–brain barrier in experimental fetal asphyxia. Acta Paediatr Scand 68:57, 1979
35. Lucey JF: The unsolved problem of kernicterus in the susceptible low birth weight infant. Pediatr 49:646, 1972
36. Maisels MJ: Neonatal jaundice. In Avery GB (ed): Neonatology: Pathophysiology and Management of the Newborn, 2nd ed. Philadelphia, JB Lippincott, 1981
37. Martin R, Roessman U, Fanaroff A: Massive intracerebellar hemorrhage in low-birth-weight infants. J Pediatr 89:290, 1976
38. Mestyan I, Jarai GB, Feket M: Surface temperature versus deep body temperature and the metabolic response to cold of hypothermic premature infants. Biol Neonate 7:230, 1964
39. Miller ME: Chemotactic function in the human neonate: Humoral and cellular function. Pediatr Res 5:487, 1971
40. Miller ME: Phagocytosis in the newborn infant: Humoral and cellular factors. J Pediatr 74:255, 1969
41. Oh W: Fluid and electrolyte management. in Avery GB (ed): Neonatology: Pathophysiology and Management of the Newborn, 2nd ed. Philadelphia, JB Lippincott, 1981
42. Oh W, Karecki H: Phototherapy and insensible water loss in the newborn infant. Am J Dis Child 124:230, 1972
43. Pape KE, Armstrong DL, Fitzhardinge PM: Central nervous system pathology associated with mask ventilation

in the very low birth-weight infant: A new etiology for intracerebellar hemorrhage. Pediatrics 58:473, 1976

44. Pape KE, Wigglesworth JS: Haemorrhage, Ischaemia and the Perinatal Brain. Philadelphia, JB Lippincott, 1979
45. Papile L, Burstein J, Burstein R et al: Incidence and evolution of subependymal hemorrhage: A study of infants with birth weights less than 1500 gm. J Pediatr 92:529, 1978
46. Rigatto H, Brady JP: Periodic breathing and apnea in preterm infants: Evidence for hypoventilation possibly due to central respiratory depression: I. Pediatrics 50:202, 1972
47. Rigatto H, Brady JP: Periodic breathing in preterm infants: Hypoxia as a primary event: II. Pediatrics 50:219, 1972
48. Robinson RJ: Assessment of gestational age by neurologic examination. Arch Dis Child 41:437, 1966
49. Saigal S, O'Neill A, Surainder Y et al: Placental transfusion and hyperbilirubinemia in the premature. Pediatrics 49:406, 1972
50. Saint-Anne Dargassies S: Neurological maturation of the premature infant of 28–41 weeks gestational age. In Falkner F (ed): Human Development. Philadelphia, WB Saunders, 1966
51. Saland J, McNamara H, Cohen MI: Navajo jaundice: A variant of neonatal hyperbilirubinemia associated with breast feeding. J Pediatr 85:271, 1974
52. Scopes JW: Metabolic rate and temperature control in the human baby. Br Med Bull 22:88, 1966
53. Scopes JW: Thermoregulation in the newborn. In Avery GB (ed): Neonatology: Pathophysiology and Management of the Newborn, 2nd ed. Philadelphia, JB Lippincott, 1981
54. Scopes JW, Ahmed I: Range of critical temperatures in sick and premature newborn babies. Arch Dis Child 41:417, 1966
55. Silverman WA, Blanc WA: The effects of humidity on survival of newly born premature infants. Pediatrics 20:477, 1957
56. Silverman WA, Fertig JW, Berger AP: The influence of the thermal environment upon the survival of newly born premature infants. Pediatrics 22:876, 1958
57. Silverman WA, Sinclair JC, Agate FJ: The oxygen cost of minor changes in heat balance of small newborn infants. Acta Paediatr Scand 55:294, 1966
58. Volpe JJ: Neonatal intracranial hemorrhage. Clin Perinatol 4:77, 1977

59. Volpe JJ: Neonatal periventricular hemorrhage: Past, present, and future. J Pediatr 92:693, 1978

60. Volpe JJ, Koenigsberger R: Neurologic disorders. In Avery GB (ed): Neonatology: Pathophysiology and Management of the Newborn, 2nd ed. Philadelphia, JB Lippincott, 1981

61. Wennberg RP, Depp R, Heinrichs WL: Indications for early exchange transfusion in patients with erythroblastosis fetalis. J Pediatr 92:789, 1978

62. Wennberg RP, Schwartz R, Sweet AY: Early versus delayed feeding of low birth weight infants: Effects on physiologic jaundice. J Pediatr 68:800, 1966

63. Williams PR, Oh W: The effects of radiant warmer on insensible water loss in newborn infants. Am J Dis Child 128:511, 1974

64. Wright WC Jr, Ank BJ, Herbert J et al: Decreased bactericidal activity of leukocytes of stressed newborn infants. Pediatrics 56:578, 1975

65. Wysowski DK, Flynt JW, Goldfield M et al: Epidemic neonatal hyperbilirubinemia and the use of phenolic disinfectant detergent. Pediatrics 61:1;65, 1978

66. Zelson C, Rubir E, Wasserman E: Neonatal narcotic addiction. Pediatrics 48:178, 1971

III·
Cardiorespiratory
Disorders
in the
Newborn

8·
Pulmonary
System
Disorders

Marlis E. Amato

Respiratory distress syndrome
Bronchopulmonary dysplasia
Meconium aspiration syndrome
Pulmonary barotrauma
Pneumonia
Apnea
Transient tachypnea of the
    newborn
Wilson–Mikity syndrome

Respiratory distress syndrome (hyaline membrane disease)

Respiratory distress syndrome (RDS) or hyaline membrane disease (HMD) is a syndrome associated with prematurity or stressed, high-risk infants. RDS is caused by insufficient amounts of pulmonary surfactant or depressed surfactant activity, leading to massive atelectasis and hypoxemia. The severity of the disease is inversely related to gestational age.

ETIOLOGY

In order for an infant to have adequate respiratory function at birth, pulmonary perfusion and alveolar expansion must be adequate to support life. At 26 to 28 weeks of gestation, alveolar ducts and respiratory bronchioles are seen, but alveoli are not distinguishable. Pulmonary capillaries are present but are not in close contact with bronchioles and ducts. Alveolar development accelerates from this point, and mature alveoli lined with Type I squamous epithelial cells are present by about 34 to 35 weeks of gestation. Pulmonary capillaries develop along with the alveoli.

In addition to adequate development of pulmonary capillary and alveolar tissue, mature pathways for the formation and secretion of surfactant must develop. Surfactant develops throughout gestation, with a surge in production of mature surfactant (lecithin) at about 34 weeks of gestation. Surfactants are secreted by Type II cells, which also line the alveoli. Thus the two major factors necessary for adequate lung function, development of adequate alveolar function and development of mature pulmonary surfactants, both peak at about the same time. Infants born before 35 weeks of gestation are thus at risk for developing RDS because of pulmonary immaturity. In addition, infants of more advanced gestational age who are stressed or whose neonatal transition has not been smooth (*e.g.*, asphyxiated infants) may have depressed production of surfactant secondary to hypoxemia and acidosis. Other high-risk factors include poorly controlled maternal diabetes and Rh incompatibility (erythroblastosis).

The gestational age that corresponds to fetal lung maturity may vary with many conditions, some of which accelerate and some of which depress fetal lung maturation. These conditions are discussed in Chapter 1.

PATHOPHYSIOLOGY

The primary disturbance in RDS is lack of surfactant, causing an increase in surface tension of the alveoli. The infant must generate tremendous intrathoracic pressures (25–30 mm Hg) to maintain patent alveoli; however, because the newborn infant has a soft, pliable chest cage, he cannot maintain the required pressures. The result is progressive atelectasis and decreased pulmonary compliance, leading to hypoxemia and metabolic acidosis. In addition, depending on the degree of prematurity, alveoli may not yet be well developed and pulmonary circulation may not be close enough to respiratory bronchioles, alveolar ducts, and alveoli to provide sufficient gas exchange, compounding the hypoxemia and metabolic acidosis. Overall, the atelectasis causes ventilation/perfusion imbalance and may lead to hypoventilation and hypercarbia. The increase in work of breathing also causes increased oxygen consumption, which decreases tissue oxygen delivery, and increased CO_2 production, which the infant may not be capable of eliminating.

Another important property of surfactant is its role in keeping alveoli dry. The fluid balance of the lung is ascertained by capillary hydrostatic and oncotic pressures and by tissue hydrostatic and oncotic pressures. The net balance in a healthy lung favors a small fluid filtration out of the capillary into the interstitium, which is cleared by the lymphatic circulation. Surface tension forces are included in interstitial hydrostatic pressure. In RDS, or surfactant deficiency, surface tension forces are greater, acting to pull fluid into the alveoli. This factor, compounded with capillary endothelial cells damaged by hypoxia and acidosis, causes fluid leakage into the alveoli. The fluid is rich in protein, and fibrin-clot formation occurs with dying epithelial cells, forming the characteristic hyaline membranes.

Histologically, the progression of RDS begins as bronchial basement membrane edema and sloughing of respiratory epithelial cells. Patchy areas of atelectasis are seen. Leakage of proteinaceous fluid, from high surface tension forces and increased capillary permeability, occurs into air spaces, forming hyaline membranes. After about 72 hours, pulmonary macrophages appear and phagocytize the haline membranes. Provided that further pulmonary damage has not occurred during treatment, resolution of the disease commonly occurs in 5 to 7 days.

In addition to respiratory effects, secondary hemodynamic problems arise. With profound hypoxemia and acidosis present, pulmonary arteriolar constriction occurs, which elevates pulmonary vascular pressures. Systemic pressures may be low, resulting in initial right-to-left shunting through fetal pathways (foramen ovale and ductus arteriosus). During treatment of the infant (oxygen therapy, fluid administration, and correction of *p*H disturbance), the shunt may suddenly switch to left-to-right through the ductus as pulmonary pressures are lowered and systemic pressures rise, resulting in pulmonary vascular congestion. This causes a further increase in pulmonary capillary leakage and pulmonary edema. Therefore, gradual correction of these imbalances is important, although left-to-right shunting may still occur.

CLINICAL PRESENTATION

The typical infant with RDS presents with signs of respiratory distress either immediately at birth or within a few hours after birth. Differential diagnosis includes a multitude of diseases, which are listed in Table 8-1. The most difficult to distinguish is Group B, Beta-hemolytic streptococcal or pneumococcal sepsis. The two diseases are almost identical in clinical presentation. If the maternal history is suspicious for infection,

Table 8-1
Differential diagnosis of RDS

Choanal atresia
Tracheal stenosis
Congenital hypoplastic lungs
Congenital pneumonias
Neonatal sepsis
Transient tachypnea of the newborn
Cyanotic congenital heart disease
Diaphragmatic hernia
Tracheoesophageal fistula

a white blood cell count with differential may be helpful. A septic infant usually demonstrates leukopenia and neutropenia with elevated bands. In addition, a gastric aspirate shake test for L/S ratio may aid in supporting the diagnosis of RDS.

Symptoms worsen progressively for 2 to 3 days after onset. Breath sounds are diminished and may exhibit dry, crackling sounds of air movement (rales). Clinical signs include nasal flaring (an attempt to increase airway diameter to increase airflow), intercostal, substernal, or suprasternal retractions, tachypnea, tachycardia, and central cyanosis. Expiratory grunting, heard in the most severely afflicted infants, is a sound created by forceful exhalation through a partially closed glottis. This maneuver is an attempt to create PEEP to aid in maintaining alveolar patency during spontaneous breathing. Paradoxical or see-saw respirations indicate the increased work of breathing, as the abdomen moves outward on inspiration and the chest cage moves inward.

As the infant becomes more hypoxic and the work of breathing increases in the first few hours after birth, peripheral vasoconstriction occurs and poor capillary refill results. The infant's color becomes pale or gray. Pitting edema may also be present, and urinary output is usually poor during the first few days.

Oxygen requirements progressively increase over the first 2 days of life. High inspired oxygen tensions are required to maintain an adequate arterial oxygen tension (50–60 mm Hg). Tissue hypoxia and poor circulatory status cause metabolic acidosis. Initially, the infant can maintain normal to low P_{CO_2}. As progression of the disease continues, acid–base status becomes a mixed respiratory and metabolic acidosis.

The clinical presentation of RDS is summarized in Figure 8-1.

RADIOLOGIC ASSESSMENT

The typical chest x-ray in RDS initially shows a diffuse, fine reticulogranular or ground-glass appearance, and air bronchograms may be seen in the periphery of the lung fields (Fig. 8-2). In severely affected infants, the chest x-ray film may show a complete white-out, demonstrating fluid-filled and atelectatic alveoli (see Chap. 5, Fig. 5-6). The lung volume is also characteristically reduced.

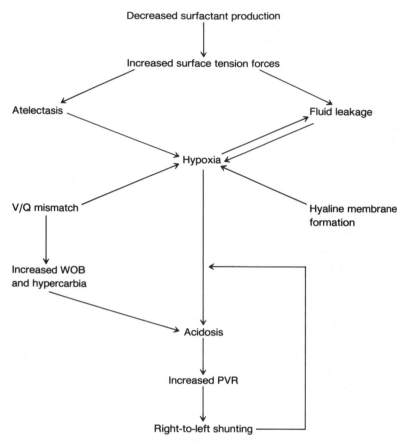

Fig. 8-1. Clinical progression of RDS.

TREATMENT

Initially, the primary goal of treatment is to maintain adequate oxygenation and acid–base balance. The Pa_{O_2} should be maintained in the 50 to 80 mm Hg range, with Pa_{CO_2} less than 60 mm Hg and *pH* greater than 7.25. If *pH* is allowed to fall to 7.0 or less, the risk of intraventricular hemorrhage is greatly increased.

Adequate hydration and a neutral thermal environment are also of prime importance. Frequent monitoring of arterial blood gases is important to maintain optimum Pa_{O_2} with the lowest possible $F_{I_{O_2}}$. Transcutaneous oxygen monitors are invaluable for monitoring these infants because changes in oxygenation can be corrected immediately and the infant's response to routine care procedures can be observed.

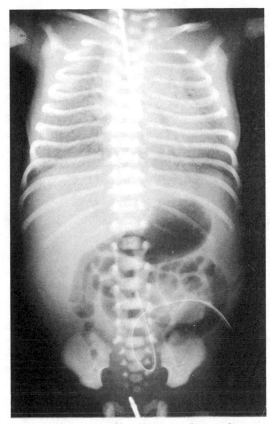

Fig. 8-2. Typical radiologic appearance of hyaline membrane disease, with diffuse bilateral reticulogranular densities, reduced lung volume, and air bronchograms. (Stahlman MT: Acute respiratory disorders in the newborn. In Avery GB [ed]: Neonatology: Pathophysiology and Management of the Newborn, 2nd ed, p. 378. Philadelphia, JB Lippincott, 1981)

As the infant's disease progresses, oxygen therapy alone may not be sufficient. Continuous distending pressure, either by CPAP or CNP (see Chap. 12), in conjunction with oxygen therapy can be used to increase functional residual capacity (FRC) and prevent further atelectasis. Some studies have shown that early intervention with nasal CPAP or CNP provides better outcome and lower mortality rate.[4,6] General guidelines for institution of CPAP are a Pa_{O_2} of 50 mm Hg or less and an FI_{O_2} of 0.60 or greater. This may vary from institution to institution, depending on experience. Nasal CPAP is usually begun at 5 to 6 cm H_2O and increased in increments of 2 cm H_2O until hypoxemia improves.

In the infant who progresses to ventilatory failure, that is, the Pa_{CO_2} is greater than 60 mm Hg with a pH of 7.20 or less, or if severe apneic episodes occur, mechanical ventilation is indicated. A time-cycled, pressure-limited ventilator is preferred because a wide range of I:E ratios, inspiratory times, inspiratory holds or plateaus, and lower pressures can be used to maintain adequate ventilation and oxygenation, thus helping to avoid some of the more serious consequences of positive pressure ventilation. Initially a 1:1 I:E ratio may be beneficial to allow more inspiratory time for oxygenation. Inspiratory hold or plateau may prove beneficial in severer disease because it allows time for equilibration of pressures and improves distribution of ventilation. Inverse I:E ratios, with inspiratory time in excess of expiratory time, may be helpful in the critical infant for the same reasons. I:E ratios of 1:1 or greater should be used judiciously and cautiously because the risk of cardiovascular effects and the incidence of air leaks are magnified by these procedures.

In addition to respiratory and ventilatory support, frequent monitoring of electrolytes, glucose, bilirubin, and urinary output is necessary. In the infant with patent ductus arteriosus (PDA), digitalis preparations or diuretics may be indicated.

COMPLICATIONS OF TREATMENT

Complications of treatment of RDS must be anticipated so that each can be quickly recognized and addressed. Pulmonary air leaks (pneumothorax, pneumomediastinum, pulmonary interstitial emphysema) occur readily in premature infants and cause rapid deterioration of the infant's clinical condition. These leaks usually occur as the infant's pulmonary status is improving, that is, as compliance is improving. Careful monitoring of the infant's ventilation status is extremely important so that modification of ventilatory parameters can be made to decrease the likelihood of air leaks. In addition to pulmonary air leaks, the administration of high oxygen tensions and mechanical ventilation can cause oxygen toxicity and bronchopulmonary dysplasia. Again, careful attention must be given to maintain the lowest ventilation pressures, PEEP levels, and $F_{I_{O_2}}$ levels.

Bronchopulmonary dysplasia

ETIOLOGY

There is much debate in the literature as to the exact causes for bronchopulmonary dysplasia (BPD). It is usually seen in infants who have RDS and who were treated with oxygen and mechanical ventilation. Specific factors that are being evaluated include high oxygen concentrations, positive pressure ventilation, endotracheal intubation, duration of therapy, and degree of prematurity. The disease is not usually seen in infants treated with negative pressure ventilation despite the use of high oxygen concentrations. Infants treated with CPAP also show a reduced incidence of BPD.[2] Infants over 1500 g birth weight are less likely to develop BPD than are infants less than 1500 g.[7] Although the exact etiology of BPD is not known at present, conservative use of oxygen and positive pressure ventilation will probably decrease the incidence and severity of this disease.

PATHOPHYSIOLOGY

Histologically, there are four stages of BPD. The first stage, or exudative phase, involves the formation of hyaline membranes in RDS. Stage II, which may be seen as early as 3 or 4 days after birth, involves regeneration and repair of alveolar epithelium, along with necrosis of alveolar epithelium and bronchiolar smooth muscle metaplasia. In Stage III, bronchiolar metaplasia continues and interstitital fibrosis is seen. Formation of emphysematous bullae also occurs at this time. In Stage IV, which usually occurs at about 1 month of age, emphysematous alveoli and bullae are present, along with bronchiolar and interstitial fibrosis and pulmonary hypertension.

The result of these pathophysiologic abnormalities is a decreased pulmonary compliance and increased airway resistance secondary to fibrosis. In addition, ventilation/perfusion mismatching occurs, resulting in increasing oxygen requirements to maintain adequate Pa_{O_2}, at a time when the infant with uncomplicated RDS should be improving clinically. Excessive mucous secretion and air trapping occur, contributing to the development of hypercarbia. Lobar atelectasis is common in these infants, secondary to mucous plugging.

Infants with BPD also demonstrate interstitial edema and excess lung fluid. Many have left-to-right shunting through a PDA which causes pulmonary congestion. The net result is hypoxemia, pulmonary hypertension, and ultimately cor pulmonale (right heart failure secondary to lung disease). Overall mortality rate is about 40%. Those who survive appear to have no serious respiratory sequelae beyond the age of 6 to 10 years.

CLINICAL MANIFESTATIONS

Clinically, it is difficult to determine when an infant actually develops BPD because the infant is usually receiving mechanical ventilation. The normal recovery phase of RDS occurs around the 4th or 5th day postonset. If the infant demonstrates a continuing need for elevated inspired oxygen tensions and for ventilatory support at this time, the onset of BPD is likely. Chest x-ray findings at this time, however, may be difficult to differentiate from those of pneumonia, pulmonary edema, or alveolar consolidation, all of which may complicate the course of recovery from RDS. The infant with BPD requires continued high oxygen concentrations to maintain adequate Pa_{O_2} and often exhibits persistent retractions and tachypnea. Increased Pa_{CO_2} requiring increased ventilatory assistance indicates the presence of air trapping and decreased compliance. The infant usually can maintain a near-normal blood *p*H by compensating metabolically for his respiratory acidosis. Mucous production is usually increased, and breath sounds may reveal diffuse rales and rhonchi indicative of edema and retained secretions in narrowed airways. With severe air trapping, the anteroposterior (A-P) diameter of the chest may be increased, causing a "barrel chest" appearance.

RADIOLOGIC ASSESSMENT

Stage I of BPD is analogous to severe hyaline membrane disease. In Stage II, diffuse haziness and opacification are seen, which may be difficult to differentiate from other causes of alveolar consolidation such as pulmonary edema or pneumonia. The chest x-ray film in Stage III, which typically occurs at about day 10, is more specific for BPD. Areas of radiolucency, indicating bullae, alternate with areas of atelectasis and give a "spongelike" appearance to the x-ray. In Stage IV, increasing size and number of emphysematous bullae and interstitial fibrosis result in a "honeycomb" appearance of the x-ray. Typical x-ray appearances of Stages II through IV are demonstrated in Figure 8-3.

TREATMENT

Treatment for BPD is primarily supportive. Adequate Pa_{O_2} and Pa_{CO_2} should be maintained with the lowest possible $F_{I_{O_2}}$ and pressures. Adequate humidification of inspired gas is of utmost importance because of the high incidence of mucous plugging of airways and endotracheal tubes. Chest physiotherapy techniques and frequent suctioning are also extremely helpful. Bronchodilators may prove beneficial in some infants but are of questionable value in patients with fibrosis. Corticosteroids have been used but without much success.[5]

Careful attention to fluid balance, along with digitalis preparations and diuretics, may be needed for those infants with excessive interstitial fluid, pulmonary congestion, and cor pulmonale. If patent ductus arteriosus is a complicating factor, surgical ligation may be helpful in weaning the infant from ventilatory support. Weaning should be slow and gradual and should be performed with close attention to the infant's arterial blood gas values. Chest x-ray improvement should not be expected because fibrotic changes do not improve rapidly. Some infants may require increased oxygen concentrations for a prolonged time after extubation, and an increasing number of these infants are sent home on oxygen therapy.

Meconium aspiration syndrome

ETIOLOGY

Meconium aspiration syndrome (MAS) is a disease seen primarily in full-term or post-term infants who have experienced some degree of asphyxia either prenatally or during the labor

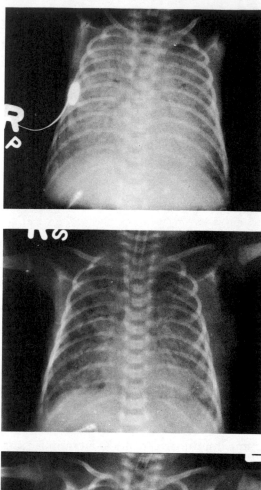

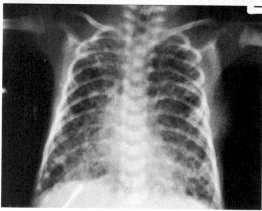

Fig. 8-3. Stage II, III, and IV of bronchopulmonary dysplasia. Note the diffuse haziness throughout the lung fields (*top*). Cystic changes result in the spongelike appearance of Stage II (*center*). Increasing cystic formation in stage IV results in a honeycomb appearance and hyperinflation (*bottom*). (Hodgman JE: Chronic lung disorders. In Avery GB [ed]: Neonatology: Pathophysiology and Management of the Newborn, 2nd ed, p 401. Philadelphia, JB Lippincott, 1981)

and delivery process. Meconium is the material contained in the fetal bowel and is composed of undigested amniotic fluid, squamous epithelial cells, and vernix. When the full-term or post-term fetus experiences *in utero* hypoxia, there is a redistribution of blood flow to vital organs (*i.e.*, the brain, heart, and placenta). Blood flow to the lungs, spleen, kidneys, and intestine is decreased,[2] promoting better oxygenation of vital organs; however, the intestinal response to hypoxia is vasoconstriction, resulting in increased peristalsis, anal sphincter relaxation, and passage of meconium into the amniotic fluid.

The normal fetus periodically exhibits rapid, shallow respirations, moving amniotic fluid in and out of the oropharynx, with the glottis remaining closed. The asphyxiated infant, however, demonstrates deep, gasping respiratory movements, and aspiration of meconium and amniotic fluid past the glottis may occur. The post-term infant is at particular risk for MAS because he has smaller amounts of amniotic fluid with which to dilute the meconium (oligohydramnios) and because of the post-term decline in placental function and consequent increase of asphyxial episodes.

The presence of meconium-stained amniotic fluid is fairly common, found in about 10% of all births. Less than half of these infants present with meconium below the vocal cords, probably because only small amounts of fluid move into upper airways *in utero*. Significant amounts of meconium, however, may be inhaled as the infant takes his first few breaths at birth, carrying the meconium into lower airways.

In addition to infants of advanced gestational age, those who are small for gestational age and those who present in the breech position are at higher risk for MAS. Infants born to toxemic, hypertensive, or obese mothers should be monitored for meconium.

PATHOPHYSIOLOGY

There are two significant sequelae to aspiration of meconium. First is the physical presence of meconium itself, a thick, tenacious substance that obstructs airways, causing a check-valve effect in which air passes the obstruction on inspiration but cannot exit on expiration as the airways narrow, resulting in air trapping and alveolar hyperinflation. In addition, pneumothorax or other air leaks commonly result from this type of obstruction. Ventilation/perfusion mismatching also occurs, leading to hypoxemia and to alveolar hypoventilation and hypercarbia in severely affected infants. With complete obstruction of an airway, absorption atelectasis occurs and an intrapulmonary shunt develops, compounding the hypoxemia.

The second possible result of MAS is a chemical pneumonitis, which is an acute inflammatory reaction in the bronchial and alveolar epithelium, resulting in mucosal and alveolar edema. A decrease in compliance occurs, resulting in alveolar underexpansion and impaired gas exchange. A decrease in diffusion may also occur, further interfering with oxygenation.

Because these infants are usually full-term or post-term and many have suffered intrauterine asphyxia, the pulmonary vascular bed may be hyper-reactive and may exhibit vasospasm or hypoxic vasoconstriction, resulting in right-to-left shunting through a PDA or foramen ovale. This occurrence of persistent fetal circulation is a relatively common complication of MAS.

CLINICAL MANIFESTATIONS

The infant with MAS generally presents with signs of postmaturity, such as long fingernails and peeling skin. The cord and nails are stained with meconium and appear yellow. Symptoms begin at birth or shortly thereafter and include tachypnea, retractions, nasal flaring, grunting, and cyanosis. The chest may be barrel shaped, reflecting severe air trapping and alveolar overinflation. Apgar scores at birth are usually low, reflecting the high incidence of associated asphyxia.

The infant with mild disease will be tachypneic and able to maintain a low Pa_{CO_2} in response to hypoxemia and compensation for the metabolic acidosis characteristic of asphyxia. A moderately affected infant may gradually develop more severe distress over a 24-hour period, with the appearance of increasing hypoxemia and hypercarbia. Severely affected infants present immediately at birth with severe metabolic acidosis, hypercarbia, and hypoxemia. Coarse bronchial breath sounds with rales and rhonchi and prolonged exhalation are heard on auscultation. Cyanosis may improve with oxygen administration, depending on the presence and degree of right-to-left shunting.

RADIOLOGIC ASSESSMENT

The typical chest x-ray in severe MAS shows areas of decreased aeration, either focal or generalized. These areas alternate with areas of hyperlucency, resulting in a pattern of irregular densities throughout the lung fields (Fig. 8-4). Consolidation is common, with no increased incidence in any particular lobe. Pleural fluid accumulation and air leaks are commonly seen, especially pneumomediastinum and pneumothorax. The diaphragms may be depressed if hyperinflation is significant, although this is uncommon.

The x-ray picture is clearly different from that of RDS; it is difficult, however, to differentiate from that of pneumonia, which may be important in the infant who develops a super-

Fig. 8-4. Meconium aspiration syndrome, resulting in irregular densities throughout both lungs. (Stahlman MT: Acute respiratory disorders in the newborn. In Avery GB [ed]: Neonatology: Pathophysiology and Management of the Newborn, 2nd ed, p 392. Philadelphia, JB Lippincott, 1981)

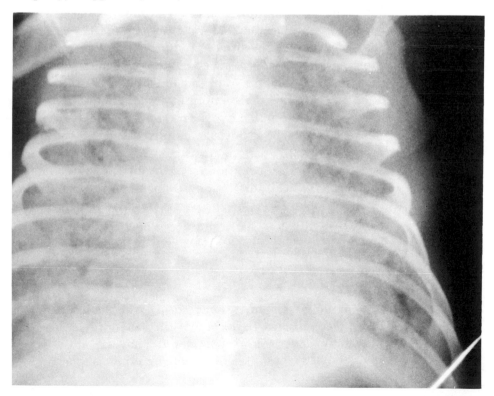

imposed bacterial infection or the infant with intrapartum pneumonia.

TREATMENT

Recognition of the infant at risk for meconium aspiration is of primary importance in the clinical management of the syndrome. When amniotic fluid is found to be meconium-stained or particulate, fetal heart rate monitoring for signs of distress is critical. In addition, monitoring of the high-risk infant may identify distress before membrane rupture. Prevention of meconium aspiration can be accomplished by immediate suctioning before the infant takes his first breath. As the head is delivered, the nasopharynx and oropharynx should be suctioned thoroughly. As soon as the infant is delivered, direct visualization and intubation should be performed. Suctioning, usually with the operator's mouth supplying negative pressure through a filter mask directly to the endotracheal tube, is then performed until all meconium has been cleared. This should be done for all infants born through particulate meconium, even if meconium is not visualized in the oropharynx. Incidence of symptoms and complicating pneumothoraces is reduced when all infants with meconium staining are suctioned, compared with those who are suctioned only when meconium is seen in the oropharynx.[3] Positive pressure ventilation should *not* be applied until the suctioning procedure has been completed because this will move the meconium to lower airways.

Once the infant is initially stabilized and transported to the intensive care area, vigorous postural drainage and percussion with frequent suctioning of the airway should be performed. Oxygen administration may be needed and, in severe meconium aspiration, mechanical ventilation is indicated. Ventilation should be avoided if possible because of the high incidence of pneumothorax associated with MAS. If ventilation is required, an I:E ratio that allows adequate time for exhalation from partially obstructed areas of the lung should be used.

Experimental studies have shown that meconium enhances bacterial growth, although this has not been demonstrated clinically.[2] The infant should have blood cultures drawn and be carefully monitored for possible superimposed infection. Antibiotic therapy may be indicated, and steroids may also be used against the inflammatory response in chemical pneumonitis.

Pulmonary barotrauma

Pulmonary barotrauma usually results from the application of positive pressure or mechanical ventilation. Many types of air leaks can develop in the neonate, including pulmonary interstitial emphysema (PIE), pneumomediastinum, and pneumothorax. Less common air leaks include pneumopericardium, pneumoperitoneum, and subcutaneous emphysema. The most common risk factors for air leak include lung immaturity, RDS, aspiration syndromes, inadvertent intubation of one bronchus, mechanical ventilation, and PEEP or CPAP. Air leaks may also occur spontaneously in the newborn.

ETIOLOGY

Infants who experience air leaks pathologically present with a pattern of atelectatic alveoli adjacent to normal alveoli. When mechanical ventilation is applied, the normal alveoli may become distended and rupture. If the disease exhibits a balanced or diffuse pattern of atelectasis, air leak is less common.

PIE occurs when air is present outside the normal airways. Air dissects along peribronchial or perivascular sheaths, interlobular septa, or visceral pleura. Preterm infants with RDS have a higher incidence of PIE than do full-term infants, which may be related to the increased distance between the alveoli and capillaries in these infants. PIE may present alone or may develop into pneumomediastinum or pneumothorax. The dissection of air into the mediastinum or pleural space actually improves the prognosis of PIE because of the relief of pressure from the interstitium and decompression of the pulmonary vessels.

Pneumomediastinum may also occur for no known reason or as a sequela of PIE. Air in the mediastinum is most commonly seen anterior to the heart and dissects along the diaphragm.

Pneumothorax is an accumulation of air in the pleural space, between the visceral and parietal layers of the pleura. It most likely occurs from distention and rupture of normal alveoli. When pneumothorax occurs in association with positive pressure ventilation, the pleural air may be under considerable pressure, resulting in the formation of a tension pneumothorax.

Infants with RDS present with pneumothorax when the initial disease is resolving and compliance is improving. The diffuse atelectasis of the initial disease process is changing to a pattern of normal alveoli next to atelectatic alveoli, and thus the incidence of pneumothorax increases at this time. Pneumothorax also occurs when airway obstruction causes peripheral distention, as in MAS.

Spontaneous pneumothorax occurs primarily in full-term infants, probably secondary to the very high negative intrathoracic pressure created with the first breath.

PATHOPHYSIOLOGY

Pulmonary interstitial emphysema, also called "air block," causes compression of pulmonary vessels, resulting in decreased pulmonary blood flow and increased pulmonary vascular resistance, and causes compression of lymphatic vessels, resulting in increased lung water. Air in the interstitium also compresses alveoli, and atelectasis follows. In addition, airways may be compressed, resulting in air trapping and distention of alveoli. If extensive enough, cor pulmonale may develop secondary to increased pulmonary vascular resistance, and right-to-left shunting (both intrapulmonary and intracardiac) will occur. Thromboembolism may form because of sluggish or obstructed capillary flow.

In pneumomediastinum, air collection above the diaphragm, when large enough, may also compress alveoli and prevent inflation. Usually, however, mediastinal air ruptures into the pleural space and results in pneumothorax.

The effects of a pneumothorax primarily depend on its size and on the pressure of the air in the pleural space. Pneumothorax causes an increased pleural pressure, compression of the great veins, increased pulmonary vascular resistance, and decreased lung volume. A decrease in venous return occurs, causing a decrease in cardiac output. A sizable tension pneumothorax is a life-threatening condition and warrants immediate removal of the extraneous air.

CLINICAL AND LABORATORY PRESENTATION

Infants with air leaks will generally present with tachypnea, cyanosis, and retractions caused by alveolar compression and diminished pulmonary blood flow. Hypoxia results from hypoventilation and V/Q mismatch. If pulmonary vascular resistance increases significantly, right-to-left shunting may occur, furthering the development of hypoxemia and resulting in decreased effectiveness of oxygen therapy. Infants with PIE may have significant air trapping, resulting in a barrel chest appearance, or increased A-P diameter of the chest.

Pneumothorax is often associated with hypotension and severe cyanosis, resulting from the drop in cardiac output, and with a shift of the mediastinum away from the involved side, manifested by a change in the location of the apical cardiac impulse. Decreased breath sounds on the involved side may be heard. Onset of symptoms may be progressive or immediate. Rapid onset usually occurs in tension pneumothorax. Severe pneumothorax results in bradypnea, bradycardia, and apnea. Arterial blood gas studies reveal acidosis, hypercarbia, and hypoxemia. Use of a high-intensity light placed against the chest wall (transillumination) may reveal increased lucency of the chest with increased pleural air. This is a valuable tool for rapid, bedside detection and evaluation of pneumothorax.

RADIOLOGIC ASSESSMENT

PIE initially presents on chest x-ray as nodular, irregular "bubbles" originating in the hilar areas and radiating outward (see Chap. 5, Fig. 5-5). Expiratory films may be helpful in demonstrating PIE, because on inspiration the bubbles may elongate and may not show very clearly on x-ray. With time, these bubbles may converge to form large cystic pneumatoceles. The x-ray picture will begin to clear around the 5th day in mild PIE.

Chest x-ray films for pneumothorax should be taken on expiration. A dense, dark area separating the lung from the chest wall, with absent lung markings, represents air in the pleural space (see Chap. 5, Fig. 5-8). Displacement of the mediastinal structures, including the heart, and of the trachea may occur, unless bilateral pneumothoraces are present. With the infant in the supine position, the air may layer out along the anterior chest wall, resulting in no obvious pleural air. The lung field on the involved side will, in this case, appear hyperlucent, with a sharp mediastinal border. Lateral or cross-table views may be helpful in detecting an anterior pneumothorax.

TREATMENT

The best treatment for pulmonary barotrauma is prevention. Ventilation should be monitored closely to avoid distention. Pressures under 30 cm H_2O are recommended to avoid PIE. In the infant who develops PIE and requires continuing ventilation, pressures should be lowered as much as possible. Administration of 100% oxygen for 10- to 15-minute intervals may facilitate reabsorption of extra-alveolar air, keeping in mind the hazards of high oxygen in the premature infant. Selective intubation of the uninvolved side in unilateral disease may also allow time for air to reabsorb. This technique should be reserved for the severely affected infant. Lobectomy has been performed in life-threatening PIE, although this is a drastic procedure for a potentially reversible disease. High-frequency ventilation has also been used with success.

Pneumothorax is best treated with chest tube placement and underwater seal drainage. Needle aspiration can be performed in an emergency to relieve pleural pressure and a needle placed in the third intercostal space until surgical placement of a chest tube can be accomplished.

Pneumonia

Pneumonias can be divided into two categories, depending on the route of acquisition and the age at onset of symptoms. Perinatal infections arise from transplacental infection and premature rupture of membranes. Prolonged labor and delivery and aspiration are also risk factors. Postnatal infection is usually nosocomial in nature, occurring beyond the 1st week of life in high-risk, low-birth-weight infants.

ETIOLOGY

The most common bacterial pathogens seen in perinatal infection are Group B, Beta-hemolytic streptococcus (normally found in the cervical and vaginal tissue), *Escherichia coli, Listeria monocytogens,* and *Treponema pallidum* (causing congenital syphilis). Viral pathogens include herpes virus (HSV), cytomegalovirus (CMV), and rubella.

In postnatal infections, the most common pathogens are coagulase-positive staphylococcus, *Klebsiella pneumoniae,* and respiratory syncitial virus (RSV).

PATHOPHYSIOLOGY

Group B, Beta-hemolytic streptococcal infection results in the development of bronchiolar and alveolar hyaline membranes, with a clinical picture virtually indistinguishable from that of RDS. The organism is spread from maternal cervicovaginal membranes to the infant. If rupture of the membranes occurs more than 12 hours before delivery, the risk of infection is increased. Symptoms of infection may present within 1 to 2 hours or may be delayed for days, particularly if infection is secondary to aspiration of contaminated amniotic fluid. Generalized sepsis may occur in the same time period, although pneumonia is the primary finding. The preterm infant is likely to have widespread alveolar involvement, whereas full-term infants may exhibit either a localized or diffuse pattern. Infants with gram-negative infection are more likely to present with sepsis.

The viral pathogens (CMV and HSV) involve multiple body systems, sometimes including the pulmonary system. CMV does not usually present for several weeks, although acquired perinatally. The clinical picture is similar to that of bronchopulmonary dysplasia. HSV infection is characterized by interstitial pneumonia.

In postnatal pneumonias, staphylococcal infection is usually caused by skin or cord stump infection. Pneumonia occurs secondary to generalized sepsis and is commonly localized to one or more lobes. Accumulation of pleural fluid is common, as is the development of pneumatoceles (thin-walled, air-filled cavities). The bacteria of most concern in postnatal infection are the gram-negative enteric bacilli, especially *Klebsiella,* which causes necrotizing pneumonia, with abscess and pneumatocele formation. RSV infection usually is transmitted by infected staff members, resulting in a diffuse pneumonitis with infiltrates.

CLINICAL AND LABORATORY PRESENTATION

Early manifestations of pneumonia and sepsis are generalized listlessness, irritability, color changes, and poor feeding. As the infection progresses, the infant becomes tachypneic, cyanotic, and hypothermic. Grunting respirations may occur, progressing to sepsis, shock, metabolic acidosis, and severe hypoxemia. Apneic episodes may also occur.

White blood cell counts in the newborn are not reliable for diagnosing infection. Leukopenia (WBC less than 5000/cm^3) usually indicates sepsis and severe infection. A left shift (greater than 15% nonsegmented neutrophils) is also a useful diagnostic sign. Arterial blood gases will initially show only hypoxemia, progressing to metabolic acidosis as sepsis develops. Blood cultures are useful in identifying the etiologic pathogen.

RADIOLOGIC ASSESSMENT

Chest x-ray film may be helpful in the differential diagnosis of some of these pathogens from other respiratory diseases in the newborn, but not particularly helpful in others. The clinical and x-ray presentation of Group B, Beta-hemolytic streptococcus infection is nearly identical to that of RDS. Staphylococcal pneumonias generally demonstrate lobar consolidation and pneumatoceles. *Klebsiella* infection is associated with lobar infiltrates and bulging fissures. General patterns of lung infection include atelectasis, which may result in a "smudged" or "dirty lung" appearance on x-ray; pleural effusions; and relative overexpansion of noninvolved areas.

TREATMENT

After cultures of blood and other sources (such as sputum and gastric aspirate) have been obtained, broad-spectrum antibiotic therapy, such as a combination of ampicillin and kanamycin, may be administered. More specific antibiotic therapy may be needed for nosocomial infection because these organisms are likely to be resistant to commonly used broad-spectrum drugs. Results of blood and other cultures will be helpful in adjusting antibiotic therapy. Oxygenation, adequate humidification, and good bronchial hygiene are important to maintain adequate pulmonary status. Mechanical ventilation should be initiated if indicated on the basis of arterial blood gas monitoring.

Apnea

Apnea is defined as absence of breathing for more than 20 seconds. This should not be confused with period breathing, which is an irregular breathing pattern associated with shorter apneic periods of 5 to 10 seconds. Periodic breathing is usually benign. Heart rate usually decreases with apnea, and color changes may be noted, along with hypoxemia. None of these are present in periodic breathing.

ETIOLOGY

The exact cause of apnea is not known, although many theories have been proposed. About 50% of premature infants experience periodic breathing, and about half of these experience apnea.

It has been shown that preterm infants have a higher resting Pa_{CO_2} and a decreased ventilatory response to CO_2, perhaps owing to an immature central nervous system. Hypoxia associated with apnea also decreases the ventilatory response to CO_2. It is currently believed that the respiratory muscles fatigue more easily in these infants, resulting in periodic breathing or apnea.

Apnea has been associated with several disorders, including intracranial bleeding, PDA, pneumonia or sepsis, and RDS. In addition, apnea may occur in association with hyperthermia, seizure disorders, and maternal narcotic use.

PATHOPHYSIOLOGY

Apnea is commonly associated with bradycardia, cyanosis, and, if it progresses to periods of 45 seconds or longer, hypotonia and unresponsiveness. Frequent apneic episodes may lead to cerebral hypoxia and ischemia, thus resulting in hypoxic–ischemic brain injury.

CLINICAL MANIFESTATIONS

Apnea presents as absence of breathing in excess of 20 seconds, associated with cyanosis, bradycardia (heart rate less than 80/min), and hypoxemia. Other clinical manifestations are associated with the underlying disorders that may predispose the infant to apnea.

TREATMENT

The first step in treating apnea involves a search for the underlying disorder, such as a septic work-up, chest x-ray, or other diagnostic procedure. If an underlying disorder is identified, it is treated appropriately. If no cause can be identified, theophylline, a methylxanthine that stimulates the central nervous system and increases ventilation, may be administered. CPAP has also been used to treat apneic episodes, and oxygen is recommended to relieve hypoxemia as both a cause and an effect of apnea. Additional measures include avoidance of elevated body temperature, use of some form of stimulation such as a rocking bed, and tactile or auditory stimulation when an apneic episode occurs.

If apnea persists despite therapy, mechanical ventilation may be needed.

Transient tachypnea of the newborn

Transient tachypnea of the newborn (TTN), also called Type II RDS or "wet lung" syndrome, presents initially with clinical symptoms similar to those of mild RDS in the first 24 to 48 hours after birth. As the name implies, the major manifestation of this disorder is tachypnea, with respiratory rates as high as 150 breaths per minute.

ETIOLOGY

Those affected with TTN are usually near-term or full-term infants of appropriate size for gestational age. History may include maternal analgesia or anesthesia during labor or an episode of intrauterine asphyxia. Maternal bleeding, maternal diabetes, C-section, and prolapsed cord have all been related to an increased incidence of TTN.

PATHOPHYSIOLOGY

The infant may be somewhat depressed at birth, resulting in an accumulation of mucus and secretions. The swallowing and cough mechanisms may also be diminished. Lack of adequate inspiratory effort or a C-section delivery may lead to delayed circulatory changeover and shunt closure, as well as to decreased absorption of fetal pulmonary liquid. Pulmonary capillary congestion with interstitial or pulmonary edema occurs.

CLINICAL AND LABORATORY MANIFESTATIONS

The typical TTN infant has good Apgar scores at birth. Several hours later, however, nasal flaring, grunting, and retractions may be noted. Cyanosis may be present but responds well to simple oxygen therapy. Tachypnea occurs, with respiratory rates as high as 100 to 150 breaths per minute. Arterial blood gas studies reveal mild hypoxemia, with possible metabolic acidosis. Breath sounds are usually clear unless significant pulmonary edema is present.

Within about 24 to 48 hours, signs of respiratory distress disappear. Absorption of lung fluid occurs because of lymphatic clearance. Oxygen requirements decrease to room air by 48 hours of age.

RADIOLOGIC ASSESSMENT

Initially, chest x-ray findings appear normal. At about 12 hours of age, signs of pulmonary congestion appear, resulting in heavy central markings (Fig. 8-5). Distention may occur, manifested by peripheral hyperlucency, flattened diaphragms, and bulging of intercostal spaces. Patchy pulmonary infiltrates may be seen in some infants.

TREATMENT

Supplemental oxygen is usually needed to maintain adequate Pa_{O_2}. CPAP may be indicated in infants who require higher $F_{I_{O_2}}$ levels. Mechanical ventilation is rarely needed.

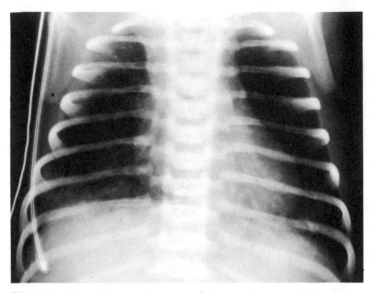

Fig. 8-5. Transient tachypnea of the newborn, with heavy central markings and signs of overinflation. (Stahlman MT: Acute respiratory disorders in the newborn. In Avery GB [ed]: Neonatology: Pathophysiology and Management of the Newborn, 2nd ed, p 389. Philadelphia, JB Lippincott, 1981)

Wilson–Mikity syndrome

The Wilson–Mikity syndrome (also known as Mikity–Wilson syndrome or pulmonary dysmaturity) is a chronic lung disease seen exclusively in preterm infants. Clinically, it is difficult to differentiate from bronchopulmonary dysplasia, although the infant's history is usually quite different.

ETIOLOGY

There is no known etiology for the Wilson–Mikity syndrome. Because it is a disease of premature infants, there is speculation that compensatory emphysematous changes occur as a result of lung immaturity. Maternal bleeding and asphyxia may be associated with its occurrence.

PATHOPHYSIOLOGY

Onset of the disease occurs within the 1st week of life. Pulmonary changes are similar to those of BPD, except that fibrosis is not present. Alternating areas of distension and atelectasis occur. On autopsy, alveolar septa have been seen to be underdeveloped, but there is no evidence of epithelial damage

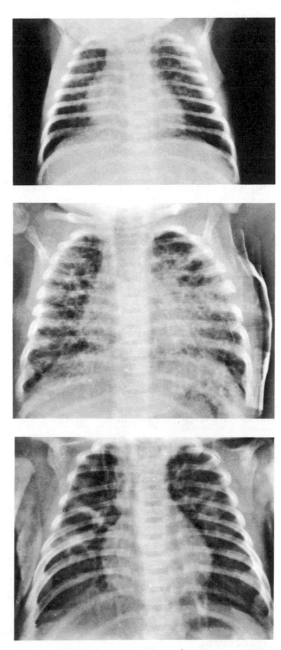

Fig. 8-6. Radiologic appearance and progression of Wilson–Mikity syndrome. Early development of streaky densities, particularly in the upper lobes (*top*). Cystic densities throughout the lung fields, similar to BPD (*center*). Streaky infiltrates persist in upper lobes during recovery, with overdistention of lower lobes (*bottom*). (Hodgman JE: Chronic lung disorders. In Avery GB [ed]: Neonatology: Pathophysiology and Management of the Newborn, 2nd ed, p 407. Philadelphia, JB Lippincott, 1981)

or fibrosis. Distension and subsequent ventilation/perfusion mismatch is the reason for clinical symptoms.

CLINICAL AND LABORATORY PRESENTATION

Onset of symptoms occurs during the 1st week of life. Tachypnea, cyanosis, and retractions are early symptoms and often progress to apnea. Ventilatory assistance may be required by the 2nd week of life, as hypercarbia and ventilatory failure follow. Arterial blood gas studies initially show hypoxemia, progressing to respiratory acidosis.

RADIOLOGIC ASSESSMENT

Initially, chest x-ray findings are essentially normal. By the end of the 1st week, there may be bilateral streaky upper lobe infiltrates (Fig. 8-6). Small cystic areas are seen in all lobes. In later stages, the cystic areas at the bases enlarge and the lower lung fields become hyperlucent because of distention. Streaky infiltrates persist in upper lobes. It is difficult to differentiate the Wilson–Mikity syndrome from Stage III or IV bronchopulmonary dysplasia on the basis of x-ray examination, but infants with BPD have a very different history, including treatment with oxygen and positive pressure ventilation.

TREATMENT

Treatment of these infants is primarily supportive. Supplemental oxygen is administered to maintain Pa_{O_2} and may be needed for long-term therapy, including home oxygen therapy. Ventilatory support may be needed for apnea or CO_2 retention. Careful attention should be given to maintenance of the lowest pressures and FI_{O_2} possible to maintain adequate ventilation and oxygenation. These factors may superimpose oxygen toxicity changes on an already chronic disease.

Objectives

Having completed this chapter, the reader should be able to do the following:

1. Discuss the etiology and risk factors associated with the development of RDS.
2. Describe the effects of lack of surfactant on lung function, fluid balance in the lung, and the cardiovascular system.

3. Describe the histologic progression of RDS.
4. Describe the clinical presentation of an infant with RDS.
5. Describe the typical x-ray pattern of RDS.
6. Discuss the treatment or treatments used for the infant with RDS, and describe the possible complications of each treatment.
7. Discuss the proposed etiology or etiologies for BPD.
8. Describe the four stages of BPD.
9. List the abnormalities in physiology that result from the development of BPD.
10. Describe the clinical presentation of an infant with BPD.
11. Discuss the typical x-ray pattern of the various stages of BPD.
12. Describe the treatment of an infant with BPD.
13. Describe the type of infant who is most likely to develop MAS.
14. Explain the mechanism by which asphyxia promotes MAS.
15. Describe the two significant sequelae of meconium aspiration, and discuss the typical results of these problems in the infant.
16. Describe the various clinical presentations of infants with MAS.
17. Describe the radiologic appearance of MAS.
18. Discuss the treatment and prevention of MAS.
19. List the various types of pulmonary barotrauma that may occur.
20. List the factors that increase the risk of barotrauma.
21. Describe the usual pathology associated with the development of air leaks in the newborn.
22. Discuss the etiology or etiologies of PIE, pneumomediastinum, and pneumothorax.
23. Describe the pathophysiologic effects of each of the above air leaks.
24. Describe the clinical and radiologic presentation of infants with PIE and infants with pneumothorax.
25. Discuss the treatment and prevention of pulmonary barotrauma.
26. List and describe the two major types of newborn pneumonia.
27. List the risk factors associated with the development of pneumonia in the newborn.
28. List the common pathogens associated with each type of pneumonia.
29. Describe the pathophysiology of pneumonia caused by Group B, Beta-hemolytic streptococcus.
30. Describe the features of other types of pneumonia.

31. Discuss the clinical and laboratory features of pneumonia in the newborn.
32. List the various x-ray abnormalities that may be seen in different types of pneumonia.
33. Describe the general treatment of pneumonia.
34. Define apnea of the newborn, and differentiate this disorder from periodic breathing.
35. Discuss the possible etiologies proposed for apnea, and list the disorders with which apnea is associated.
36. Discuss the clinical manifestation, consequences, and treatment of apnea.
37. Compare the presentation of TTN to that of RDS.
38. Discuss the etiology, pathophysiology, and clinical presentation of TTN.
39. Describe the clinical and radiologic appearance of TTN.
40. Discuss the treatment of TTN.
41. Describe the Wilson–Mikity syndrome, including possible etiology, pathophysiology, clinical presentation, and radiologic appearance.
42. Compare the Wilson–Mikity syndrome with BPD.
43. Discuss the treatment of the Wilson–Mikity syndrome.
44. Define the following terms:

RDS	PIE
HMD	air block
BPD	TTN
MAS	Type II RDS
Meconium	

References

1. Berg TJ, Pagtakhan RD, Reed MH et al: Bronchopulmonary dysplasia and lung rupture in hyaline membrane disease. Pediatrics 55:51, 1975
2. Brady J: Management of meconium aspiration syndrome. In Thibeault D, Gregory G (eds): Neonatal Pulmonary Care. Menlo Park, CA, Addison–Wesley, 1979
3. Fletcher M: Respiratory distress syndrome and other respiratory diseases in neonates. In Burton G, Hodgkin J (eds): Respiratory Care. A Guide to Clinical Practice, 2nd ed. Philadelphia, JB Lippincott, 1984
4. Gerard P, Fox WW, Outerbridge EW et al: Early versus late introduction of continuous negative pressure in the management of idiopathic respiratory distress syndrome. J Pediatr 87:591, 1975
5. Hodgman J: Chronic lung disorders. In Avery GB (ed):

Neonatology: Pathophysiology and Management of the Newborn, 2nd ed. Philadelphia, JB Lippincott, 1981

6. Krouskop RW, Brown EG, Sweet AY: The early use of continuous positive airway pressure in the treatment of IRDS. J Pediatr 87:263, 1975

7. Shannon D: Chronic complications of respiratory therapy in the newborn. In Thibeault D, Gregory G (eds): Neonatal Pulmonary Care. Menlo Park, CA, Addison–Wesley, 1979

Bibliography

Bancalari E, Berlin J: Meconium aspiration and other asphyxial disorders. Clin Perinatol 87:591, 1975

Brady J: Management of meconium aspiration syndrome. In Thibeault D, Gregory G (eds): Neonatal Pulmonary Care. Menlo Park, CA, Addison–Wesley, 1979

Fletcher M: Respiratory distress syndrome and other respiratory diseases in neonates. In Burton G, Hodgkin J (eds): Respiratory Care. A Guide to Clinical Practice, 2nd ed. Philadelphia, JB Lippincott, 1984

Hodgman J: Chronic lung disorders. In Avery GB (ed): Neonatology: Pathophysiology and Management of the Newborn, 2nd ed. Philadelphia, JB Lippincott, 1981

Mannino F, Gluck L: The management of respiratory distress syndrome. In Thibeault D, Gregory G (eds): Neonatal Pulmonary Care. Menlo Park, CA, Addison Wesley, 1979

Monin P, Vert P: Pneumothorax. Clin Perinatol 5:2, 1978

Plenat G, Vert P, Didier F, Andre M: Pulmonary interstitial emphysema. Clin Perinatol 5:2, 1978

Rigatto, H: Apnea. In Thibeault D, Gregory G (eds): Neonatal Pulmonary Care. Menlo Park, CA, Addison–Wesley, 1979

Shannon D: Chronic complications of respiratory therapy in the newborn. In Thibeault D, Gregory G (eds): Neonatal Pulmonary Care. Menlo Park, CA, Addison–Wesley, 1979

Stahlman M: Acute respiratory disorders in the newborn. In Avery GB (ed): Neonatology: Pathophysiology and Management of the Newborn, 2nd ed. Philadelphia, JB Lippincott, 1981

St Geme J Jr: Pulmonary infection in the newborn. In Thibeault D, Gregory G (eds): Neonatal Pulmonary Care. Menlo Park, CA, Addison–Wesley, 1979

Thibeault D: Pulmonary barotrauma: Interstitial emphysema, pneumomediastinum, and pneumothorax. In Thibeault D, Gregory G (eds): Neonatal Pulmonary Care. Menlo Park, CA, Addison–Wesley, 1979

9.
Cardiovascular Disorders

Marlis E. Amato

Persistent fetal circulation

Persistent fetal circulation (PFC) is a syndrome usually affecting full-term or post-term infants that is characterized by severe hypoxemia and cyanosis. Right-to-left shunting through a patent ductus arteriosus (PDA) and foramen ovale secondary to pulmonary hypertension is responsible for the hypoxemia. Usually there are no signs of intrinsic lung disease. This syndrome has also been called persistent pulmonary hypertension, persistent transitional hypertension, or persistent pulmonary vascular obstruction.

ETIOLOGY

The full-term newborn has increased amounts of smooth muscle in pulmonary arterioles. The pulmonary vascular bed, therefore, is more reactive, and pulmonary vascular resistance (PVR) may increase dramatically secondary to hypoxia and acidosis, both of which cause pulmonary vasoconstriction. PFC develops when PVR fails to drop at birth. Infants who develop PFC usually have Apgar scores of 5 or less at 1 and 5 minutes. About 50% have a history of perinatal asphyxia. Chronic intrauterine hypoxia may result in PFC secondary to medial hypertrophy of pulmonary arteries and polycythemia. Increased hematocrit values have been shown to increase PVR and to decrease cardiac output.

Severe bacterial or viral pneumonias, aspiration sydromes, and septicemia with pulmonary involvement are also associated with pulmonary hypertension. Transient tachypnea of the newborn (TTN; RDS Type II) may also result in mild pulmonary hypertension if hypoxia and hyperinflation of the lungs are severe.

Congenital lung malformations such as lobar emphysema and diaphragmatic hernia may increase PVR owing to hypoxia and increased blood flow to the noncompressed lung.

Central nervous system disease may result in hypoxia, atelectasis, and hypoventilation, caused by intracranial hemorrhage secondary to birth trauma, asphyxia, and meningitis.

PATHOPHYSIOLOGY

The primary hemodynamic characteristic of PFC is pulmonary hypertension. When PVR increases to the point where pulmonary artery pressures become higher than systemic arterial pressures, right-to-left shunting through the ductus arteriosus will occur. Because of decreased pulmonary venous return to the left atrium, right atrial pressures may exceed left atrial pressures and cause interatrial shunting across the foramen ovale. The end result is severe hypoxemia and cyanosis, without hypercarbia, which is poorly responsive to oxygen administration. Resolution of the syndrome varies from a few days to a few weeks.

CLINICAL MANIFESTATIONS

In most cases of PFC, certain characteristic clinical features are present that lead to the diagnosis. The differential diagnosis includes active pulmonary disease, respiratory distress syndrome (RDS), and congenital heart disease. To aid in the diagnosis of PFC, it is first necessary to rule out these other possibilities in a step-wise fashion (Table 9-1). The first test to differentiate parenchymal disease from cardiac disease is the hyperoxia test. The infant is placed in an oxyhood at 100% oxygen for about 10 minutes. If parenchymal disease resulting in V/Q mismatch is present, the Pa_{O_2} will be greater than 100 mm Hg at the end of the 10 minutes. If the Pa_{O_2} is equal to or less than 50 mm Hg, a fixed right-to-left shunt is probably present, indicating either PFC or a cyanotic congenital heart

Table 9-1
Differential diagnosis of PFC

---

1. Perform hyperoxia test (place infant in 100% hood).
    a. Pa_{O_2} > 100 mm Hg: parenchymal lung disease
    b. Pa_{O_2} = 50 to 100 mm Hg: either parenchymal disease or cardiovascular disease
    c. Pa_{O_2} < 50 mm Hg: fixed right to left shunt
2. If fixed right-to-left shunt is present or suspected, obtain preductal and postductal arterial samples.
    a. > 15 mm Hg difference in Pa_{O_2} values: ductal shunting
    b. <15 mm Hg difference in Pa_{O_2} values: no ductal shunting
3. Perform hyperoxia–hyperventilation test: mechanically hyperventilate infant with 100% oxygen until Pa_{CO_2} of 20 to 25 mm Hg is reached.
    a. Pa_{O_2} > 100 mm Hg with hyperventilation: PFC
    b. Pa_{O_2} < 100 mm Hg with hyperventilation: R/O congenital heart disease with echocardiography or other diagnostic technique
        (1) Abnormal echo: congenital heart disease
        (2) Normal echo: probably PFC

---

defect. If the hyperoxia test shows a right-to-left shunt, a check for ductal shunting should be done. Simultaneous arterial blood samples obtained preductally (right radial or temporal arteries) and postductally (umbilical artery) are drawn with the infant breathing 100% oxygen. A difference of 15 mm Hg or greater between preductal and postductal Pa_{O_2} measurements indicates ductal shunting; however, this does not necessarily rule out or diagnose PFC because about 50% of infants with PFC have significant ductal shunting.

The next test in the differential diagnosis of PFC is the hyperoxia–hyperventilation test. Mechanical hyperventilation with 100% oxygen is accomplished using a resuscitator bag and pressure manometer to assess the most effective ventilation pressure. The infant is assessed for good chest excursion, breath sounds, and color during manual ventilation. Arterial blood samples are drawn, and Pa_{CO_2} is maintained in the range of 20 to 25 mm Hg, a range that has been shown to promote optimum pulmonary vasodilation. The Pa_{O_2} should show a significant increase to 100 mm Hg or greater if PFC is present. Transcutaneous oxygen and CO_2 monitors are extremely helpful in observing the infant during these tests because sudden changes in the infant's condition, as well as the effectiveness of ventilation, can be assessed immediately. This test is fairly definitive to rule out congenital heart disease because in most cases shunting is unaffected by changes in PVR secondary to hyperventilation. The "critical P_{CO_2}" concept is important in clinical management of these infants to produce the best Pa_{O_2} and to aid in the selection of ventilator settings to minimize barotrauma associated with mechanical ventilation.

The typical PFC infant is a full-term or post-term infant who presents with tachypnea, mild to moderate respiratory distress, and hypoxemia with or without cyanosis that is poorly responsive to oxygen therapy. Symptoms usually begin within the first 24 hours of life. Chest x-ray findings will usually be normal, with normal to decreased pulmonary vasculature, ruling out the diagnosis of active pulmonary disease. Occasionally, signs of heart failure may be present. On chest examination, breath sounds will be normal and a holosystolic murmur will be present. A right ventricular heave or systolic sternal lift may be present, resulting from the increased right ventricular load. Echocardiography should rule out the possibility of congenital heart disease, showing a structurally normal heart.

TREATMENT

The primary goal in treating PFC is to decrease PVR. The infant should be placed in an oxygen hood at high oxygen concentrations initially; high inspired oxygen concentrations will aid in pulmonary vasodilation. A neutral thermal environment should be maintained to minimize oxygen consumption.

If respiratory assistance is needed, usually because of a poor response to oxygen therapy by hood, mechanical ventilation can be instituted. Ventilating pressures should be kept low to prevent barotrauma; however, if the infant has a history of asphyxia, acidosis, and hypoxia, decreased lung compliance as a result of surfactant deficiency may be a complicating factor, requiring variations in ventilating pressures. Critical P_{CO_2} is the therapeutic index for clinical management. Hyperventilation to maintain an arterial P_{CO_2} of 25 to 30 mm Hg and a *p*H of about 7.5 is recommended to promote pulmonary vasodilation. PEEP should not be used because the essentially normal lungs may transmit pressure quite well and cause cardiovascular side-effects, in addition to increasing the risk of barotrauma.

Infants with PFC have an extremely labile Pa_{O_2} secondary to pulmonary vasospasm. A small change in P_{CO_2} may cause dramatic drops in P_{O_2} (*e.g.*, 40–50 mm Hg). Minimal handling is essential in routine care of the infant with PFC. Additionally, continuous monitoring using transcutaneous O_2 and CO_2 monitors or oximetry at a preductal site (for best indication of cerebral and retinal oxygenation) and CVP monitoring for fluids and right heart strain are of critical importance.

In addition to mechanical hyperventilation, intravenous administration of vasodilators such as tolazoline (Priscoline) may be indicated. The infant must be carefully monitored for side-effects, including systemic hypotension and renal or intestinal hemorrhaging. These agents are generally reserved for infants who do not respond to ventilatory management.

Congenital heart disease

Embryologically, the heart is structurally developed by 8 weeks of gestation. Congenital heart disease results from inadequate formation of specialized tissues in this time period. The etiology of these defects is not always clear and is probably multifactorial. Some defects may be familial in incidence, and some defects are more predominant in one sex than the other. Males, for example, are more likely to have coarctation, aortic stenosis, and transposition, whereas females are more prone to atrial septal defect and PDA. Chromosomal syndromes, maternal diabetes, and maternal rubella are also associated with an increase in defects. A high index of suspicion can be established from maternal and familial history.

Certain signs and symptoms may lead to the suspicion of congenital heart disease. Cyanosis may be present either due to shunting of deoxygenated blood directly to the left heart or secondary to pulmonary congestion and fluid-filled lungs. Tachypnea will be present in response to hypoxemia. Murmur, frequent respiratory infections, and clubbing may also be present. Fatigue and exercise intolerance may be exhibited, manifested in the infant by feeding and sucking difficulties with cyanotic episodes during feeding. Failure to thrive or gain weight appropriately for his age and sex may be a sign of left-to-right shunting.

Congenital diseases are generally categorized in two ways: the left-to-right shunts, or acyanotic diseases, where oxygenated blood is shunted from the left heart to the right heart, resulting in pulmonary congestion; and the right-to-left shunts, or cyanotic heart diseases, where deoxygenated blood is shunted from the right heart to the left heart, resulting in severe hypoxemia. Either of these types of shunts results in hemodynamic disturbances.

Three basic hemodynamic consequences of congenital heart disease affect overall circulation. First is volume overload, when more than the normal amount of blood enters the ventricle. The result is increased ventricular work, ventricular hypertrophy, and, if severe enough, ventricular failure. Second is a pressure overload. When an obstruction to outflow of blood from a ventricle is present, there is, again, increased ventricular work, hypertrophy, and failure. Third is desaturation or a lowered arterial oxygen content secondary to a right-to-left shunt, which leads to poor tissue oxygenation and acidosis, further decreasing cardiac efficiency. Some defects may cause only one of these disturbances, whereas others may lead to a combination of problems from all three hemodynamic alterations.

Patent ductus arteriosus

ETIOLOGY

The ductus arteriosus is present in the fetus between the left pulmonary artery and the descending aorta and causes blood to bypass the pulmonary circulation (Fig. 9-1). This structure functionally closes during the first day of life when PVR drops. If the ductus does not constrict when pulmonary artery pressures drop and aortic pressures increase, there will be left-to-right shunting through the duct.

PDA may be present as an isolated defect or in combination with other congenital heart defects. As an isolated structure, it is the most common heart defect found in congenital rubella syndrome and is present in about 4% of all

Fig. 9-1. Patent ductus arteriosus. Note the persistence of the fetal channel connecting the descending aorta and the pulmonary artery.

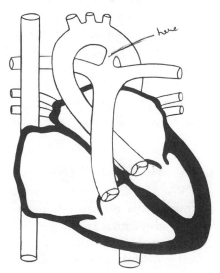

newborns with symptomatic heart disease. PDA is also a frequent complication of RDS, prematurity, and low birth weight and is more prevalent in females.

PATHOPHYSIOLOGY

The normal stimuli that cause ductal closure include rising arterial oxygen tensions and bradykinin release. The amount of smooth muscle present is also a factor when assessing a premature infant. If the infant has a low arterial P_{O_2} at birth, he is at a higher risk for PDA since this is a primary stimulus for closure.

The magnitude of shunting across the ductus depends on the size of the ductus. If the ductus is small, there will be little hemodynamic consequence. If the ductus is of moderate size, however, the amount of blood being shunted into the pulmonary circulation will be significant enough to cause a volume overload of the left ventricle, resulting in elevation of left atrial pressure. This in turn leads to pulmonary congestion, interstitial and alveolar edema, and congestive heart failure (CHF).

In the premature infant, CHF may appear earlier. The premature infant has immature development of smooth musculature of the pulmonary arterioles; therefore PVR is lower. This increases the amount of shunting across the ductus.

If the size of the ductus is large, pulmonary hypertension may develop owing to a pressure overload reflected from the high pressure aorta. Right ventricular failure will result. Pulmonary hypertension is also a long-term effect of uncorrected PDA secondary to intimal proliferation of pulmonary vessels. If pulmonary pressures become high enough, the direction of the shunt may reverse to a right-to-left shunt and the infant or child will exhibit severe cyanosis.

CLINICAL MANIFESTATIONS

A continuous murmur is usually heard, particularly in the very small premature infant. The murmur can also be a crescendo systolic murmur that can obliterate the diastolic sound. Because of the increased left ventricular volume, stroke volume increases, causing increased systolic pressures, bounding pulse, and wide pulse pressures.

Signs and symptoms include failure to thrive, recurrent respiratory infection, and signs of CHF. Heart failure in the newborn does not usually occur until several weeks of age except in the premature infant, in whom it can occur much earlier.

Chest x-ray findings may reveal a prominent pulmonary artery knob and increased pulmonary vascular markings, resulting from the volume overload. Cardiac enlargement will be seen in CHF, as will interstitial and alveolar edema patterns.

Echocardiography may be performed and will reveal the left ventricular volume overload and left heart enlargement.

TREATMENT

The infant with CHF is treated with digitalization to increase contractility and with diuretics if necessary. Oxygen should be administered to maintain adequate arterial P_{O_2}; if the infant requires ventilatory support because of hypercarbia, mechanical ventilation should be instituted. PEEP may be indicated in the infant with pulmonary edema.

Indomethacin, a prostaglandin synthesis inhibitor, may be used to induce constriction of the ductus arteriosus. Results with indomethacin are mixed, however, and it seems to be more effective in infants of more advanced gestational age. Side-effects of indomethacin include transient renal failure, necrotizing enterocolitis, and intracranial hemorrhage, since it both decreases blood flow to the kidneys and gastrointestinal tract and decreases platelet function.

In the infant with significant left-to-right shunting, surgical ligation of the ductus is indicated, particularly if pulmonary hypertension is present. Ligation is accomplished by tying off the ductus with suture ties and is done through a left thoracotomy. Associated mortality is low. Complications of surgical ligation include recanalization and reappearance of murmur and shunting. Surgical division can also be performed by clamping and cutting the duct and oversewing the pulmonary artery and aortic edges.

Complications of surgery for PDA include phrenic nerve

damage and diaphragmatic paralysis, recurrent laryngeal nerve damage, transient hypertension, and atrial fibrillation.

Ventricular septal defect

Ventricular septal defect (VSD) occurs with the greatest frequency of any of the congenital heart defects (Fig. 9-2). It may occur as an isolated defect or in combination with other defects. The septal defect is usually found in the membranous portion of the intraventricular septum and can vary in size and number. Severity of symptoms in isolated VSD depends on the size of the communication between the ventricles.

PATHOPHYSIOLOGY

The infant with a small VSD will be asymptomatic, and spontaneous closure of the defect is common. With a larger defect, when PVR decreases after birth, a left-to-right shunt develops through the defect and causes both a volume and pressure overload of the right ventricle. Most infants with larger defects will become symptomatic by the 2nd week of age, but symptoms may be delayed until 3 months of age or more. Appearance of symptoms depends on the rapidity of the drop in PVR. Premature infants with VSD will present with symptoms earlier than will full-term infants because of lower PVRs secondary to underdeveloped smooth musculature.

Increased pulmonary blood volume, resulting in CHF, is the major hemodynamic consequence of significant left-to-right shunting through a VSD. The results of increased pulmonary blood flow and pulmonary congestion are increased left atrial volumes and pressures. Pulmonary congestion causes decreased lung compliance and makes the infant more susceptible to respiratory infection and respiratory distress. In addition, an increase in pulmonary artery and left atrial size may cause mechanical bronchial obstruction and atelectasis. The pressure and volume overloads also cause right ventricular hypertrophy and failure. In uncorrected VSD, the child will develop an increased PVR owing to intimal proliferation that is irreversible. In some cases, clinical improvement occurs because the defect becomes smaller or pulmonary infundibular stenosis develops.

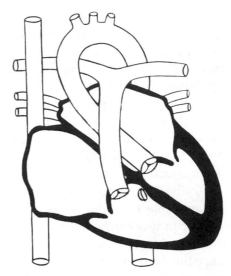

Fig. 9-2. Ventricular septal defect. Note the opening in the wall between the right and left ventricles.

CLINICAL MANIFESTATIONS

Signs and symptoms of VSD depend on the size of the defect. A systolic murmur can be heard with intraventricular shunting. The infant with significant pulmonary congestion or CHF will present with tachypnea, tachycardia, feeding difficulties, and diaphoresis. Arterial blood gas studies reveal respiratory acidosis and hypoxemia. The older infant or child will have a history of recurrent respiratory infection and failure to thrive.

Chest x-ray findings reveal cardiac enlargement and prominent pulmonary vasculature. Pulmonary edema may be present. Echocardiography will reveal left and right ventricular hypertrophy, while the ventricular defect itself can be seen with two-dimensional echocardiography.

TREATMENT

The asymptomatic infant or child with a small VSD usually requires no treatment but should be followed closely. Those in CHF or with signs of pulmonary hypertension are usually treated with digitalization and diuresis. Antibiotics and, if tolerated, chest physical therapy are indicated when pulmonary infection is present. Oxygen therapy may be needed if pulmonary congestion is significant.

If the infant is stable and controlled with medical management, surgical repair may be avoided. Spontaneous closure or diminution of the defect occurs in many infants. If necessary, corrective surgery of a small defect is accomplished by simple suture of the closure during open heart surgery. A Teflon or Dacron patch may be sutured in place to close a larger defect. Postoperative mortality in corrective surgery is between 1% and 10%. Those with CHF at the time of surgery are at higher risk and will have an increased risk of failure postoperatively.

Palliative surgery can be performed on infants who are too unstable to undergo open heart procedures. Pulmonary artery banding can be done by wrapping and tightening Teflon or Dacron tape around the pulmonary artery, which will reduce the amount of pulmonary blood flow and decrease the left-to-right shunt. CHF will not be as severe and should allow the infant to stabilize and grow until open heart surgery with definitive repair can be performed at less risk. The pulmonary artery band is then removed at the time of corrective surgery.

Atrial septal defect

There are three types of atrial septal defects (ASD). The most common type is the osteum secundum defect, located high in the interatrial septum at the site of the foramen ovale (Fig. 9-3). In infants, the septum secundum has not developed sufficiently to act as the "flap valve" to cover the foramen, resulting in a septal defect. An osteum primum defect is located in the lower portion of the interatrial septum and is often associated with mitral or tricuspid valve clefts. The sinus venosus ASD has the lowest rate of occurrence. Located high in the septum near the superior vena cava, this form of ASD is often associated with abnormal pulmonary venous drainage into the right atrium or superior vena cava.

PATHOPHYSIOLOGY

Hemodynamic alterations are not as severe in ASD as in other left-to-right shunts because atrial pressures are relatively low. Left-to-right shunting through the defect may occur, resulting

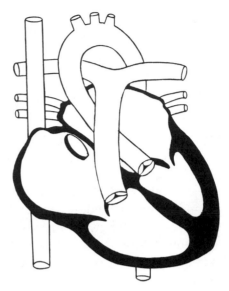

Fig. 9-3. Atrial septal defect. Note the opening in the wall between the right and left atria.

in a volume overload of the right ventricle and pulmonary circulation. There is usually no added burden on the left ventricle, and in some cases the left ventricle may actually be smaller than normal in size. The resultant pulmonary pressures are not usually excessive unless the defect is very large.

Most children with ASD are asymptomatic until adulthood, when right atrial and ventricular hypertrophy become apparent. Atrial arrhythmias are not uncommon as the child matures. Pulmonary hypertension may occur as well, with prolonged increased pulmonary blood flow leading to anatomic changes in the pulmonary vasculature.

CLINICAL MANIFESTATIONS

Depending on the size of the defect, the affected child may be somewhat smaller than normal for his age. In larger shunts the infant or child will present with cardiomegaly and increased pulmonary vascular markings on chest x-ray. The pulmonary artery knob may also be prominent. A systolic pulmonary valvular murmur can be heard secondary to the increased pulmonary blood flow; this is often the reason that

ASD is detected at an early age. Splitting of S2 occurs secondary to delayed closure of the pulmonary valve.

TREATMENT

In the child who is symptomatic from increased pulmonary blood flow, it may be necessary to correct the defect surgically. Open heart surgery is performed, followed by either simple suture closure or suture of a pericardial or Dacron patch over the defect.

Mortality of ASD repair is less than 1%. Postoperative complications include arrhythmias, especially in repair of sinus venosus defect, because the patch is close to the SA node and injury could lead to heart block. If the left ventricle is small, failure may occur when an increase in left ventricular blood volume must be accepted following surgical repair.

Tetralogy of Fallot

Tetralogy of Fallot is a right-to-left shunt characterized by four defects: a large VSD, pulmonic or right ventricular infundibular stenosis, an aorta that overrides the VSD, and right ventricular hypertrophy (Fig. 9-4). Pulmonary atresia may be present or may develop from severe pulmonic or infundibular stenosis. A ductus arteriosus is patent in cases of pulmonary atresia to provide pulmonary arterial blood flow. Tetralogy is a very serious defect, with an overall mortality rate of about 35% within the 1st year of life.

PATHOPHYSIOLOGY

Pulmonary or infundibular stenosis represents an outflow obstruction to the right ventricle, causing increased right ventricular pressures and decreased pulmonary blood flow. The high right ventricular pressures cause right-to-left shunting through the VSD; between right and left ventricular pressures there may be full equilibration. The magnitude of the outflow obstruction determines the amount of shunting and pulmonary blood volume. There may be a PDA or aortopulmonary collateral vessels present to increase pulmonary blood flow.

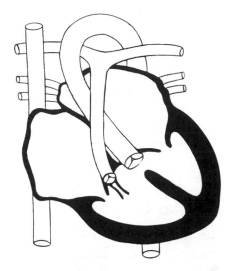

Fig. 9-4. Tetralogy of Fallot. Note the large opening in the ventricular septum, the narrowing of the entrance to the pulmonary artery as it leaves the right ventricle, and the position of the aorta as it overrides the opening in the ventricular septal wall.

Hypoxemia and severe cyanosis are present with the decreased pulmonary flow. Hypoxemia causes pulmonary vasoconstriction and pulmonary hypertension, which also decreases left atrial volumes and systemic pressure, further increasing the right-to-left shunt. If the ductus arteriosus closes or infundibular spasm occurs, a further drop in pulmonary blood flow and severer hypoxemia will occur, leading to acidosis and decreased myocardial function. This often occurs on exertion and presents in the infant or child as "hypoxic spells," causing fainting spells and exertional dyspnea.

CLINICAL MANIFESTATIONS

Severe cyanosis is present in the newborn with tetralogy unless the infant has sufficient ductal and aortopulmonary collateral circulation. In these cases, the infant is prone to develop CHF. The cyanotic infant will become more cyanotic with exertion, such as crying or feeding, and may exhibit syncope.

Arterial blood gas studies reveal low Pa_{O_2} with normal or low Pa_{CO_2}, and a metabolic acidosis. A loud systolic ejection murmur can be heard, and there is a single S2 sound. A continuous murmur may be heard if a PDA is present.

Chest x-ray shows decreased pulmonary vasculature with normal heart size. The left ventricular apex is tilted upward because of increased right ventricular size, resulting in the appearance of a "boot-shaped" heart. Echocardiography will show right ventricular hypertrophy and the overriding aorta. Cardiac catheterization reflects right ventricular systolic pressure equal to systemic systolic pressure, with normal pulmonary artery pressure.

TREATMENT

The newborn with mild cyanosis should be monitored closely and given oxygen therapy to stabilize Pa_{O_2}. Hypoxic spells are treated with oxygen, morphine sulfate, and sodium bicarbonate to relieve metabolic acidosis. To improve pulmonary blood flow, prostaglandin E_1 can be administered to the infant to maintain a PDA.

Hypoxic spells in the infant indicate the need for immediate surgery. The defect may be totally corrected initially, or a palliative procedure can be performed to allow the infant to grow with less postsurgical risk. Recently, corrective surgery has been performed in infancy with excellent results.

Three types of palliative procedures can be performed to increase pulmonary blood flow. The Waterston–Cooley shunt is an anastomosis between the ascending aorta and the right pulmonary artery. The Pott's shunt connects the descending aorta to the left pulmonary artery. The Blalock–Taussig shunt involves diversion of the subclavian artery and anastomosis to the pulmonary artery and is the most commonly performed shunt procedure for palliation of tetralogy.

Corrective surgery involves closure of the palliative shunt and pulmonary infundibular resection. The pulmonary valve may need to be enlarged by incision or by suturing a pericardial patch to form a monocusp. Closure of the VSD is accomplished by suturing a Dacron patch in place.

Transposition of the great vessels

Complete transposition of the great vessels (TGV), also known as dextrotransposition, is the most common cyanotic congenital defect of the newborn period and is associated with an overall mortality rate of about 50%. In TGV, the aorta arises from the right ventricle, and the pulmonary artery from the left ventricle, resulting in parallel rather than sequential circulations. Venous returns to the atria are normal (Fig. 9-5).

PATHOPHYSIOLOGY

Oxygenated blood circulates from the pulmonary veins to the left atrium and left ventricle to the pulmonary arteries. The systemic circulation returns to the right atrium and right ventricle and out through the aorta. Thus the two circulations (pulmonary and systemic) are completely separate. A PDA, ASD, or VSD is essential to provide a mixture of systemic and pulmonary blood. The newborn becomes severely cyanotic when the foramen ovale and ductus arteriosus closures occur shortly after birth, eliminating mixture of the two circulations. If a VSD is present, the infant will be less cyanotic. These infants may not be diagnosed until a few months of age, when the VSD diminishes in size and cyanosis appears. The VSD

Fig. 9-5. Transposition of the great vessels. Note the origin of the aorta in the right ventricle and the main pulmonary artery in the left ventricle, which is the reverse of normal. Also present are an atrial septal defect and a patent ductus arteriosus, which allow the pulmonary and systemic circulations to mix.

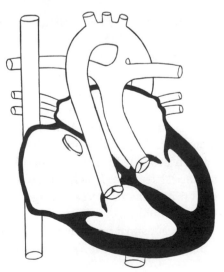

also imposes a volume and pressure overload on the left ventricle, resulting in CHF.

CLINICAL MANIFESTATIONS

The infant with no VSD develops severe cyanosis shortly after birth. Tachycardia and tachypnea will be present secondary to severe hypoxemia. Murmur may not be present unless there are associated septal defects or PDA.

Initially, chest x-ray findings may be normal, until CHF ensues. Evidence of cardiac enlargement and increased pulmonary vascular markings will then be apparent. Additionally, two-dimensional echocardiography may be very helpful in establishing the diagnosis.

Administration of 100% oxygen will result in little improvement in the infant's condition over that seen while breathing room air. This refractory hypoxemia is evidence of right-to-left shunting.

Cardiac catheterization shows systemic pressures in the right ventricle, with low oxygen saturation unless a VSD is present. With no VSD present, left ventricular pressure will be consistent with normal right ventricular pressures. If a VSD is present, left ventricular pressure is higher. Oxygen saturation of the pulmonary artery is higher than that in the aorta.

TREATMENT

Administration of prostaglandin E_1 may be helpful in the severely cyanotic infant to maintain a PDA. A balloon septostomy or Rashkind procedure may be performed to create an ASD and provide a mixture of the two circulations. A balloon-tipped catheter is passed through the foramen ovale. The balloon is inflated and then forcibly withdrawn through the foramen, rupturing the flap valve and creating an enlarged opening in the atrial septum. If this procedure fails, a Blalock–Hanlon procedure is performed by resecting a portion of the interatrial septum. It is hoped that this will stabilize the infant until 6 months to 1 year of age, when corrective surgery can be performed.

The Mustard procedure is the corrective surgery for TGV. A pericardial baffle is created, which acts as a shunt to direct vena caval blood flow from the right atrium to the left atrium. This allows deoxygenated systemic blood to be directed to the left ventricle and thus into the pulmonary circulation, since the pulmonary artery arises from the left ventricle. Blood return from the pulmonary circulation is then directed to the right ventricle and out into the aorta and systemic circulation.

The infant should be supported with oxygen therapy and normalization of *p*H. Digitalization and diuretic therapy are administered in those infants with CHF.

Total anomalous pulmonary venous return

Total anomalous pulmonary venous return (TAPVR) occurs in a very small percentage of infants with CHD (Fig. 9-6). Anatomically, pulmonary venous drainage may be in one of three locations. Supracardiac venous return empties into the

Fig. 9-6. Total anamolous pulmonary venous return. Note the connection of the pulmonary veins to the venous drainage system and thus into the right atrium of the heart, rather than to the left atrium.

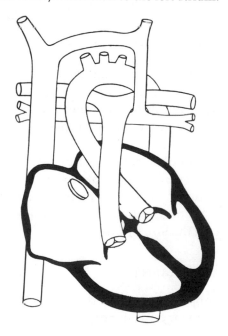

superior vena cava, intracardiac into the coronary sinus in the right atrium, and subdiaphragmatic into the inferior vena cava. A patent foramen ovale or ASD must be present for left atrial and systemic blood supply.

There are two types of TAPVR: obstructed and nonobstructed. The severity of hemodynamic disturbance is related to the type of anomalous drainage. In the nonobstructed type, pulmonary venous flow is directly into the right heart circulation, causing increased oxygen saturation in that area. A patent foraman ovale or ASD then allows shunting of this blood to the left heart and provides a moderate saturation to be delivered to the systemic circulation. Mild cyanosis is the result. A volume and pressure overload of the right ventricle occurs, leading to hypertrophy, pulmonary hypertension, and failure.

In obstructed TAPVR, often a long, common pulmonary venous channel is present that causes an increased resistance to blood flow. If this is not the case, there may be localized obstruction to flow. The increased resistance causes significant pulmonary venous and arterial hypertension, pulmonary edema, and severe cyanosis. Interatrial shunt is present; however, because of a reduced pulmonary blood flow, systemic oxygenation is compromised.

CLINICAL MANIFESTATIONS

Infants with nonobstructed TAPVR usually are not symptomatic until after the neonatal period. At that time, PVR normally drops, and there is an increase in the blood volume to the right heart. Symptoms of heart failure occur, along with cyanosis.

In obstructed TAPVR, signs of CHF, tachypnea, and severe cyanosis present within the 1st week of life. Chest x-ray findings show pulmonary edema, and a continuous murmur is heard. Cardiac catheterization must be performed to ascertain the site of obstruction.

TREATMENT

Supportive oxygen therapy or mchanical ventilation may be necessary in obstructed TAPVR. Medical treatment should include digitalization and diuresis for treatment of CHF. Surgical treatment is required immediately in infants with CHF and significant pulmonary hypertension. This is accomplished by redirection of pulmonary venous drainage to the left atrium.

Coarctation of the aorta

Coarctation of the aorta occurs in about 7% of infants with severe congenital heart disease and is either simple or complex. Simple coarctation involves a constriction of the aorta just at or below the site of the ductus arteriosus, resulting in an increase in left ventricular afterload and left-to-right shunting. Complex coarctation involves a narrowing of the aortic arch, PDA, and a variety of left-side abnormalities that may include VSD, aortic stenosis, mitral stenosis, and left ventricular hypoplasia. A PDA contributes most of the systemic blood flow in these infants.

PATHOPHYSIOLOGY

In simple coarctation, as PVR decreases in the neonatal period, a left-to-right shunt develops across the ductus arteriosus. Pulmonary congestion, pulmonary edema, and pulmonary hypertension then occur, leading to right ventricular failure. In addition, the increase in resistance to left ventricular outflow causes a pressure overload, left ventricular failure, and pulmonary edema.

Complex coarctation also involves a PDA and usually a VSD. The VSD causes a left-to-right shunt, whereas the PDA supplies the systemic circulation. Biventricular failure occurs because of pressure and volume overloads. If ductal closure occurs after birth, peripheral circulation is impaired, peripheral pulses diminish, and shock may result.

CLINICAL MANIFESTATIONS

Infants with simple coarctation commonly present with CHF after the 1st month of age, whereas those with complex coarctation present very early. Femoral pulses are diminished and delayed when compared to brachial pulses. Systolic pressures are higher in upper extremities than in lower extremities.

Signs of biventricular failure are present and include pulmonary and peripheral edema. Chest x-ray findings show cardiac enlargement and increased vascular markings.

TREATMENT

Supportive medical therapy for CHF should be administered, including digitalis and diuretics. Infants with simple coarctation may not require surgery if significant pulmonary hypertension is not present and will respond well to medical therapy for CHF.

Surgical procedures for coarctation vary according to size and location of the constriction. They include resection and anastomosis of the coarctation and construction of a conduit bridging past the coarcted (constricted) area. Pulmonary artery banding may be necessary if there is associated VSD, and division or ligation of the PDA may be needed. Surgical correction in complex coarctation improves mortality from 85% to 50%.

Hypoplastic left heart syndrome

Hypoplastic left heart syndrome includes a mixture of cardiac anomalies, such as aortic and mitral atresia or stenosis and hypoplasia of the left ventricle. It is also found as part of complex coarctation of the aorta. Familial incidence is known to occur.

PATHOPHYSIOLOGY

The left heart chamber is small in hypoplastic left heart, and, with associated atresia or severe obstruction to outflow, a severely diminished blood flow to the systemic circulation results. Venous return to the right heart and pulmonary circulation are normal; however, pulmonary venous return to the left atrium must be shunted back to the right atrium by means of an ASD or patent foramen ovale, resulting in increased pulmonary blood flow. The systemic circulation is supplied by means of a PDA. If constriction of the ductus occurs after birth, shock and immediate death result.

CLINICAL MANIFESTATIONS

Onset of signs and symptoms occurs quickly upon constriction of the ductus arteriosus. The infant becomes ashen pale with poor peripheral pulses and presents with a picture of shock secondary to diminished systemic blood supply. The ductus may "flip-flop," and thus the infant may experience episodes of shock.

Chest x-ray findings reveal right ventricular hypertrophy and increased pulmonary vascular markings. Echocardiography is helpful in revealing a left ventricle that is smaller than normal, and atresia. Definitive diagnosis is by means of cardiac catheterization, revealing the same oxygen saturations in the right ventricle and in the aorta.

TREATMENT

There is no corrective surgery for hypoplastic left heart syndrome at present. Mortality is 98% within 1 year of birth, depending on the severity of mitral or aortic stenosis or atresia.

Objectives

Having completed this chapter, the reader should be able to do the following:

1. Define PFC and state several other names for this disorder.
2. Discuss the possible etiology of PFC.
3. List diseases other than PFC that may result in pulmonary hypertension in the newborn.
4. Describe the pathophysiology of PFC.
5. Describe the differential diagnosis of PFC, including the types of diagnostic tests that are performed and the interpretation of the results of each test.
6. Describe the typical infant who presents with PFC.
7. Describe the major treatment methods for PFC, including the rationale for each and the consequences of each.
8. Explain the term "labile" in relation to PFC.

9. List the common signs and symptoms of congenital heart disease.
10. Differentiate between cyanotic and acyanotic heart defects.
11. Discuss the major hemodynamic consequences of congenital heart disease.
12. Define PDA, VSD, ASD, tetralogy of Fallot, TGV, TAPVR, and coarctation of the aorta, and describe the clinical presentation of each.
13. Describe the medical and surgical treatment of each of the above congenital defects, including the rationale for each treatment and common complications.
14. Discuss the pathophysiology of PDA in relation to ductal size, prematurity, and oxygenation.
15. Discuss the pathophysiology of VSD, including influence of size of defect, major hemodynamic consequences, and long-term sequelae.
16. Describe the three major types of ASD and state which occurs most commonly.
17. Discuss the pathophysiology of ASD and compare the hemodynamic alterations in this disorder to other types of congenital heart disease.
18. Discuss the pathophysiology of tetralogy of Fallot, including an explanation of "hypoxic spells."
19. Describe the pathophysiology of TGV, and explain the importance of intracardiac shunting in this disorder.
20. Describe the pathophysiology of both obstructed and nonobstructed TAPVR.
21. Differentiate between simple and complex coarctation of the aorta.
22. Discuss the possible anomalies that may occur in hypoplastic left heart syndrome, its pathophysiology, its clinical presentation, and the usual outcome.

Bibliography

Benzing G: Congenital heart disease and pulmonary insufficiency. In Thibeault D, Gregory G (eds): Neonatal Pulmonary Care. Menlo Park, CA, Addison–Wesley, 1979

Duara S, Gewitz M, Fox W: Use of mechanical ventilation for clinical management of pulmonary hypertension of the newborn. Clin Perinatol 11:3, 1984

Emmanouilides G: Persistence of fetal circulation. In Thibeault D, Gregory G (eds): Neonatal Pulmonary Care. Menlo Park, CA, Addison–Wesley, 1979

Fyler D, Rosenthal A: Neonatal heart disease. In Avery GB (ed): Neonatology: Pathophysiology and Management of the Newborn, 2nd ed. Philadelphia, JB Lippincott, 1981

Hallman G, Cooley D: Surgical Treatment of Congenital Heart Disease, 2nd ed. Philadelphia, Lea & Febiger, 1975

Lyrene R, Phillips J: Control of pulmonary vascular resistance in the fetus and newborn. Clin Perinatol 11:3, 1984

Sanderson R: Congenital heart disease. In Sanderson R, Kurth C: The Cardiac Patient, 2nd ed. Philadelphia, WB Saunders, 1983

Sanderson R: The surgical cardiac patient. In Sanderson R, Kurth C (ed): The Cardiac Patient, 2nd ed. Philadelphia, WB Saunders, 1983

Wood R: Pharmacology of tolazoline. Clin Perinatol 11:3, 1984

10·
Congenital Anomalies That Cause Respiratory Distress

Marlis E. Amato

Choanal atresia

The choanae are the two openings in the posterior portion of the nasal cavity, directing airflow into the nasopharynx. The choanae are separated by the posterior nasal septum. Choanal atresia results from choanal stenosis, a bony choanal septum, or a complete membrane obstructing the nasal passage. The primary result is occlusion or blockage of the airway between the posterior nasal passage and the nasopharynx. This anomaly occurs in approximately 1 in 7000 births.

Choanal atresia may be bilateral or unilateral. About 40% of infants with choanal atresia have unilateral atresia. A 12.5% mortality rate from respiratory failure is associated with choanal atresia.

PATHOPHYSIOLOGY

Newborn infants are obligate nose breathers. If an obstruction prevents air passage through the nose, the infant will demonstrate signs of respiratory distress. In bilateral choanal atresia, the infant will present soon after birth with severe cyanosis and inability to ventilate and will become asphyxiated unless an airway is established.

In unilateral choanal atresia, the infant has less severe symptoms, and the diagnosis of choanal atresia may actually be delayed for several years.

CLINICAL PRESENTATION

The infant with bilateral choanal atresia presents immediately after birth with cyanosis and retractions. In unilateral or partial obstruction, labored nasal breathing or inspiratory stridor may be heard. A high inspiratory resistance causes the soft, pliable extrathoracic airways to collapse, causing stridor on inspiration. If the obstruction is not relieved, pulmonary hypertension secondary to hypoxia and acidosis lead to right heart failure. In complete, bilateral obstruction, the infant becomes severely cyanotic and dies of asphyxiation unless relieved by insertion of an oral airway.

Cyanosis and inability to ventilate properly occur during sucking or feeding, leading to the suspicion of partial or unilateral choanal atresia. Diagnosis is made by attempting passage of a fairly large catheter (No. 8 French) through the nares. Instillation through the catheter with a radiopaque contrast medium and lateral x-rays will reveal the obstruction. Because nasal edema may mimic choanal atresia, a topical nasal decongestant can be administered before the x-ray procedure to decrease edema and to rule out this possibility.

TREATMENT

Treatment for choanal atresia involves provision of a patent airway. Tracheotomy was performed in the past, but management is now more conservative. Insertion of an oral airway to position the tongue anteriorly will allow the infant to breathe through the oropharynx and relieve symptoms. A McGovern nipple or a nipple with the end cut off will also relieve symptoms.

Early surgical repair is indicated. A transnasal approach is used, and the obstruction is enlarged or perforated. Large-bore plastic tubes are then inserted and kept in place for several months. It is important to keep the tubes clear of secretions to prevent obstruction. The infant can be fed as soon as one nare is patent. The infant can be discharged once the parents have been trained in suctioning. Long-term postoperative complications include scarring and closure of the choanae so that further dilation may be necessary.

Pierre–Robin syndrome

Pierre–Robin syndrome is characterized by glossoptosis (downward displacement of the tongue) and micrognathia (small jaw). The tongue is large in comparison to mandible size, predisposing the infant to airway obstruction. This defect is associated with cleft palate in about 50% to 70% of cases and occurs in about 1 in 2000 births.

PATHOPHYSIOLOGY

Micrognathia, or hypoplasia of the mandible, causes the tongue position to be more posterior than normal. Airway obstruction then occurs secondary to the tongue's falling back to the hypopharynx. During sucking and swallowing the negative pressure that is created pulls the tongue upward into the cleft palate and obstructs the nasopharynx. The obstructed airway causes respiratory distress and insufficiency.

CLINICAL MANIFESTATIONS

Symptoms of Pierre–Robin syndrome vary from minor respiratory distress to severe airway obstruction depending on the extent of the anomaly or other anomalies present. In severe obstruction, sternal retractions are seen, as are intercostal, substernal, and suprasternal retractions. The infant has choking and gagging episodes with feeding and may hyperextend his neck in an attempt to relieve the obstruction. Cyanotic episodes occur and may be severe enough to cause brain damage and death.

As the infant grows, the glossoptosis and feeding problems may diminish in severity by the age of 6 months.

TREATMENT

To alleviate the airway obstruction, the infant should be placed in the prone position with his face down. Towel rolls are placed under the shoulders and forehead to maintain this position; this keeps the tongue more anterior and prevents obstruction of the airway. A nasotracheal tube may be inserted that will maintain a patent airway and also prevent the pulling upward of the tongue during sucking. The tube can be kept in position until the infant has grown or can have surgical correction. The infant is fed by means of a nasogastric feeding tube or gastrostomy tube. Particular attention must be given to positioning because the risk of aspiration is high.

Surgery can be performed to relieve airway obstruction. A heavy suture is sewn through the base of the tongue out to traction or tied around a button attached to the skin of the chin. This, or the nasotracheal tube, will maintain the child until the mandible has grown sufficiently. Tracheostomy may be indicated for very severe problems and life-threatening episodes of obstruction. If cleft palate is present, a surgical repair may be done when the child is 12 to 15 months of age.

Congenital diaphragmatic hernia

Congenital diaphragmatic hernia occurs in about 1 in 3000 births. The syndrome is caused by a failure in the posterolateral portion (foramen of Bochdalek) of the diaphragm to close properly, or failure of the pleural peritoneal membrane to develop. Mortality rate is about 85%.

PATHOPHYSIOLOGY

Seventy percent of congenital diaphragmatic hernias occur on the left side. It is thought that right-sided defects occur more rarely because the liver partially occludes the diaphragmatic defect and prevents intestinal herniation. Symptoms of right-sided hernias are less severe and mortality rate is lower.

The intestinal contents enter through the hernia at about 8 weeks in gestational development. The lung on that side, therefore, has less than the normal number of alveoli, retarded pulmonary capillary development, and cuboidal cells lining the endothelial tissue. After birth the intestines in the thoracic cavity prevent expansion of the lung, causing respiratory insufficiency and decreased cardiac performance. A mediastinal shift to the unaffected side impinges on inflation of the developed lung. Dextrocardia is seen in the most common form of diaphragmatic hernia, secondary to the mediastinal shift.

Secondary to the underdeveloped pulmonary capillary bed and intestinal impingement on the capillaries, a high pulmonary vascular resistance is maintained after birth. Persistent fetal circulation and right-to-left shunting may result and further complicate the respiratory insufficiency. Severe hypoxia and acidosis continue until the intestines are surgically removed from the thoracic cavity.

CLINICAL PRESENTATION

The infant born with congenital diaphragmatic hernia presents immediately after birth with respiratory distress. Barrel-shaped chest and a scaphoid abdomen may be present, since the intestines are in the thoracic cavity rather than in the abdominal cavity. Right-sided heart sounds represent dextrocardia, confirmed on chest x-ray. Breath sounds will be decreased or absent, and bowel sounds will be heard in the chest. After birth, gas enters and dilates the bowel, compromising ventilation and cardiac status.

Diagnosis is made by chest x-ray (Fig. 10-1). The gas-filled bowel will be visualized in the thoracic cavity and the abdominal cavity will be airless. Dextrocardia will be seen if the intestines are on the left side. Contrast media are not needed to confirm the diagnosis.

Arterial blood gas studies reveal a respiratory and metabolic acidosis from hypoventilation and severe hypoxia.

TREATMENT

Immediate surgery is indicated for congenital diaphragmatic hernia. The infant must be carefully monitored, intubated, and ventilated before surgery. Bag-mask ventilation should not be used because this is likely to increase the amount of air in the intestines and further compromise ventilation. Once an artificial airway has been established, low ventilating pressures must be used because of severe bilateral restriction of lung expansion, and incidences of pneumothorax and barotrauma are high. A nasogastric tube is inserted to decrease gas distention of the intestines and allow some expansion of the lung.

Metabolic acidosis may persist even though the infant is ventilated. A slow, careful infusion of sodium bicarbonate may be necessary to correct this.

Surgery is performed as soon as possible by the abdominal approach. The intestines are carefully withdrawn, and the diaphragmatic defect is sutured closed. Because the abdomen has not accommodated the intestines throughout gestational development, a pouch may have to be created to hold the intestines. If the intestines are replaced into the small abdominal cavity, an increase in pressure on the diaphragm will prevent adequate ventilation postoperatively. The pouch can be repaired after the infant grows and stabilizes.

Cautious use of the ventilator is important. The lung on the affected side is underdeveloped and will resist re-expansion. Pneumothorax may occur easily and is an unwanted complication in an already severely compromised infant. Ventilation should be administered using the lowest possible pressures to maintain an adequate P_{CO_2}. A high FI_{O_2} may be

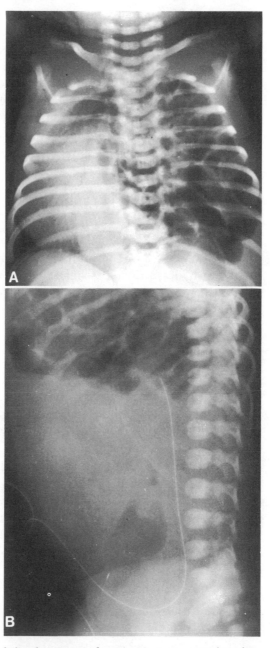

Fig. 10-1. Congenital diaphragmatic hernia. Anteroposterior view (*A*) reveals loops of bowel in the left chest cavity, along with shift of the mediastinal structures to the right. Lateral view (*B*) of the same infant. (Fletcher MA: Respiratory distress syndrome and other respiratory diseases in neonates. In Burton GG, Hodgkin JE: Respiratory Care: A Guide to Clinical Practice, 2nd ed, p 740. Philadelphia, JB Lippincott, 1984)

required. PEEP is usually not indicated for these infants, but, if it becomes necessary, low levels should be used.

Pulmonary hypertension and persistent right-to-left shunting complicate the postoperative course of these infants. Tolazoline (Priscoline) may be used to vasodilate and decrease pulmonary vascular resistance. The usual treatment for persistent right-to-left shunting includes hyperventilation, but this may be difficult to accomplish in these infants because of pulmonary hypoplasia and a high incidence of pneumothorax.

Tracheoesophageal fistula

Tracheoesophageal fistula (TEF) occurs in about 1 in 3000 births. About 34% of the infants are premature. A maternal history of hydramnios is associated with about 33% of these infants. In approximately 50% of TEF defects, other anomalies are present, such as imperforate anus and congenital heart defects.

PATHOPHYSIOLOGY

TEF presents in one of five different forms (Fig. 10-2). The most common is a blind esophageal pouch with the lower esophagus attached to the trachea. The rarest form is the double fistula. Signs and symptoms are very similar in all types of TEF and will be addressed here generally.

The central clinical problem in TEF is aspiration of saliva and reflux of gastric acid into the trachea. A chemical aspiration pneumonitis results. When crying, the infant closes the glottis, which forces air into the fistula, dilates the stomach, and causes respiratory insufficiency that results from elevation of the diaphragm. Management of these infants is directed primarily at prevention of aspiration.

CLINICAL PRESENTATION

The infant presents with symptoms early after birth. Excess salivation and drooling are seen first. Episodes of choking, gagging, and dyspnea occur, especially with feeding. When crying or coughing, the infant has a distended abdomen and

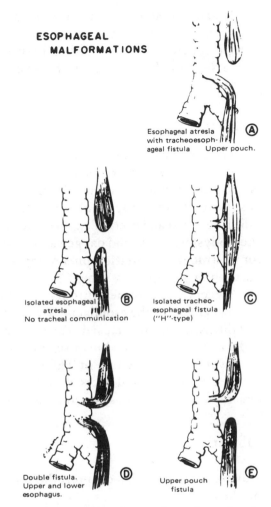

ESOPHAGEAL MALFORMATIONS

Esophageal atresia with tracheoesophageal fistula   Upper pouch. Ⓐ

Isolated esophageal atresia
No tracheal communication Ⓑ

Isolated tracheoesophageal fistula ("H"-type) Ⓒ

Double fistula. Upper and lower esophagus. Ⓓ

Upper pouch fistula Ⓔ

Fig. 10-2. Representations of the various forms of esophageal malformations associated with tracheoesophageal fistula. (Nardi GL, Zuidema GD: Surgery, 3rd ed, Boston, Little, Brown & Co, 1972)

demonstrates respiratory distress. Chest x-ray reveals atelectasis and an elevated diaphragm. Chest and abdominal x-rays show a dilated esophageal pouch and either presence or absence of air in the abdomen, depending on the type of fistula. Chemical pneumonitis may be present on chest x-ray if the infant has aspirated. Contrast media may be used to outline the blind pouch but must be suctioned out immediately to prevent aspiration.

Diagnosis can also be ascertained by the inability to pass a large catheter slowly into the esophagus. A fairly large, inflexible catheter must be used to prevent coiling within the pouch, leading the examiner to believe it has passed into the stomach.

TREATMENT

Surgery for TEF is usually delayed because the infant is often a high risk owing to prematurity, other anomalies, or aspiration pneumonia. The infant should be kept in a 30° upright position to decrease the chance of gastric reflux. A nasogastric tube is inserted and suction applied. Adequate humidification, chest physiotherapy, and oxygen administration are indicated for treatment of aspiration pneumonitis. The infant is fed by means of a gastrostomy tube.

Surgery is performed through a right thoracotomy. The lower segment of the esophagus is detached from the trachea and the fistula sutured closed. The blind pouch is then opened and anastomosed to the lower segment of the esophagus.

Overall mortality rate of TEF is 39%. If there are no associated anomalies or defects, survival improves to 78%. The major complication is aspiration pneumonia.

Objectives

Having completed this chapter, the reader should be able to do the following:

1. Define the following terms:
   choanae   micrognathia
   choanal atresia   dextrocardia
   glossoptosis
2. List the causes of choanal atresia.
3. Discuss the pathophysiologic effects, clinical presentation, diagnosis, and treatment of both unilateral and bilateral choanal atresia.
4. Describe the pathophysiology of Pierre–Robin syndrome, and state the most common other congenital defect associated with this disorder.
5. Discuss the pathophysiology, clinical manifestations, and treatment of Pierre–Robin syndrome.

6. State the causes of congenital diaphragmatic hernia and the most common location of this defect.
7. Discuss the effects of congenital diaphragmatic hernia on the cardiac and pulmonary systems.
8. Describe the clinical and x-ray presentation of congenital diaphragmatic hernia.
9. Discuss the use of bag-mask ventilation in infants born with congenital diaphragmatic hernia.
10. Discuss the problems associated with mechanical ventilation of infants with congenital diaphragmatic hernia, both preoperatively and postoperatively.
11. Describe the surgical treatment of congenital diaphragmatic hernia.
12. State three major features of the history of infants born with TEF.
13. List and describe the five types of TEF.
14. Discuss the general problems, clinical and x-ray presentation, and treatment of TEF.

Bibliography

DeLuca F, Wesselhoeft C: Surgically treatable causes of neonatal respiratory distress. Clin Perinatol 5:2, 1978

Platzker A: Congenital anomalies causing respiratory failure. In Thibeault D, Gregory G (eds): Neonatal Pulmonary Care. Menlo Park, CA, Addison–Wesley, 1979

Randolph JG, Altman RP, Anderson KD: Surgery of the neonate. In Avery GB (ed): Neonatology: Pathophysiology and Management of the Newborn, 2nd ed. Philadelphia, JB Lippincott, 1981

IV·
Respiratory
Therapeutics
for the
Newborn

11·
Oxygen Therapy

Daniel V. Cleveland

Oxygen has been the most widely used therapeutic agent in respiratory care for decades. Despite this fact, many of the physiologic effects of oxygen have been identified only recently, and there is great potential for misuse. It is now common knowledge that prolonged exposure to elevated concentrations of oxygen may cause toxic side-effects. Infants, especially premature infants, are particularly susceptible to these toxic effects, and extreme caution must be used in administering and monitoring oxygen therapy.

Indications for administration

The major indication for oxygen therapy is to relieve arterial hypoxemia, thus relieving tissue hypoxia. There are four basic categories of hypoxia, not all of which are responsive to oxygen therapy. Table 11-1 summarizes the major categories of hypoxia.

TYPES OF HYPOXIA

Hypoxic hypoxia occurs with any condition that causes desaturation of arterial blood. Intrapulmonary ventilation–perfusion mismatching, diffusion defects, right-to-left shunt-

Table 11-1
Categories of hypoxia

Type	Causes	Response to oxygen
Hypoxic hypoxia	Intrapulmonary ventilation–perfusion mismatching, diffusion defects, right-to-left shunting, decreased inspired oxygen	Responds without a large shunt
Circulatory hypoxia	Shock, heart failure, vascular occlusion, hypothermia	No response to increased oxygen once arterial blood is fully saturated
Histotoxic hypoxia	Tissues unable to utilize oxygen (cyanide poisoning, sepsis)	No response to increased oxygen once arterial blood is fully saturated
Anemic hypoxia	Anemia, carbon monoxide poisoning	Some acute anemias may respond

ing, and a decrease in the fractional concentration of inspired oxygen (FI_{O_2}) may all cause hypoxic hypoxia. This type of hypoxia will respond to oxygen therapy unless shunting is severe.

Circulatory hypoxia occurs when tissue oxygen demands exceed the ability of the circulatory system to provide adequate oxygen supply. Shock, heart failure, vascular occlusion, and hypothermia may all lead to circulatory hypoxia. Assuming that arterial blood is fully saturated with oxygen, circulatory hypoxia will not respond to further increases in FI_{O_2}.

Histotoxic hypoxia occurs when body tissues cannot use available oxygen supplies. Cyanide poisoning and sepsis are examples of histotoxic hypoxia. Like circulatory hypoxia, histotoxic hypoxia does not respond to oxygen administration.

Anemic hypoxia is caused by a decrease in the oxygen carrying capacity of the blood, secondary to a decrease in hemoglobin concentration. Anemia and carbon monoxide poisoning are examples of anemic hypoxia. Acute anemias will respond to oxygen therapy to the degree that blood oxygen saturation is increased by this treatment, but prolonged oxygen treatment may worsen anemia by retarding the production of red blood cells by the bone marrow.[1]

Stress is also an important factor that contributes to the development of tissue hypoxia. Constant stimulation for "routine" care procedures, excessive noise levels, hypothermia, and hyperthermia may cause unnecessary stress and transient hypoxia.

SIGNS OF HYPOXIA

The signs of hypoxia include tachypnea, tachycardia, retractions, grunting, cyanosis, and, in some cases, a fall in rectal temperature. If hypoxia is prolonged, bradycardia and apnea may follow. These signs will vary in severity among infants and are dependent upon the degree and duration of hypoxia.

Cyanosis is a blue discoloration of the skin and mucous membranes that occurs when at least 5 g % of reduced hemoglobin is present in capillary blood. It is important to differentiate between peripheral and central cyanosis when evaluating oxygenation status. Peripheral cyanosis is a poor indicator of oxygenation, since it may be caused by external factors such as cold environmental temperature, which causes peripheral vasoconstriction, and circulatory impairment. Central cyanosis, which occurs in warm, well-perfused areas of the body, is a better indicator of hypoxia but still may be unreliable. The presence of 5 g % of reduced hemoglobin corresponds to an arterial oxygen saturation of about 80% or an arterial oxygen pressure (Pa_{O_2}) of about 50 mm Hg. Fetal hemoglobin has an increased affinity for oxygen, and cyanosis may not occur in infants with high levels of this type of hemoglobin until the Pa_{O_2} drops to 30 or 40 mm Hg or lower.

Principles of oxygen administration

Normal arterial blood gas values for a newborn initially show a metabolic acidosis and arterial hypoxemia when compared with normal adult blood gas values (*e.g.*, pH 7.37, Pa_{CO_2} 33 mm Hg, Pa_{O_2} 73 mm Hg). During the first weeks of life, these values go through a gradual transition toward normal adult values. It would be a great disservice to the newborn to maintain normal adult values in a premature or otherwise compromised newborn.

The Pa_{O_2} of an infant receiving oxygen therapy is normally maintained between 50 and 80 mm Hg.[3] At this level adequate tissue oxygenation can generally be maintained while decreasing the risks of developing toxic effects of oxygen therapy. One notable exception to this "rule of thumb" is the infant who is being treated for persistent fetal circulation, in whom hyperoxyenation is maintained to decrease pulmonary vasoconstriction.

The therapy for each infant must be individually tailored. Infants may have remarkable mechanisms for compensating for hypoxia, including polycythemia, increased cardiac output, decreasing affinity of hemoglobin for oxygen, and preferential shunting of blood to vital organs.[3] The individual's ability to compensate should be considered when providing oxygen therapy. Some infants may be maintained comfortably at a relatively low Pa_{O_2} as long as metabolic acidosis from lactic acid production, tachycardia, or other signs of hypoxia are not present.

In the past, the presence or absence of cyanosis has often been used as a guide to oxygen administration in the newborn.

As previously discussed, cyanosis is not a reliable sign of oxygenation, and this practice is discouraged. In the term infant, who is not particularly likely to develop toxic effects from short-term oxygen administration, cyanosis may be useful as a guide if blood gas determinations cannot be done. In the preterm infant, who is much more susceptible to oxygen's harmful effects, blood gas monitoring is essential.

Methods of oxygen administration

Oxygen from a cylinder or wall source is cold and dry and must be warmed and humidified before therapeutic application. Many devices have been used to deliver oxygen to infants, including funnels, masks, nasal cannulas, nasal catheters, oxygen hoods, and incubators. Many of these devices have inherent disadvantages and are not routinely used for oxygen delivery in the newborn. Funnels, masks, cannulas, and catheters all produce an unknown F_{IO_2} that is dependent on the infant's inspiratory flow rate and minute ventilation. With

Table 11-2
Oxygen delivery devices

Device	Advantages	Disadvantages
Mask		CO_2 buildup with inadequate flow; pressure necrosis; inaccurate F_{IO_2}, difficult to fit and maintain on infant
Cannula/catheter	Good for long-term care in chronic disease; usually tolerated well	Inaccurate F_{IO_2}; insufficient humidity; insertion difficulties with catheter
Isolette	Warmed and humidified gas; good for low oxygen levels in stable infants	Varying F_{IO_2}; long stabilization time; risk of bacterial contamination
Oxyhood	Warmed and humidified gas at any F_{IO_2} when used with oxygen blender Stable F_{IO_2} not interrupted by routine care of infant	Overheating can cause apnea and dehydration; underheating will cause increased oxygen consumption; inadequate flow will cause CO_2 buildup; noise may lead to hearing loss

the realization of the importance of an accurately controlled inspired oxygen concentration, these devices have fallen out of favor, although they may still be useful for short-term emergency administration or for long-term use in the chronic but stable patient. In addition, these devices employ oxygen tubing with a small diameter lumen (small bore) that can easily become occluded with condensate if these devices are attached to a heated humidifying device. Oxygen delivery devices used in the care of the newborn are summarized in Table 11-2.

Masks and related devices are also difficult to maintain on an active infant and are not always available in the proper sizes. Inadequate flow to an oxygen mask may cause the buildup of carbon dioxide. Additionally, if masks are strapped on too tightly, pressure necrosis of the facial area may occur.

Isolettes and Incubators

Modern isolettes or incubators may be used with varying degrees of success to deliver low concentrations of oxygen. Two common examples are the Ohio Incubator (Ohio Medical Products, Madison, WI) and the Air Shields Isolette (Air Shields Inc., Hatboro, PA).

The Ohio Incubator has two nipples to which to attach oxygen supply tubing. Flow through one inlet provides an oxygen level of 40% or below; flow through the other inlet provides an oxygen level of nearly 100% by eliminating room air entrainment. Because the incubator is essentially a large, leaky box, it is difficult to obtain and maintain high oxygen levels even when the 100% inlet is used.

The Air Shields Isolette has an inlet nipple to which to attach oxygen supply tubing and a red "flag" lever attached to a cover that can occlude the air entrainment ports. When the flag is raised, the entrainment ports are occluded, and oxygen in the range of 60% to 70% is provided in the isolette. When the flag is lowered, the entrainment ports are open and the oxygen is lowered to 40% or less.

It is possible to add an enriched oxygen source directly into the isolette or incubator itself, rather than using the oxygen delivery system of the equipment; for example, large-bore tubing from a large-reservoir jet nebulizer may be directed into the interior of the isolette. The oxygen concentration may be adjusted either by adjusting the air entrainment port of the nebulizer or by attaching the nebulizer to a blender.

There are several disadvantages associated with the use of isolettes or incubators for oxygen delivery. The oxygen concentration delivered is not precise and therefore not appropriate for critical care. Each time the isolette is opened for nursing care or other procedures, the air within is diluted with room air, causing frequent fluctuations in $F_{I_{O_2}}$. High oxygen tensions are difficult to produce and to maintain, and stabilization of oxygen percentage requires several minutes. In addition, there is increased risk of bacterial growth within the isolette because the oxygen is humidified, thus providing a warm, moist atmosphere for microorganisms in the interior of the isolette.

Oxygen Hoods

The oxygen hood is a preferred method for oxygen delivery in the newborn. An oxygen hood, also called an oxyhood, is a clear plastic box or cylinder that usually incorporates a removable lid. The hood has a port for connecting large-bore corrugated delivery tubing. Opposite this port is an opening for the infant's neck, which is often padded with a soft rubber or foam material. Figure 11-1 illustrates an oxygen hood in use.

An oxygen blender is used with the oxyhood for precise control of F_{IO_2}. Flow from the blender is warmed and humidified by a heated humidifier (cascade-type, wick, and passover are all useful) or a large-volume nebulizer and delivered to the hood through corrugated tubing. Oxygen percentage inside the hood is monitored using one of various oxygen analyzers. Continuous monitoring is preferred over intermittent sampling whenever possible, particularly in the unstable infant. Many oxygen analyzing devices now incorporate alarms to warn of changes in inspired oxygen concentration. In addition, the temperature in the hood should be monitored to avoid overheating or underheating the infant.

The oxyhood maintains a stable F_{IO_2} at any concentration around the infant's head while leaving the body accessible for care. Oxyhoods can be used inside isolettes so that the infant may be maintained in a neutral thermal environment without the disadvantage of changing oxygen concentration whenever the isolette is opened.

The use of an oxyhood is not without possible hazards. Overheating of the gas may cause apnea and dehydration, whereas underheating may cause increased oxygen consumption in the infant. If an oxyhood is used inside an isolette, care should be taken to maintain the hood temperature and the isolette temperature at the same level so that a neutral thermal environment for the infant can be sustained. In addition, flow must be maintained at a level adequate to flush ex-

Fig. 11-1. Oxygen hood in use. Note the temperature probe through the lid of the hood and the oxygen analyzer placed near the infant's face. (Avery GB: Neonatology: Pathophysiology and Management of the Newborn, 2nd ed, p 418. Philadelphia, JB Lippincott, 1981)

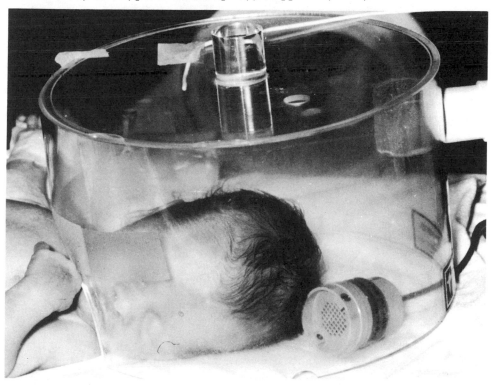

haled gas with its elevated carbon dioxide content from the hood. A flow of 5 liters-minute is usually adequate for this purpose.

Noisy equipment or careless noise by care providers may cause hearing loss in the infant. Hoods should not be attached to devices that use air entrainment to adjust oxygen concentration because these devices will produce excessive noise levels within the hood. Care must also be taken to avoid pressure necrosis around the infant's neck from a hood that is not properly sized.

Cannulas and Catheters

Oxygen cannulas and catheters attached to bubble humidifiers are used for long-term supplemental oxygen in the treatment of chronic diseases such as bronchopulmonary dysplasia (BPD). Flow meters for infants using these devices should be calibrated in small increments such as quarters or tenths of a liter per minute. Excessive flow through nasal cannulas or catheters may yield extremely high oxygen percentages and may also cause drying and sinus damage.

Hazards of oxygen therapy

Several studies published around 1940 noted that oxygen therapy reduced apnea, cyanosis, and brain injury in preterm infants.[4,5,9] This finding led to indiscriminate use of oxygen therapy in the 1940s and 1950s and a subsequent increase in the incidence of retrolental fibroplasia (RLF), consequent loss of vision, and the development of BPD.[2] Since then, our understanding of the pathophysiology of the toxic effects of oxygen has improved, and technological advances have improved our ability to monitor infants receiving oxygen therapy. The knowledge base is still incomplete, however, and the design of controlled human studies is difficult at best.

When initiating oxygen therapy, it is better to give too much than too little. The dangers of hypoxia far outweigh the dangers of temporary hyperoxia. Excessive FI_{O_2} levels revealed by arterial blood analysis following establishment of oxygen therapy may be decreased by the use of noninvasive monitoring or serial blood gas sampling.

RETROLENTAL FIBROPLASIA

RLF occurs when the Pa_{O_2} in the blood vessels supplying the retina is maintained at an elevated level (usually greater than 100 mm Hg). RLF develops primarily in premature infants with immature retinal vasculature. Rare cases of RLF have been reported in full-term infants, but after retinal vessels have matured and extended to the periphery of the retina, RLF will not occur regardless of Pa_{O_2} or duration of oxygen therapy.[8]

The first stage of RLF is characterized by constriction of immature retinal vessels in response to excessive oxygen tension. If constriction lasts for several hours, it may not be reversible and vessels will be obliterated. The second, proliferative stage is characterized by the formation of new vessels in an attempt to oxygenate the retina. As these new vessels proliferate, they may extend into the vitreous, and retinal hemorrhaging may occur. These factors combine to cause retinal detachment and blindness.[8] RLF may result in varying degrees of sight loss, and the eyes of infants exposed to oxygen in the nursery should be examined before discharge, with regular follow-up if there is any sign of abnormality.

The three major factors that contribute to the development of RLF are arterial oxygen tension, maturity of retinal vessels, and duration of hyperoxia. Blood samples must be obtained frequently from an arterial site that represents blood supply to the head (peripheral artery or umbilical artery in the absence of a ductal shunt; right radial, brachial, or temporal artery if ductal shunting exists) to determine the oxygen tension in the retinal vessels. Additionally, transcutaneous oxygen monitoring or oximetry should be used whenever possible for critically ill premature infants. Infants often demonstrate frequent swings in Pa_{O_2} that may not be detected by isolated blood gas measurements. Although noninvasive monitoring of oxygenation using transcutaneous electrodes or oximetry has limitations, it remains an effective method for guiding oxygen therapy in most cases.

BRONCHOPULMONARY DYSPLASIA

BPD occurs primarily in premature infants who have had prolonged treatment with increased $F_{I_{O_2}}$ and positive pressure ventilation. Table 11-3 summarizes the factors that contribute to the development of BPD. The pulmonary destruction seen with this disorder is believed to be caused by oxygen free radicals produced in the reduction of molecular oxygen. These radicals injure alveolar epithelium. The etiology, pathophys-

Table 11-3
Factors that contribute to development of BPD

1. Duration of exposure to increased oxygen tension
2. Level of inspired oxygen used
3. Duration of exposure to positive pressure ventilation
4. Amount of positive pressure used
5. Endotracheal intubation
6. Development of pulmonary interstitial edema or other air leaks

iology, diagnosis, and treatment of BPD are discussed in detail in Chapter 8.

VITAMIN E THERAPY

Vitamin E is one member of a group of naturally occurring defenses against oxygen free radicals, a group that includes various enzymes, vitamins, and other antioxidants that may be deficient in premature infants. Some researchers have reported a decrease in the incidence of BPD following vitamin E administration.[6] Research into the possible effects of vitamin E in preventing RLF is also underway.[7] Although vitamin E is commonly used and appears to be a safe supplement to neonatal care, further study is needed before we understand its full role in the prevention of toxic effects of oxygen.

Objectives

Having completed this chapter, the reader should be able to do the following:

1. Describe the major indication for administration of oxygen.
2. List and describe the types of hypoxia, and discuss the use of oxygen therapy in each type.
3. List the signs of hypoxia in the newborn.
4. Discuss the significance of both central and peripheral cyanosis in the newborn, and describe the use of this sign as a guide to oxygen therapy.
5. Discuss the general principles used to guide the administration of oxygen in the newborn.
6. Discuss the operation, advantages, and disadvantages of

the various methods of oxygen therapy that may be used for the newborn.

7. Describe the etiology, pathophysiology, and prevention of retrolental fibroplasia.
8. List the factors that contribute to the development of BPD.
9. Discuss the use of vitamin E in the newborn.

References

1. Bancalari E: Pulmonary function testing and other diagnostic laboratory procedures. In Thibeault DW, Gregory GA (eds): Neonatal Pulmonary Care. Menlo Park, CA, Addison–Wesley, 1979
2. Bland R: Special considerations in oxygen therapy for infants and children. Am Rev Respir Dis 122(5):45, 1980
3. Burgess W, Chernik V: Respiratory Therapy for Newborn Infants and Children. New York, Thieme–Stratton, 1981
4. Clifford SH: The effects of asphyxia on the newborn infant. J Pediatr 18:567, 1941
5. Clifford SH et al: Round table discussion of neonatal asphyxia. Proceedings of the 10th Annual Meeting of the American Academy of Pediatrics. J Pediatr 19:258, 1941
6. Ehrenkranz DA et al: Prevention of BPD with vitamin E administration during the acute stages of respiratory distress syndrome. J Pediatr 95:873, 1979
7. Kisling JA, Schreiner RL: Oxygen. In Schreiner RL, Kisling JA (eds): Practical Neonatal Care. New York, Raven Press, 1982
8. Meyer CL, Schreiner RL: Oxygen toxicity. In Schreiner RL, Kisling JA (eds): Practical Neonatal Respiratory Care. New York, Raven Press, 1982
9. Schreiber F: Apnea of the newborn and associated cerebral injury; a clinical and statistical study. JAMA 111:1263, 1938

12·
Continuous
Distending
Pressure

Daniel V. Cleveland

Continuous distending pressure (CDP) is a mode of therapy intended to maintain an increased transpulmonary pressure throughout the ventilatory cycle in spontaneously breathing patients. The result is an increased functional residual capacity (FRC) at end-expiration. CDP may be accomplished either with continuous positive airway pressure (CPAP) or with continuous negative pressure (CNP).

Grunting is one of the cardinal signs of respiratory distress in the newborn and appears to be a natural attempt to produce the same physiologic effect as CDP. By partially closing the glottis on expiration, the infant maintains a positive pressure in the airways. Harrison and co-workers noted a decreased alveolar oxygen tension when grunting was eliminated by endotracheal (ET) intubation.[8] The Pa_{O_2} in infants suffering from hyaline membrane disease (HMD) improved after extubation and restoration of grunting, whereas the spontaneous minute volume decreased.

The increase in FRC is most likely due to expansion of previously atelectatic alveoli and stabilization of alveoli with a tendency to collapse.[14] According to LaPlace's Law, the pressure (P) within a sphere varies with changes in the surface tension (ST) and the radius (R) of the sphere, as follows:

$$P = \frac{2 \times ST}{R}$$

In other words, as the radius of a sphere (alveolus) becomes smaller, or as the surface tension increases, the pressure that tends to collapse the alveolus becomes greater.

In newborn respiratory distress syndrome (RDS) or HMD, there is a primary surfactant deficiency, resulting in higher surface tension. As alveoli become smaller, they reach a critical volume where surface tension destabilizes the alveoli and atelectasis occurs.[14]

For these reasons, CDP has become a cornerstone of treatment for RDS, decreasing morbidity and mortality from this disease.[5,7,14]

Effects on the pulmonary system

Table 12-1 summarizes the physiologic effects of CPAP. CPAP increases FRC, decreasing intrapulmonary shunting and improving Pa_{O_2}. This allows the clinician to decrease the fractional concentration of inspired oxygen (FI_{O_2}) to nontoxic levels in many cases while maintaining acceptable Pa_{O_2} levels. The risks of bronchopulmonary dysplasia, retrolental fibroplasia, and other toxic effects of oxygen are thus reduced (see Chap. 11). CNP has essentially the same effects on FRC and oxygenation.

Unless excessive levels of CPAP are applied, the static compliance (Cs) will improve and the work of breathing will decrease. Work of breathing may increase to two to four times normal in infants with RDS, an energy expenditure that the compromised newborn cannot afford. With excessive levels of CPAP, the Cs may be decreased, secondary to distention of alveoli, resulting in an increased work of breathing. CNP also acts to improve static compliance and decrease the work of breathing.

Improved oxygenation will also relieve hypoxic vasoconstriction in the pulmonary vascular bed and decrease pulmonary vascular resistance (PVR), resulting in increased pulmonary blood flow, decreased shunting, and increased Pa_{O_2}.

There is always a risk of barotrauma when applying any

Table 12-1
Physiologic effects of CPAP

Organ system	Beneficial effects	Risks
Pulmonary	Increased FRC	Barotrauma (pneumothorax, pneumomediastinum, PIE); increased PVR; increased work of breathing; decreased static compliance
	Decreased shunt	
	Increased Pa_{O_2}	
	Decreased PVR	
	Increased static compliance	
	Decreased work of breathing	
Cardiovascular		Decreased venous return and consequent decrease in cardiac output
Other		Reflex secretion of ADH causing decreased urine output and renal clearance; obstruction of lymph drainage through the thoracic duct

form of positive pressure, including CPAP. The infant must be monitored closely for signs of pneumothorax and pneumomediastinum. Pulmonary interstitital emphysema may also occur (see Chap. 8).

Effects on the cardiovascular system

CPAP causes an increase in thoracic pressure that may decrease venous return to the heart and consequently decrease cardiac output. The risk of cardiac compromise depends on the amount of pulmonary disease present. When none is present, as much as 50% of CPAP may be transmitted to the cardiovascular system, but in RDS, where Cs is dramatically reduced, most of the pressure may be absorbed in the lung, with little or no negative effect on cardiac output.[5,14] Because CNP does not involve the application of positive pressure to the lungs, there is no danger of diminishing cardiac output in this manner; however, CNP may result in venous pooling in the extremities, as the negative pressure is applied to the entire trunk of the infant, and thus may also impede venous return and cardiac output.

Distention of alveoli with excessive amounts of CPAP may result in compression of alveolar vessels, which will in turn increase PVR.

Effects on other body systems

CPAP, as with other forms of positive pressure, may stimulate a reflex secretion of antidiuretic hormone (ADH), leading to decreased urine output and renal clearance.[2,4,11,12] CPAP may also obstruct flow from the thoracic duct, impeding lymph drainage and contributing to fluid overload.[13] Hemodynamic function, including accurate assessment of fluid and electrolyte balance, must be monitored closely in infants being treated with CPAP.

Methods

The advantages and disadvantages associated with all methods of providing CDP are discussed below. Methods for applying CPAP are summarized in Table 12-2.

CPAP

CPAP may be applied by means of an ET tube, nasal cannula or prongs, nasopharyngeal (NP) tube, face mask, head box, or head bag. CPAP by means of an ET tube is a relatively safe, reliable method used by many newborn care centers. The ET tube provides a patent airway and allows attachment of a manual resuscitator or mechanical ventilator when needed. In addition, there is little chance for dissipation of positive pressure in the upper airway, and thus more of the CPAP is applied to the desired site: the alveoli. The disadvantages of this method are primarily those associated with the intubation process and with the presence of an artificial airway (see Chap. 15). Trauma to airway mucosa, infection, tracheal stenosis, and vocal cord damage make up a partial list of potential hazards. Most of the problems associated with ET tubes can be avoided by using proper techniques of insertion and maintenance.

Table 12-2
Comparison of CPAP methods

Method	Advantages	Disadvantages
ET tube	Patent airway; easy attachment to resuscitator or mechanical ventilator; easily stabilized and controlled	Hazards associated with intubation
Nasal prongs	Eliminates need for intubation; easily applied	Pressure necrosis and trauma; loss of CPAP with crying or leaks; false pressure reading with high flows; positioning difficult to maintain
NP tube	Eliminates need for intubation; easily inserted	Pressure necrosis and trauma; loss of CPAP with crying or leaks
Mask	Eliminates need for intubation; easily applied	Mouth care difficult; leaks; danger of increasing CO_2 with inadequate flow; pressure necrosis; danger of aspiration
Head chamber	Eliminates need for intubation; easily applied	Leaks; compression of neck vessels; tissue necrosis; excessive noise levels; access for resuscitation difficult; mouth and head care difficult

Once the airway has been established, a warmed, humidified supply of oxygen-enriched gas is delivered to the ET tube. This gas may be provided from a heated large-volume jet nebulizer or from a heated humidifier attached to an oxygen blender. Use of the blender allows the jet mixing device on the nebulizer to be closed (100% setting) so that no pressure is lost to the atmosphere. Gas flow is delivered through corrugated large-bore aerosol tubing attached to a T-piece (Briggs adaptor). Expiratory flow from the T-piece is directed to some device that will prevent the pressure from falling to atmospheric levels at the end of exhalation, such as submersion of the expiratory line under water to the depth at which the desired CPAP is achieved (underwater seal method). Alternative methods include passing the expiratory line through an anesthesia bag with an adjustable clamp to vary the size of the exhalation orifice (orificial resistor) or adding one of several types of threshold resistors available for creating PEEP (water column, weighted ball, spring-loaded valve, or magnetic valve).[9]

The use of an orificial resistor was first described by Gregory and colleagues in the initial application of CPAP to infants with RDS in 1971.[7] An anesthesia bag with a controlled leak is used to generate CPAP. The desired pressure is achieved by titrating the flow into the bag and the leak out of the bag's tailpiece. A pressure manometer and underwater seal pressure relief system are also used (Fig. 12-1). The bag may be used for resuscitation or hyperoxygenation during suctioning pressures, since it fills with premixed gas and acts as a readily available reservoir.

Since the introduction of CPAP for infants with RDS by Gregory and colleagues, many other systems have been proposed. In 1974, Carden and colleagues described the use of an inverted Venturi device for applying CPAP, referred to as the "Carden valve."[3] The Emerson PEEP valve, which involves a diaphragm weighted by a column of water (Emerson Co., Cambridge, MA), has also been used to create CPAP. More recently, a series of disposable CPAP valves have become available (Vital Signs, Inc., Totowa, NJ). These valves contain a spring-loaded diaphragm to maintain positive pressure on exhalation and are readily adapted to a CPAP circuit.

In addition to a warmed, humidified, blended gas source and a method of creating end-expiratory pressure, an in-line

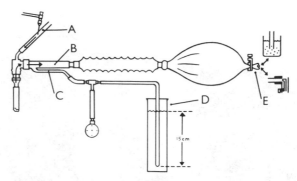

Fig. 12-1. Continuous-flow CPAP system using orificial resistor as originally described by Gregory. (A) Premixed and humidified source gas to patient connector inlet; (B) expiratory line; (C) attachment to pressure manometer and to (D) underwater-seal pressure pop-off system; (E) screw clamp on tail of anesthesia bag used to vary size of orifice and adjust PEEP level. (Blodgett D: Manual of Pediatric Respiratory Care Procedures, p 129. Philadelphia, JB Lippincott, 1982)

pressure manometer should always be used to monitor the level of CPAP and should be connected as close as possible to the airway, with no significant sources of resistance between the manometer and the patient. If an orificial resistor system is used, some form of pressure relief should also be incorporated because the PEEP level is flow-dependent and may vary.

Most infant ventilators provide a "CPAP" mode (see Chap. 13) that allows warmed, humidified gas to be delivered through the ventilator circuit and positive end-expiratory pressure to be generated by the ventilator's mechanical circuitry at the exhalation valve of the circuit. This is a commonly used and convenient technique. Ventilator alarms may be used to monitor airway pressures in some ventilators, and the ventilator is readily available should the infant's condition deteriorate.

Another method of delivery of CPAP is by means of a specially designed nasal cannula or nasal prongs.[10] These nosepieces are manufactured with a standard 15 mm adaptor for connection to any of the gas delivery systems described above. In the Argyle device (Sherwood Medical Industries), two short tubes that extend into the nares are surrounded by a padded gasket at their base that protects the skin and helps maintain a seal (Fig. 12-2). In the Jackson–Reese tube, prongs extend through a straight piece of plastic that has an inspi-

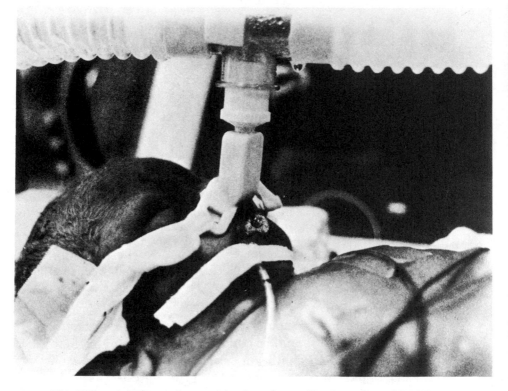

Fig. 12-2. Argyle nasal prongs in place for application of nasal CPAP. (Reproduced by permission of Sherwood Medical Industries)

ratory and expiratory port. Recently, ET tubes that have been cut off at the patient connector end and inserted through the external nares into the nasopharynx have been used (nasopharyngeal or NP tubes). All of these methods avoid the hazards associated with intubation but have their own limitations. Examples of nasal prongs and a modified ET tube (NP tube) are seen in Figure 12-3.

The use of nasal cannulas or prongs and NP tubes to establish CPAP in the neonate is based on newborns being obligate nose breathers. If the infant fails to breathe through his nose (*e.g.*, when crying) or if the prongs are displaced, the CPAP is "lost." Positioning of the cannula may be difficult to maintain, particularly in larger, more active infants. The cannula may be anchored by a sling applied around the head or by an Angel Frame (DeVilbiss Co., Somerset, PA) that supports the tubing and cannula, taking the weight off the infant. When using a sling, there is a risk of compressing blood vessels in

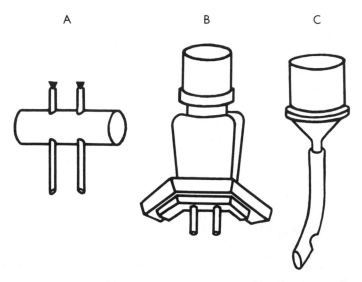

Fig. 12-3. Examples of devices used to establish nasal CPAP. (*A*) Jackson–Reese tubes; (*B*) Argyle nasal cannula (prongs); (*C*) endotracheal tube modified for nasopharyngeal application (NP tube). (Blodgett D. Manual of Pediatric Respiratory Care Procedures, p 133. Philadelphia, JB Lippincott, 1982)

the head and neck, causing increased intracranial pressure and risk of hemorrhage. Other risks associated with the use of nasal prongs include pressure necrosis and infection. Falsely high pressures may be recorded on the manometer with excessive flows into the small openings of the cannula. There is also some question as to how much of the pressure is actually transmitted to the lungs, as opposed to the upper airway, when prongs are used. On the positive side, the prongs avoid excessive PEEP levels because the mouth acts as a "pop-off."

NP tubes may provide some advantages over prongs because they are less easily dislodged and may transmit more pressure to the lower airway. Damage to the nasal mucosa may occur because of the presence of the tube, particularly if attached equipment is not well supported.

Another way to deliver CPAP to an infant is with a mask. This method is not popular because it is very difficult to maintain a seal. The tight-fitting mask makes mouth care difficult and may set the stage for aspiration if the infant should vomit. Adequate flow must be used to flush carbon dioxide from the "dead space" under the mask. Damage to facial tissue may also occur.

In the past, CPAP has been delivered with a head chamber or bag.[1,7] A bag fitted over the patient's head with a drawstring closure at the neck is filled by a flow of gas. The positive pressure generated within is controlled by the amount of leak out of the bag. The head chamber is a Plexiglas or metal chamber that functions similarly to the head bag with a seal around the neck opening of the chamber.

These two systems have several disadvantages. Maintaining a seal is difficult, and leaks will cause loss of pressure; attempts to prevent leaks may lead to tissue necrosis or ulceration at the neck or compression of cerebral blood vessels. Care for the head, face, and mouth and resuscitation efforts are seriously impeded. Head chambers transmit noise that may damage an infant's hearing. Finally, prolonged pressure on the cervical spine may cause brachial plexus palsy, resulting in upper limb paralysis. These devices are rarely used.

CNP

CNP is accomplished by applying a subatmospheric pressure to the chest wall that is transmitted to the pleural space. This negative intrapleural pressure tends to hold alveoli open. CNP eliminates the risk of barotrauma and other problems associated with positive pressure but has several disadvantages of its own. CNP may be provided with the Isolette Respirator (Air Shields Co.), which is designed to function as a negative pressure ventilator (see Chap. 13).

The Isolette Respirator consists of two Plexiglas chambers connected by an iris diaphragm. The smaller chamber receives the head of the infant through the diaphragm, which is then tightened to create a seal around the neck. A negative pressure is maintained in the body chamber by a vacuum motor. The Isolette uses a servo-thermostat to regulate the temperature of the environment within the chambers.

This system is cumbersome, and access to the infant is difficult. The pump must be turned off before breaking the seal, or rapid cooling of the infant will occur as cooler room air is drawn into the vacuum. While the body chamber is open, CPAP must be applied by another method (mask) at the same time that care is provided. The seal around the access door and between the two chambers is difficult to maintain, and room air drawn into the head chamber will decrease inspired oxygen concentration. The seal around the neck may lead to obstruction of blood vessels or necrosis of neck tissue. Negative pressure applied to the entire trunk may interfere with blood return to the chest, resulting in peripheral venous pooling.

CNP tends to produce better results in larger infants with less serious lung disease, such as infants of diabetic mothers, and allows an easier transition to an oxygen hood during weaning from the ventilator.

Clinical application of CDP

CDP is indicated for infants with reduced lung compliance and hypoxemia. Some success has also been documented using CPAP to treat apnea in the newborn. In the past, CDP was not initiated until more traditional methods of oxygen delivery had failed; for instance, CPAP might be introduced when Pa_{O_2} fell below 50 mm Hg with an $F_{I_{O_2}}$ of 1.0. Recent studies indicate a decrease in morbidity and mortality with intervention earlier in the course of RDS. Early initiation allows the $F_{I_{O_2}}$ to be decreased earlier so that the risks of oxygen toxicity are decreased. CPAP or CNP should be started when Pa_{O_2} is less than 50 mm Hg on moderate levels of oxygen support ($F_{I_{O_2}}$ 0.40–0.60). Starting at 4 to 6 cm H_2O of CPAP, using the last $F_{I_{O_2}}$ level before CPAP was instituted, the pressure should be increased in increments of 1 to 2 cm until a Pa_{O_2} between 50 and 90 mm Hg is achieved. If it is also necessary to increase $F_{I_{O_2}}$, this should be done in 5% to 10% increments. Only one parameter (CPAP or $F_{I_{O_2}}$) should be changed at a time, and results should be monitored with arterial blood gas determinations after each change. Continuous monitoring with a transcutaneous oxygen monitor or oximeter should be done if available because infants suffer desaturation easily with routine procedures such as suctioning and handling. While on CPAP, the infant should be manually sighed periodically to prevent atelectasis. This should be done before, during, and after suctioning of the airway.

Chest x-ray, blood gas determinations, and clinical condition should show stabilization and resolution before weaning of oxygen and CDP. The $F_{I_{O_2}}$ should be decreased first, until nontoxic levels (less than 0.40) produce acceptable blood gas results (Pa_{O_2} greater than 50 mm Hg). CPAP may then be decreased slowly in 1 to 2 cm decrements. If the patient is intubated, CPAP should not be decreased below 2 cm H_2O because the small diameter lumen of the infant ET tube may cause increased airway resistance and increased work of breathing. Once extubated, the infant should be placed in an oxygen hood at the same $F_{I_{O_2}}$ or slightly higher (*e.g.*, 10%).

The effectiveness of CPAP or CNP may be assessed by noting a decrease in signs of distress, such as tachypnea, retractions, cyanosis, and see-saw respirations, and by blood gas changes. CPAP therapy should be considered a failure if high levels (15 cm H_2O) have been applied and a toxic level (greater than 0.40) of oxygen is still required to maintain an acceptable Pa_{O_2} (greater than 50 mm Hg). At this point, positive pressure ventilation should be considered.

Optimal CPAP has been defined as the level at which "Pa_{O_2} increases significantly."[14] Other investigators have measured esophageal pressures to determine the optimal CPAP level.[4,15] Further increases above the optimal level will not affect Pa_{O_2} significantly and may cause an increase in arterial carbon dioxide tension (Pa_{CO_2}) by increasing PVR and diverting blood flow from ventilated areas of the lung. A rising arterial carbon dioxide tension may be used to indicate overapplication of CPAP. Other risks associated with the application of positive airway pressure would not justify attempts to improve oxygenation by further increases in CPAP.

Any infant being treated with CDP should receive intensive care with close observation by professionals who have a sound knowledge of the equipment and principles of administration. Continuous hemodynamic and blood gas monitoring should be available, and special attention should be given to bronchial hygiene and nutritional, fluid, and electrolyte status.

Objectives

Having completed this chapter, the reader should be able to do the following:

1. Define and state the objectives of continuous distending pressure (CDP).

2. State two general methods of providing CDP.
3. Discuss the relation between grunting and CDP.
4. State LaPlace's Law, and explain how it is related to the need for CDP.
5. Describe the beneficial and adverse effects of CDP on the pulmonary system, the cardiovascular system, and other body systems.
6. List the methods used for applying CDP, and discuss the advantages and disadvantages of each method.
7. Describe the requirements of a continuous flow CPAP system.
8. Describe the Gregory CPAP system, and compare this system to other methods of applying CPAP.
9. Explain the rationale for using nasal CPAP in newborns.
10. Describe the indications and setup of CPAP in the newborn.
11. Discuss the methods used to wean infants from CPAP.
12. List the ways in which the effectiveness or ineffectiveness of CPAP may be evaluated.
13. Define the term "optimal CPAP," and relate this concept to arterial carbon dioxide tensions.

References

1. Banta BW, Yany R, Warshan JB, Motoyama EK: Determination of optimal continuous positive airway pressure for the treatment of IRDS by measurement of esophageal pressure. J Pediatr 91:449, 1977
2. Baratz RA, Ingraham RC: Renal hemodynamics and antidiuretic hormone release associated with volume regulation. Am J Physiol 198:565, 1960
3. Carden E, Levin K, Fisk G, Vidyasagar D: A new method of providing continuous positive pressure breathing in infants. Pediatrics 53:757, 1974
4. Gammanpila S, Bevan DR, Bhudu R: Effect of positive and negative expiratory pressure on renal function. Br J Anaesth 49:199, 1977
5. Gregory GA: Continuous positive airway pressure (CPAP). In Thibeault DW, Gregory GA (eds): Neonatal Pulmonary Care. Menlo Park, CA, Addison–Wesley, 1979
6. Gregory GA: Continuous positive airway pressure for neonatal respiratory distress. Hosp Pract 7:100, 1972
7. Gregory GA, Kitterman JA, Phibbs RH, Tooley WH, Hamilton WK: Treatment of idiopathic respiratory dis-

tress syndrome with continuous positive airway pressure. N Engl J Med 284:1333, 1971

8. Harrison VC, Hesse H, Klein M: The significance of grunting in hyaline membrane disease. Pediatrics 41:549, 1968

9. Kacmarek RM, Dimas S, Reynolds J, Shapiro BA: Technical aspects of positive end-expiratory pressure (PEEP): Part I. Physics of PEEP devices. Respir Care 27:1478, 1982

10. Kattwinkel J, Nearman HS, Fanaroff AA, Katona PG, Klaus MH: Apnea of prematurity, comparative therapeutic effects of cutaneous stimulation and nasal continuous positive airway pressure. J Pediatr 86:588, 1975

11. Khambatta HJ, Baratz RA: IPPB, plasma ADH and urine flow in conscious man. J Appl Physiol 33:362, 1972

12. Kumar W, Pontoppidan H, Baratz RA, Lever MB: Inappropriate response to increased plasma ADH during mechanical ventilation in acute respiratory failure. Anesthesiology 40:215, 1974

13. Pilon RN, Bittar DA: The effect of positive end expiratory pressure on thoracic duct lymph flow during controlled ventilation in anesthetized dogs. Anesthesiology 39:607, 1973

14. Stevens DC, Fenton LJ, Wellman LR: Continuous distending airway pressure. In Schreiner RL, Kisling JA (eds): Practical Neonatal Respiratory Care. New York, Raven Press, 1982

15. Tanswell AK, Clubb RA, Smith BT, Barton RW: Individualized continuous distending pressure applied within six hours of delivery in infants with respiratory distress syndrome. Arch Dis Child 55:33, 1980

13·
Mechanical
Ventilation

Over the past several years, the ability to ventilate new-born infants successfully has improved dramatically, owing to the development of ventilators specifically designed for use in neonates, the clinical investigation of the use of mechanical ventilation for the problems commonly encountered in this age group, and improved understanding of the pathophysi-ology of these problems. With few exceptions, ventilators de-signed for use in infants are very similar in their operation and application, although the adjustment of specific settings may vary widely depending on the type and severity of disease and on the individual experience of the clinical staff respon-sible for care of the infant. In this chapter I shall discuss the mechanical function of ventilators either specifically designed or commonly used for infant ventilation; I shall also review the specific clinical considerations involved in the application of mechanical ventilation to the newborn.

Basic terminology of mechanical ventilation

POSITIVE AND NEGATIVE PRESSURE VENTILATION

There are two ways to deliver a volume of gas to the lungs of a patient: Positive pressure applied directly to the airway may force air down the airway and into the lungs; and negative pressure applied to the chest cage will change the pressure dynamics so that gas flows from the relatively positive at-mosphere to the relatively negative air spaces. Both techniques are used in infant ventilation, although positive pressure ven-tilation is used more commonly by far. Negative pressure ventilation avoids many of the complications associated with positive pressure ventilation and with the presence of an en-dotracheal tube, which is not required for this technique. This type of ventilator, however, appears to be limited in its ability to ventilate very small and very sick neonates successfully.

MODES OF VENTILATION

Ventilatory mode usually refers to the way in which a venti-lator begins the inspiratory phase; this may include modes in which only spontaneous breathing efforts take place, modes in which only mechanical breaths are given, or a combination of these.

Controlled mechanical ventilation

In controlled mechanical ventilation (CMV), all breaths are initiated and delivered by the mechanical ventilator, with the patient taking no active role in the ventilatory cycle. In general, this is reserved for patients who do not have sufficient ventilatory drive, although occasionally it may be necessary to eliminate the patient's drive with pharmacologic agents and to institute controlled ventilation. This is often encountered when it is necessary to ventilate infants at very high rates, for example, in the treatment of persistent fetal circulation (see Chap. 9).

Augmented modes

Augmented modes are those in which the patient plays a significant role in the initiation of a breath, and include *assisted ventilation* and *intermittent mandatory ventilation (IMV)*, sometimes referred to as intermittent mechanical ventilation. In assisted ventilation, the machine senses when the patient begins inspiration and responds by delivering a mechanical breath according to the ventilator settings. All breaths that the patient receives are initiated by the patient but delivered by the ventilator. This mode is seldom used in infant ventilation because it has been technically difficult to design a ventilator that is sensitive to infant inspiratory demands, and because this mode appears to have no advantages over others that are easier to design and apply. IMV is a mode in which some breaths are delivered by the ventilator (mechanical breaths) at preset intervals and some breaths are spontaneous breaths taken by the patient on his own, with no support from the ventilator. For these breaths, the ventilator simply acts as a source of humidified and oxygen-enriched gas. A variation of this mode, synchronized IMV (SIMV), allows the mechanical breaths to be given on patient demand (*i.e.*, "synchronized" to the patient's ventilatory pattern). As with the assist mode, it has been difficult to develop this ability in infant ventilators, and most of these machines deliver IMV only, not SIMV.

Continuous positive airway pressure

A third type of pattern may be delivered through infant ventilators, although technically this is not a ventilator mode at all because no mechanical breaths are given. This is usually referred to as continuous positive airway pressure (CPAP). The infant breathes spontaneously through the ventilator circuit and exhales against a mechanical device designed to keep the airway pressure above atmospheric pressure at the end of expiration (positive end-expiratory pressure [PEEP]). In this case, the ventilator again acts as a gas supply source and is not really functional. CPAP may also be supplied with systems that do not incorporate mechanical ventilation, although using the ventilator is often the most convenient method.

Pressure support

A new mode of ventilation, pressure support, has recently been developed and used with some success in both infants and adults. In this mode, the patient breathes spontaneously and controls the breathing rate, length of inspiration, and length of expiration. A variable pressure setting allows the clinician to augment spontaneous inspiratory efforts over a wide range of pressures. The flow rate of gas and the tidal volume generated in this mode will be a product of the interaction between the patient and the pressure setting. This mode may be used by itself, so that all breaths are initiated by the patient and pressure-supported by the ventilator, or it may be used in combination with IMV, so that the patient receives some mechanical breaths and some pressure-supported spontaneous breaths. Clinical investigations of this mode are ongoing in both the infant and adult populations. Anecdotal reports, however, indicate that this mode may prove extremely helpful in the patient who is difficult to wean from mechanical ventilatory support.

I:E RATIO

I:E ratio refers to the relationship between inspiratory time ("I") and expiratory time ("E"). Conventionally, inspiratory time is expressed as "1" in this relationship; for instance, if inspiratory time is 1 second and expiratory time is 2 seconds, the I:E ratio is expressed as 1:2. If the times are reversed, however, such that inspiratory time is 2 seconds and expiratory time is 1 second, the I:E ratio is expressed as 1:0.5 (not 2:1). There is some variability in this convention from ventilator to ventilator. The "normal" I:E ratio is usually considered to be about 1:2. In infant ventilation, ratios in which inspiratory time is prolonged in comparison to expiratory time are used with some frequency and are referred to as reversed ratios. This terminology is used regardless of whether the numbers are mathematically reversed; for instance, an I:E ratio of 1:1 is considered a reversed ratio clinically, although mathematically it is not. The clinical application of reversed ratios will be discussed in a later section of this chapter.

SENSITIVITY

Sensitivity refers to the ease with which a ventilator can sense the patient's demand for a breath and is usually expressed as the amount of negative pressure a patient must create in order for the ventilator to respond. As previously mentioned, most infant ventilators have no capability of sensing breaths, and therefore have no need for sensitivity. In ventilators that can sense breaths, sensitivity is usually adjustable to allow for patient and system variations. It is sometimes possible to set the sensitivity so high that the ventilator cycles without sensing *any* negative pressure. This phenomenon is referred to as "chattering" or "self-cycling."

POSITIVE END-EXPIRATORY PRESSURE

Positive end-expiratory pressure (PEEP) is a mechanical technique that prevents the pressure in the patient's lungs from returning to atmospheric levels (conventionally referred to as "0") at the end of an expiration. This technique is widely used in both infants and adults as a mechanism for avoiding alveolar collapse at the end of each breath, and thus avoiding the need to use high pressures or high patient effort to re-expand with the next breath. It has found its widest application in the newborn in the treatment of respiratory distress syndrome (hyaline membrane disease), a disorder that involves inadequate surfactant and widespread alveolar collapse, although it can be helpful in other disorders that are diffuse and that involve alveolar patency (*e.g.*, pulmonary edema). Because its use results in constant positive pressure in the lungs, PEEP may accentuate the problems associated with positive pressure ventilation, which will be discussed in a later section of this chapter. This technique may be used with either positive or negative pressure ventilation.

DEMAND AND CONTINUOUS FLOW

As previously described, most infant ventilators incorporate IMV and CPAP modes of ventilation, meaning that they must have some system for supplying gas for spontaneous breathing, either for all breaths (CPAP) or for some (IMV). Most infant ventilators use a continuous flow system in which gas flows constantly through the breathing circuit. The patient can inhale from this gas flow at any time. The flow is also used to supply gas for mechanical breaths in IMV or control modes. Some ventilators incorporate a demand flow system instead of a continuous flow. In this system, the machine must sense when the patient wants a spontaneous breath and supply flow at that time. One new ventilator, the Infant Star, which is microprocessor controlled, incorporates demand flow as well as continuous flow.

SERVO-CONTROLLED

The term "servo-controlled" simply means that the function of some device is controlled by feedback from sensors. The simplest example is a servo-controlled humidifier, which incorporates an external temperature probe that senses gas temperature, usually close to the patient airway connection. The probe feeds back information to the humidifier heater, which turns off and on as needed to maintain a set temperature at the patient interface. Servo-control may also be used within a ventilator to control valves, volume delivery, airway pressure, or other parameters.

PRESSURE LIMITS AND POPOFFS

For those clinicians who were first trained in adult ventilatory care, the terminology of infant ventilation can be confusing.

The term *pressure limit* in adult care usually refers to a mechanism that terminates the inspiratory cycle at a preset pressure level. In infant ventilation, however, the term usually does *not* imply termination; rather, pressure limiting refers to a technique in which the highest pressure that can be met during the inspiratory cycle is preset. If this level is met before the inspiratory time has ended, inspiration will continue with pressure held at the preset level. This creates, in effect, a pressure hold or pressure plateau and is often referred to as "square-wave" pressure ventilation, which describes the physical appearance of the pressure waveform. Inspiration is *not* aborted when this pressure limit is met. A better definition, then, for the term "pressure limit" would be "the highest pressure that can be reached during the inspiratory cycle." How the ventilator is adjusted to react when this pressure is met is variable, depending on both the ventilator and the patient. To distinguish between the two possibilities (holding at a preset pressure, or aborting at a preset pressure), different terms have been used in infant ventilation. The term "pressure limit" generally refers to a pressure hold mechanism, and the terms *pressure popoff* and *pressure relief* refer to an aborting mechanism. If a ventilator has both a limiting and a popoff mechanism, whichever pressure level is reached first will become operative. Many infant ventilators incorporate only a pressure limit with no popoff or relief mechanism. The relative settings of these two pressure levels depend on the underlying pathophysiology of the patient being treated and will be discussed in a later section of this chapter.

Classification of ventilators

In order to compare the operation of available ventilators, it is helpful to understand the terminology used in their description. Although various classification systems have been proposed, the "four-phase" classification system appears to be the most widely used, easily understood, and universally applicable system. In this classification scheme, a ventilator is classified according to the methods by which it accomplishes the four phases of the ventilatory cycle: beginning inspiration (ending expiration); accomplishing inspiration (delivering a breath); ending inspiration (beginning expiration); and accomplishing expiration (modifying the normally passive expiratory phase).

BEGINNING INSPIRATION

The terms used to classify the way in which a ventilator begins inspiration have historically been limited to a description of the stimulus for beginning a pressurized (mechanical) breath. With the advent of modes of ventilation that incorporate spontaneous breathing (IMV, CPAP, pressure support), however, the terminology has been expanded to include all available options. In general, the terms used to classify this phase of ventilator operation are the same as those used for description of modes. If a ventilator can respond to patient demands by delivering a mechanical breath, it is an *assister*. If it cannot respond to patient breaths but can deliver machine breaths at preset intervals, it is a *controller*. If it can do both, it is an *assister–controller*. Because it is confusing to classify a ventilator as an "assister, controller, assister–controller," we sometimes use the term *guarantor* to describe a machine that can assist the patient on demand but can also "guarantee" a preset ventilator rate because it is also a controller. Thus a machine that can both assist and control would be classified as "assistor–controller–guarantor."

In addition to the way in which machine breaths are initiated, we also describe the ability of the ventilator to respond to patient demands for spontaneous breaths in this classification phase. Thus additional possibilities include IMV, SIMV, CPAP, and pressure support, all of which are described above.

ACCOMPLISHING INSPIRATION

The terminology used to describe the inspiratory phase is related to the flow pattern that the ventilator generates. This, in turn, is related to the mechanism by which a ventilator delivers gas to the patient. These mechanisms include high-pressure gas sources, low-pressure gas sources, and pistons. In addition, the flow of gas may be modified at any point during its delivery to the patient. These various combinations of mechanical factors result in three basic types of gas flow patterns: decelerating flow (machines that decelerate flow during inspiration are usually called pressure generators); constant flow (square-wave) generators; and nonconstant flow (accelerating or sine-wave) generators.

Pressure generators

A pressure generator utilizes a relatively low pressure to drive gas to the patient. If the patient has fairly normal lungs, with little resistance to flow through the airways and little resistance to expansion of the lung–thorax itself, the flow of gas to the patient will be relatively constant. If, however, the patient generates back pressure ("resists" delivery of gas) by offering narrowed airways or stiff lungs, or both, the machine will not be able to overcome this "resistance" to flow and expansion, and flow will slow down (decelerate) during inspiration. The rate of deceleration and the point to which deceleration occurs will depend on the specific pressure generated by the ventilator itself and on the back pressure generated by the patient. The difference between these two pressures (machine and patient) is referred to as the *driving pressure.* The lower the driving pressure (*i.e.*, the closer the machine and patient pressures are to one another), the more likely that flow will decelerate.

Constant flow generators

For a ventilator to deliver a constant flow of gas to the patient, the driving pressure must be fairly high. This is usually accomplished by either a high-pressure gas source or by an electrically powered linear-driven piston. Such ventilators do not respond to patient-generated back pressures; flow remains constant at a preset rate determined by the operator. Most infant ventilators are constant flow generators.

Nonconstant flow generators

A nonconstant flow generator is very similar to a constant flow generator in that driving pressure must be high and the flow pattern of gas delivered to the patient is not influenced by patient characteristics (airway resistance and lung–thorax compliance). A mechanical mechanism, however, is incorporated that alters the flow during inspiration. This may include a rotary-driven piston (Emerson ventilators) or a mechanism that adjusts flow during inspiration (*e.g.*, "scissors" valves, Siemens ventilators). One type of flow pattern produced by a nonconstant flow generator is a sine wave, where flow accelerates at the beginning of inspiration, reaches its peak around midinspiration, and decelerates at the end of inspiration. Although this pattern most closely approximates that of a normal breath, there is no evidence that ventilation with this flow pattern is superior to other types. Another type of nonconstant flow pattern is accelerated flow, in which flow increases at the beginning of inspiration and then levels off and remains constant for the remainder of the breath.

ENDING INSPIRATION

Three basic mechanisms terminate the inspiratory phase: time, volume, and pressure. This is usually referred to as the "cycling mechanism" of the ventilator. If a ventilator ends inspiration at the end of a preset time interval, it is classified as *time cycled*. Most infant ventilators fall into this classification. If a ventilator ends inspiration when a preset volume has been delivered, it is classified as *volume cycled*. Most adult ventilators are volume cycled. If a ventilator ends inspiration when a preset pressure is met, it is classified as *pressure cycled*. Few pressure-cycled ventilators are in widespread use at present, although they were the first type of positive pressure ventilator to be used widely.

ACCOMPLISHING EXPIRATION

Most of the time, expiration occurs passively when pressure is released from the lungs. There are, however, various ways to alter the pattern either before, during, or after passive exhalation. Once a volume of gas has been delivered to the lungs, it is possible to hold that volume in the lungs for a preset time interval. This is referred to as *inspiratory hold*. A similar pattern can be generated by use of the pressure-limiting mechanism on most infant ventilators. This is not a common feature in this group of machines. Another modification of the expiratory phase that has been discussed previously is PEEP, which is found in every ventilator currently manufactured, both infant and adult. It is also possible to narrow the expiratory port and slow the expiratory gas flow. This is referred to as *expiratory retard* and is seldom used, although incorporated in some ventilators. This mechanism may be used to

Table 13-1
Characteristics of common infant ventilators

Ventilator model	Integral blender	Maximum flow (liters/ min)	Maximum rate (breaths/ min)	Maximum pressure and PEEP (cm H_2O)	Built-in high/low pressure alarms	Pressure relief
Babybird	No	30	100	65/30	High (preset)	Preset at 65 cm H_2O
Babybird 2A	No	30	150	80/30	High	Adjustable
Bear Cub BP 2001	Yes	30	150	72/20	High and low	Adjustable
Bio-Med (Cavitron)	Yes*	12	120	70/18	No	Preset at 80 cm H_2O
Bourns BP 200	Yes	20	150	80/20	No	No
Healthdyne Model 100	No	50	100	100/20	No	No
Healthdyne Model 102	No	60	150	100/20	No	No
Healthdyne Model 105	Yes	60	150	70/20	High and low	No
Healthdyne Model 200	No	15	150	60/20	High and low (preset)	No
Infant Star	Yes	40	150	90/24	High and low	Adjustable
McGaw CV 200	Yes	12(I) 40(E)	85	100/25	High and low	Adjustable
Newport	Yes	80	60	80/25	High and low	Adjustable
Sechrist	Yes	32	200	70/15	Low	No
Siemens 900B	No	–	60	100/50	High†	Adjustable
Siemens 900C	No	–	120	120/50	High†	Adjustable
Bourns LS104-150	No	12	80	100/18	High and low	Adjustable

* Bio Med Ventilator has air and oxygen flowmeters that are used to blend gas and to achieve desired oxygen concentration.

† Siemens ventilators have low volume rather than low pressure alarms incorporated.

produce PEEP in the system in infants, although it is dependent on flow to maintain a specific PEEP level. Many other devices have been developed that can generate PEEP with more safety and less variability.

Infant ventilators

Three basic types of infant ventilators are in use today: time-cycled, pressure-limited ventilators; volume-cycled ventilators; and negative-pressure ventilators. The time-cycled ventilators are the most commonly used and will be discussed first. The reader should note that this discussion focuses on the clinically relevant aspects of each ventilator and does not attempt to provide a detailed analysis of the internal mechanical function of the ventilator. Such discussion can be found in several excellent textbooks that are listed in the bibliography of this chapter. Some characteristics of common infant ventilators are summarized in Table 13-1.

TIME-CYCLED VENTILATORS

BABYbird Ventilator

Classification: The BABYbird Ventilator (Fig. 13-1) is classified as a controller with IMV and CPAP (continuous flow), constant flow generator, time cycled and pressure limited, with PEEP.

Operation: IMV mode is used for IMV or control breathing, whereas spontaneous mode is used for CPAP. The ventilator is designed to be used with a separate blender supplied by pressurized oxygen and air and is fully pneumatic, requiring no electrical power for its operation. Flow is adjustable up to 30 liters/minute, allowing for a wide range of patient applications. Inspiratory and expiratory times are separately adjustable and allow for rates up to 100 breaths/minute and a wide variety of I:E ratios covering the clinically useful range. Because there is no mechanism for determining inspiratory time or rate other than the operator's watch, the addition of a digital monitor is extremely helpful. Clinicians who use this ventilator frequently, however, find that they soon can make precise adjustments without this additional technology. PEEP (up to 30 cm H_2O) is established in this ventilator by the adjustment of a restricted orifice on the exhalation port and is thus flow dependent.

Alarms and displays: Alarms for disconnect must be added. A pressure popoff preset for 65 cm H_2O is supplied.

Special features: The BABYbird Ventilator is designed to be used with a Bird nebulizer for humidification, although other humidification systems may be substituted. When using the Bird nebulizer, up to 12 liters/minute of the main gas flow may be diverted through the jet of the nebulizer, allowing for adjustment of humidification level. The ventilator also has an expiratory flow gradient control, which is designed to facilitate flow through the exhalation valve, thus preventing the back-up of pressure in the system and the development of "inadvertent PEEP." It is particularly helpful in the larger child or with high ventilator rates, where high flows are required. A manual resuscitator is incorporated into the ventilator and may be used to deliver manual breaths at any time.

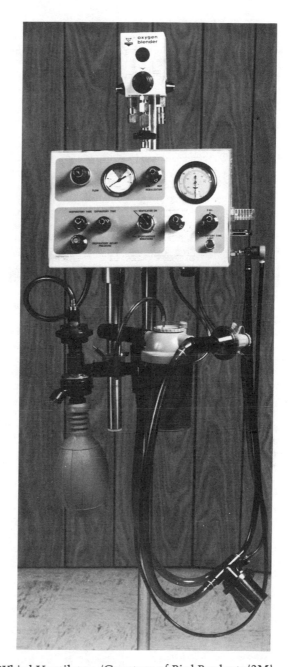

Fig. 13-1. The BABYbird Ventilator. (Courtesy of Bird Products/3M)

Babybird 2A Ventilator

Classification: The Babybird 2A Ventilator is a controller with IMV and CPAP, constant flow generator, time cycled and pressure limited, with PEEP.

Operation: The Babybird 2A Ventilator is electronically controlled and pneumatically powered. The ventilator does not have an integral oxygen blender and is usually supplied with the Bird Hi–Low Flow Oxygen Blender. There is no mode selector. With the rate set, the ventilator will deliver controlled ventilation or IMV ventilation, depending on the presence of patient spontaneous breathing. With the frequency setting turned to the off position, CPAP can be delivered by adjusting flow and PEEP/CPAP settings. Gas flow is adjustable to 30 liters/minute. Peak inspiratory pressure is adjustable to 80 cm H_2O and PEEP to 30 cm H_2O. Frequency (to 150 breaths/minute) and inspiratory time are adjusted to determine I:E ratio. A manual breath control provides pressurized breaths in any mode and is operative during power failure conditions.

Alarms and displays: Alarms include low source pressure, incompatible timer setting (expiratory time less than 0.2 seconds), inspiratory time failure (longer than 4.25 seconds), and electrical power failure. The Babybird 2A Ventilator has a calibrated pressure pop-off that is adjustable from 15 to 80 cm H_2O. When the pressure set on this control (relief pressure) is met, the ventilator will reduce circuit pressure to zero, and audible and visible alerts will be activated. The ventilator is designed to be used with the Bird P-7 Scanner Monitor/Alarm, an electronic, microprocessor controlled monitor that has either automatic or adjustable alarm limits for peak inspiratory pressure (PIP), mean airway pressure (Paw), and PEEP/CPAP. These parameters, as well as inspiratory time, expiratory time, ventilator frequency, and I:E ratio, are digitally displayed. An "autoset" switch allows the operator to set pressure alarm limits 20% above or below their latest readings automatically. A disconnect alarm is automatically set at 25% plus 2 seconds above total cycle time (inspiratory time plus expiratory time). All alarms can be adjusted to other settings if the operator wishes to do so. The monitor can be set to scan and display sequentially all seven monitored parameters, to hold the display of any given parameter, or to monitor the CPAP mode. If an alarm condition is met, the monitor provides audible and visible warnings. These alarms will self-cancel if the alarm condition is corrected, but the alarmed parameter will automatically be placed in the "hold" mode so that the operator can determine the nature of the alarm condition. A 60-second alarm silence is incorporated in the monitor.

Bear Cub Infant Ventilator Model BP 2001

Classification: The Bear Cub (Fig. 13-2) is a controller with IMV and CPAP (continuous flow), constant flow generator, time cycled and pressure limited, with PEEP.

Operation: Mode selections include CMV/IMV and CPAP. The ventilator has an integral air/oxygen blender that requires pressurized air and oxygen sources and is electronically controlled. Flow rates to 30 liters/minute are available, with maximum inspiratory pressure of 72 cm H_2O, maximum PEEP/CPAP of 20 cm H_2O, and maximum rate of 150 breaths/minute. Manual breaths are available in either mode. Inspiratory time and breathing rate settings determine I:E ratio.

Alarms and displays: Digital displays of rate, inspiratory time, expiratory time, I:E ratio, and mean airway pressure are integral to the ventilator. A low inspiratory pressure alarm, adjustable to 50 cm H_2O, and a low PEEP/CPAP alarm, adjustable to 20 cm H_2O, are incorporated, with both audible and visible displays. Additional alarms and alerts include prolonged inspiratory pressure, which is automatically set at 10 cm H_2O above the low PEEP/CPAP alarm setting and which alarms when inspiratory pressure is greater than this automatic pressure setting for longer than 3.5 seconds; low air and oxygen pressure alarms; and rate/time incompatibility, which indicates that the rate and inspiratory time settings do not allow sufficient expiratory time (0.25 seconds in this ventilator). Alarms may be silenced for 30 seconds, and a visual display indicates that alarms are silenced. An adjustable inspiratory pressure relief control with audible alarm is incorporated in this ventilator.

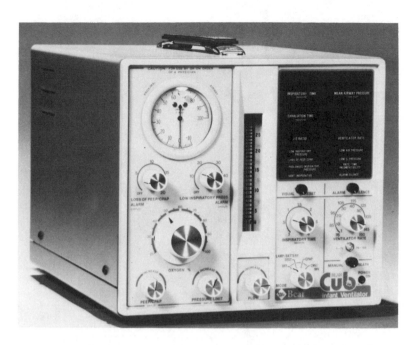

Fig. 13-2. The Bear Cub BP 2001 Ventilator. (Courtesy of Bear Medical Systems)

Bio-Med Flodisc MVP-10 Pediatric Respirator

Classification: The Bio-Med MVP-10, also marketed as the Cavitron PV-10, is a controller with IMV and CPAP, constant flow generator, time cycled and pressure limited, with PEEP.

Operation: The Bio-Med Respirator incorporates air and oxygen flowmeters, which must be supplied with pressurized gas sources. Each flowmeter is adjustable to 6 liters/minute. Delivered oxygen is controlled by the amount of air and oxygen set on each flowmeter, as is total flow to the patient. Because flow to the patient and oxygen concentration are interdependent, this ventilator is not ideal for continuous use; however, the unit is fully pneumatic and very small and is thus ideal for transport situations. It can also be attached to the side of an incubator to con-serve floor or counter space in the intensive care unit, operating room, or emergency room. Control mode or IMV may be selected by setting the ventilator on the cycle setting; CPAP setting is also included. Rate is adjustable to 120 breaths/minute by adjusting separate inspiratory and expiratory time controls. These adjustments also determine I:E ratio, which is infinitely variable over the clinically useful range. Maximum pressure is adjustable to 70 cm H_2O, with a backup pressure relief valve preset at 80 cm H_2O and PEEP to 18 cm H_2O. Gas consumption for automatic functions is low (3 liters/minute), allowing extended transport periods. Manual breaths are incorporated.

Alarms and displays: None.

Bourns BP-200 Infant Pressure Ventilator

Classification: The Bourns BP-200, commonly referred to as the "Pressure Bourns" (Fig. 13-3) to distinguish it from its predecessor (the "Volume Bourns"), is classified as a controller with IMV and CPAP (continuous flow), constant flow generator, time cycled and pressure limited, with PEEP.

Operation: Modes of operation include

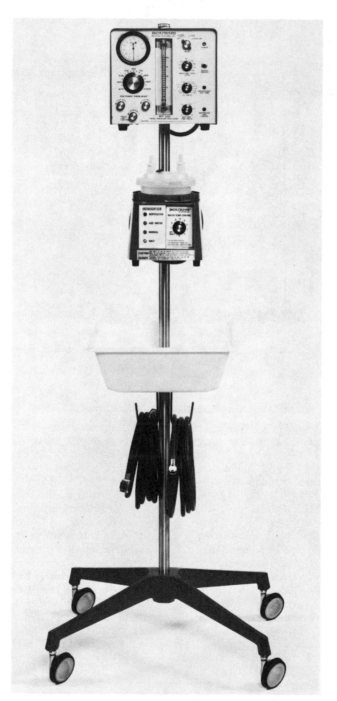

Fig. 13-3. The Bourns BP 200 Ventilator. (Courtesy of Bear Medical Systems)

IPPB/IMV and CPAP. The flow is adjustable up to 20 liters/minute, which prevents its use in larger infant or pediatric patients without modification. A blender is built into the machine and must be supplied with pressurized air and oxygen. The BP-200 also requires an electrical power source to accomplish its automatic functions. Peak inspiratory pressure is adjustable to about 80 cm H_2O. The rate is adjustable from 1 to 150 breaths/minute. A wide range of I:E ratios is available (4:1 to 1:10). PEEP of up to 20 cm H_2O is supplied by the force of a Venturi jet against the internal exhalation valve and is adjusted by the PEEP/CPAP control. A manual breath control will deliver a breath at the parameters set on the ventilator during the CPAP mode only.

Alarms and displays: There is no pressure popoff nor a disconnect alarm, which must be added. Alarms include low gas supply pressures and electrical failure. Flashing lights alert the operator to conditions that produce expiratory times of about 0.4 seconds or less, and to conditions in which the inspiratory time limit is overriding the rate and I:E ratio controls.

Special features: Inspiratory time is determined by one of two methods: normally, the rate and I:E ratio are set by the operator, and these determine inspiratory time; however, a second control can be set to override the I:E ratio control. This control, the inspiratory time limit, allows for reasonable inspiratory times at very low ventilating rates. The use of two separate methods of controlling inspiratory time can be confusing to the operator.

Healthdyne Infant Ventilators

Model 100. Classification: The Healthdyne 100 (Fig. 13-4) is a controller with IMV and CPAP (continuous flow), constant flow generator, time cycled and pressure limited, with PEEP.

Operation: Mode settings include IPPB/IMV and CPAP. The ventilator is pneumatically operated and electronically controlled using a microprocessor system and requires a blended gas source because no blender is built into the ventilator. Total flows in excess of 50 liters/minute can be delivered through a dual flowmeter system, with rates up to 100 breaths/minute available. The manual breath control is operative in both mode settings. Rate and inspiratory time are set using digital selector switches and together determine I:E ratio. PEEP is adjustable to 20 cm H_2O and peak inspiratory pressure to 100 cm H_2O.

Alarms and displays: Alarms for insufficient expiratory time (less than 0.5 seconds), maximum inverse I:E ratio (greater than 4:1), low inlet pressure, power failure, and system failure are incorporated. A disconnect alarm must be added. I:E ratio is digitally displayed.

Special features: The Healthdyne 100 has a ventilation computer that allows the operator to calculate inspiratory and expiratory times, IPPB/IMV flow rate, and CPAP flow rate. These calculations are totally independent of the operation of the ventilator, a fact that must be clear to all who operate this equipment. Input of ordered parameters for ventilator rate and I:E ratio will result in digital readouts of inspiratory and expiratory times. Input of desired tidal volume or maximum pressure, system compliance, and inspiratory time will give an approximate required setting for flow in the IMV/IPPB mode.

Finally, input of infant weight in kilograms and respiratory rate will give an approximate required setting for CPAP flow. This feature is a useful tool for teaching or for those institutions in which infant ventilation is a relatively uncommon occurrence and ability to perform routine calculations may be seldom practiced. A battery pack option allows the ventilator to be transported easily.

Model 102. Classification: The Healthdyne 102 is classified identically with the Healthdyne 100.

Operation: The operation of the Healthdyne 102 is identical to that of the Healthdyne 100, with the following exceptions: The maximum flow is increased to 60 liters/minute or more; the maximum rate is increased to 150 breaths/minute; the ventilator adapts to either infant ventilator circuits (⅜ inch) or adult ventilator circuits (22 mm), allowing

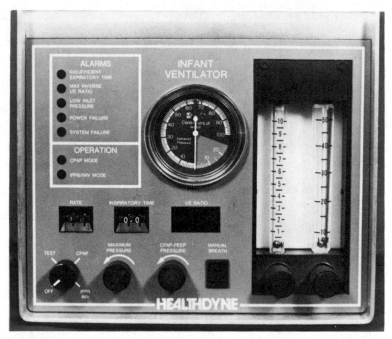

Fig. 13-4. The Healthdyne 100 Ventilator. (Courtesy of Healthdyne Corporation)

for a wide range of patient applications in both the infant and the pediatric patient population; and the minimum expiratory time is reduced to 0.3 seconds.

Alarms and displays: The Healthdyne 102 has the same alarms and displays as does the Healthdyne 100. In addition, the ventilator has a high/low pressure alarm to monitor for leaks and disconnects and to supply a warning of higher pressures than desired, although no popoff is included.

Special features: The Healthdyne 102 uses the same microprocessor-based computer as does the Healthdyne 100, as well as the battery pack option. When used with the Healthdyne Model 145 patient circuit kit, inadvertent PEEP is minimized

Model 105. Classification: The Healthdyne 105 is classified as a controller with IMV and CPAP (continuous flow), constant flow generator, time cycled and pressure limited, with PEEP.

Operation: Mode selections include IPPB/IMV and CPAP. The Healthdyne 105 is microprocessor controlled and incorporates a blender that is supplied with high-pressure air and oxygen. Dual flowmeters supply flows in excess of 60 liters/minute through either infant or adult circuits, as in the Healthdyne 102. Rates up to 150 breaths per minute are available, with minimal flow resistance and inadvertent PEEP. Inspiratory time and rate adjustments allow a wide range of I:E ratios, which are displayed on the ventilator panel. A manual breath control is functional in both modes. Adaptation to a battery pack for transport use is available. A maximum PEEP of 20 cm H_2O and a maximal inspiratory pressure of 70 cm H_2O are provided.

Alarms and displays: Alarms are the same as those in the Healthdyne 100 and 102 models, with a change in the minimal expiratory time to 0.2 seconds. Additional alarms for high pressure and for low pressure, with an adjustable time delay of up to 90 seconds, are integral to the ventilator. I:E ratio is digitally displayed.

Model 200 Transport Ventilator. Classification: The Healthdyne 200 is a controller with IMV and CPAP (continuous flow), constant flow generator, time cycled and pressure limited, with PEEP.

Operation: The Healthdyne 200 is electrically powered from an internal rechargeable battery that supplies up to 8 hours of continuous operation. The ventilator requires blended pressurized gas, with flow adjustable to 15 liters/minute. IMV/IPPB or CPAP mode may be selected. Inspiratory and expiratory times are independently adjustable in increments of 0.1 seconds, with rates to 150

breaths/minute available. I:E ratio, which can be set for almost any value, is not displayed and must be calculated from inspiratory and expiratory times. PEEP to 20 cm H_2O and maximum inspiratory pressure to 60 cm H_2O are featured.

Alarms and displays: Audible and visible high- and low-pressure alarms are built in. The high-pressure alarm is preset at 65 to 70 cm H_2O and the low-pressure alarm, at 2.5 cm H_2O. The alarm delay is adjustable to 40 seconds. A low battery alarm (LED) is also supplied.

Special features: A low bleed flow of blended gas (3 liters/minute) helps to conserve cylinder gas during transport.

Infrasonics Infant Star Ventilator

Classification: The Infant Star is classified as a strict controller with IMV and CPAP (either demand or continuous flow), constant flow generator, time cycled and pressure limited, with PEEP.

Operation: The Infant Star is electrically powered and includes an automatic recharging battery. The battery powers the ventilator at all times; when the ventilator is connected to an electrical outlet, the battery recharges as power is used. Ventilator functions are controlled by two microprocessors: one that controls operations and one that provides information for display. These two microprocessors "monitor" one another. If either malfunctions, the ventilator will vent the circuit to the atmosphere and the "ventilator inoperative" alarm will sound and light. An internal blender requires pressurized sources of oxygen and air. Four modes of ventilation are available: CPAP (continuous flow); CPAP (demand flow); IMV (continuous flow); and IMV (demand flow). Flow rate is adjustable in 2 liter increments up to 40 liters/minute. Rate is adjustable up to 150 breaths/minute, in one breath increments up to 60 breaths/minute, two breath increments up to 130 breaths/minute, and five breath increments up to 150 breaths/minute. Peak pressure is adjustable to 90 cm H_2O and PEEP to 24 cm H_2O. The peak pressure must be set at least 8 cm above the PEEP setting. The inspiratory time is adjustable in 0.01 second increments up to 3 seconds and, with the rate setting,

determines the I:E ratio. A manual breath control is operative in all modes.

Alarms and displays: Digital displays of flow, frequency, peak pressure, inspiratory time, I:E ratio, expiratory time, and PEEP/CPAP settings are incorporated into the ventilator. A low-pressure alarm for disconnects and leaks may be set, and the set value will also be displayed. The ventilator also displays peak and PEEP/CPAP pressures measured at the patient airway and computes and displays mean airway pressure values. I:E ratio and expiratory time are also displayed. An adjustable pressure popoff control is also included.

An obstructed tube alarm is activated if the proximal airway pressure exceeds the peak inspiratory pressure (pressure limit) setting by 5 cm H_2O. When this condition is met, the exhalation valve is opened and the circuit vented to ambient pressure. If proximal pressure exceeds the pressure limit by 10 cm H_2O, an additional internal vent valve is activated to decrease pressure. If the internal pressure is sensed as more than 15 cm above the pressure limit setting, the internal vent valve will also open. Both of these circumstances also set off the obstructed tube alarm, which detects problems that cause pressures to exceed the set pressure limit or PEEP/CPAP setting and problems that interfere with active exhalation. When this alarm is activated, additional information in the form of a code will appear in the windows which usually display mean pressure, peak pressure, and I:E ratio/expiratory time. Interpretation of this coded message allows the operator to determine more precisely the nature of the problem. The reader is referred to the ventilator operating manual for a more detailed description of obstructed tube alarm conditions.

A low PEEP/CPAP alarm is automatically adjusted by the microprocessor, depending on the PEEP/CPAP setting. The pressure difference between set and measured PEEP/CPAP values required to activate this alarm varies from 2 cm H_2O at low PEEP/CPAP settings to 5 cm H_2O at high settings. Alarm activation is based on the average PEEP/CPAP level over a 25-second time interval. An airway leak alarm detects leaks that are too small to be detected by the low PEEP/CPAP alarm. An insufficient expiratory time alarm indicates expiratory times of less than 0.3 seconds for rates below 100 and 0.2 seconds for rates above 100. Low air and oxygen pressure alarms are also incorporated into the system, as is a power loss alarm. The power loss alarm will flash alternately with the internal battery alarm when the battery is nearing full discharge, and alternately with the ventilator in-

operative alarm when the battery is fully discharged. The internal battery indicator will light whenever no external electrical power is supplied. The ventilator inoperative alarm indicates that the ventilator electronics have detected a potential unsafe condition and the ventilator has been shut down. A 60-second alarm silence is incorporated and will silence all except the power loss and ventilator inoperative alarms. Audible alarm intensity is adjustable.

Special features: The microprocessor controlled design of this ventilator allows software updates to be used so that new features may be added in the future. The ventilator can be interfaced with a personal computer to collect, review, and display data. With the addition of a printer, this information can be retained as a permanent record. In addition, the ventilator can be connected to a strip chart recorder and analogue pressure waveforms generated. Gas waste from the blender bleeding system is less than 2 liters/minute. When demand flow is used, gas consumption is reduced even further. A jet Venturi system is included in the exhalation valve block and is designed to minimize inadvertent PEEP.

McGaw CV200 Infant Ventilator

Classification: The McGaw CV200 (originally markéted as the Veriflo CV200) is an assister–controller–guarantor with IMV, SIMV and CPAP, constant flow generator, time cycled, with PEEP.

Operation: The CV200 has three operating modes: continuous flow/spontaneous breathing (CPAP); assist/control; and control–IMV. In addition, SIMV or IMV may be selected. The ventilator is pneumatically powered, with an integral air/oxygen blender. Inspiratory and expiratory times are adjusted independently to determine rate and I:E ratio. Rates to 85 breaths/minute can be achieved. A chart on the front panel allows the operator to determine the appropriate expiratory time setting for a given rate and inspiratory time. Flows during the inspiratory and expiratory phases are independently adjustable. Inspiratory flow may be adjusted to 12 liters/minute and expiratory flow to 20 liters/minute. Peak pressures to 100 cm H_2O and PEEP to 25 cm H_2O are available. The ventilator incorporates a pressure limit, but this control

is designed to function as an alarm rather than to establish a pressure plateau. A sensitivity adjustment (inspiratory effort) is included and is adjustable from 0 to 8 cm H_2O below baseline, automatically referenced to the PEEP level. This control is operative in assist or SIMV modes. A manual start button is provided.

Alarms and displays: When the pressure limit is met, an audible alarm is activated and pressure cannot exceed this setting. A visual indicator ("inspiratory effort") is activated when the patient triggers the ventilator or when the manual start button is operated. A low pressure/apnea alarm is built in. The alarm pressure is adjustable, and the alarm delay time is 10 to 12 seconds (factory preset).

Special features: The McGaw CV200 may be set for either IMV or SIMV. Gas for spontaneous breaths is supplied by adjusting the continuous expiratory flow. An additional 20 liters/minute of gas can be obtained from a demand valve that opens with an inspiratory effort of 1.0 cm H_2O. In the SIMV mode, the ventilator will "wait" for the patient's spontaneous effort before delivering a pressurized breath but will automatically initiate the breath if no spontaneous effort is sensed. The waiting period is determined by the expiratory time setting on the ventilator. An exhalation assist is included to compensate for inadvertent PEEP in high continuous flow situations.

Newport Ventilator

Classification: The Newport Ventilator is classified as an assister–controller–guarantor with IMV and CPAP, constant flow generator, time cycled or pressure cycled, with PEEP.

Operation: The Newport Ventilator is designed to ventilate patients of all sizes and to operate in various modes. The ventilator is pneumatically powered with an integral air/oxygen blender and requires electrical power for its controlling functions. The ventilator may be set to time cycle or to pressure cycle. Time cycling is usually preferred for infant ventilation. Under these conditions, the ventilator has a maximum peak pressure of 80 cm H_2O and a maximum PEEP of 25 cm H_2O, with flow adjustable to 80 liters/minute. Respiratory rates up to 60 breaths/minute may be obtained, and inspiratory time is adjustable to 3 seconds. A sensitivity adjustment is included for assisted ventilation and may be referenced to the PEEP level by the operator. A manual breath control is operative in all modes.

Alarms and displays: Audible and visible alarms for high and low pressure are incorporated into the unit, as are a visual alarm for excessive inspiratory time and audible alarms for low air or oxygen inlet pressures and for power failure. A 55-second alarm silence is provided. A pressure relief valve (popoff) adjustable to 80 cm H_2O is also integral to the ventilator.

Special features: The Newport is easily adapted for transport with a gel cell battery, which provides up to 6 hours of operation. In addition, because of its wide variety of modes, including time cycled, constant flow to provide volume ventilation, and its wide range of rates and flows, this ventilator can be used for almost any patient—infant, pediatric, or adult.

Sechrist IV-100B Infant/Pediatric Ventilator

Classification: The Sechrist (Fig. 13-5) is classified as a controller with IMV and CPAP (continuous flow), constant or nonconstant flow generator, time cycled and pressure limited, with PEEP.

Operation: Mode selections include IMV and CPAP. The ventilator uses a sophisticated fluidic and microprocessor-controlled system to accomplish its gas delivery functions. A blender is supplied with, but not incorporated into, the ventilator. Electrical power must also be supplied. Inspiratory and expiratory time are adjusted to determine rate and I:E ratio, with LED displays of all parameters to facilitate adjustment. Rate is adjustable to 200 breaths/minute, and all clinically useful I:E ratios can be obtained. Maximum pressure is 70 cm H_2O and maximum flow, 32 liters/minute. PEEP is adjustable to 15 cm H_2O by pressurizing the exhalation valve with gas flow. A manual breath button is operative in either mode.

Alarms and displays: LED displays of inspiratory and expiratory times, I:E ratio, and ventilator rate are featured. No pressure popoff is present. A low-pressure alarm with adjustable delay time is incorporated into the ventilator for both audible and visual monitoring of leaks, disconnects, or other patient emergencies.

Special features: The Sechrist has a waveform modifier that adjusts the rate at which the exhalation valve is opened and closed by controlling the rate of gas flow to pressurize the exhalation valve. If the wave-form control is fully open, flow to the exhalation valve will be high, and the valve will close and open abruptly, resulting in a square-wave (constant) flow pattern. If flow is decreased to the exhalation valve, the valve will open and close more slowly, resulting in a gradual acceleration and deceleration of inspiratory gas flow (sine-wave or nonconstant flow pattern). The PEEP can be adjusted in the negative pressure range to accelerate expiratory flow and avoid inadvertent PEEP, much like the BABYbird Ventilator.

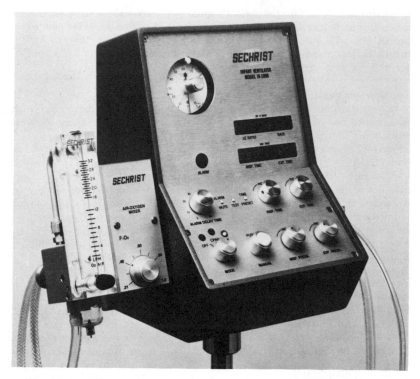

Fig. 13-5. The Sechrist Ventilator. (Courtesy of Sechrist Corporation)

Siemens–Elema Servo Ventilator 900B

Classification: The Siemens 900B (Fig. 13-6) is classified as an assister–controller-guarantor with SIMV and CPAP (demand flow), constant flow generator, nonconstant flow generator, or pressure generator, time cycled and pressure limited, with PEEP, inspiratory hold and expiratory retard.

Operation: The Siemens 900B is pneumatically powered from an external blender and electronically controlled. The 900B may be set to deliver controlled ventilation, to assist the patient's spontaneous ventilations, to deliver IMV breaths at various intervals, or to deliver no pressurized breaths (CPAP); it is useful for a wide variety of patients, from neonates to adults. The breathing rate is adjustable to 60 breaths/minute. Minute volume is adjustable from 0.5 liters/minute to more than 30 liters/minute. This setting may be modified to a range of 0.5 to 2.5 liters/

minute for use in neonates.[13] Tidal volume is determined by dividing the minute volume by the rate setting. The flow pattern may be selected by a toggle switch as either accelerating (nonconstant) or constant flow. Alteration of this setting results in variation in the rate of opening of the inspiratory valve. As with all ventilators, the flow pattern is determined by the driving pressure, which is the difference between patient-generated back pressure and machine-generated working pressure. Working pressure in the 900B is adjustable from 10 to 100 cm H_2O. If patient back pressure approaches the set working pressure, flow will be likely to decelerate, regardless of flow pattern selected. This would produce a flow pattern that decelerates in the face of increasing back pressure, which we have previously defined as characteristic of a pressure generator. PEEP is adjustable to 50

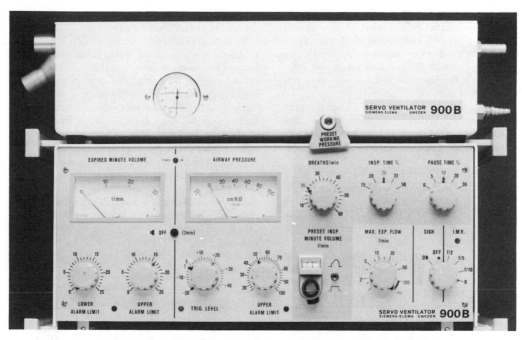

Fig. 13-6. The Siemens 900B Ventilator. (Courtesy of Siemens–Elema Corporation)

cm H_2O with the addition of the overpressure valve to the exhalation port.

Inspiratory time is determined by the inspiratory time percent control, which determines what portion of total cycle time will be used to deliver the tidal volume and is adjustable from 15% to 50%. Total cycle time is determined by the rate control. The inspiratory time control and the minute volume control determine the necessary flow rate. The ventilator will use the flow rate necessary to deliver the set volume in the set time. In addition, the ventilator will compensate for decelerating flow and consequent loss of volume by opening the inspiratory valve and delivering more flow until accurate volume delivery occurs. This mechanism of volume compensation is *not* operative in the IMV mode. Inspiratory hold may be accomplished by setting pause time of 5% to 30% of the total cycle time, which results in delayed opening of the exhalation valve and creates an inspiratory pressure plateau. Inspiratory time percentage and pause time percentage

determine total inspiratory time; in conjunction with the rate control, these controls then determine I:E ratio.

SIMV ventilation may be selected by setting the ventilator for the f/2, f/5, or f/10 setting on the IMV control. Each of these settings divides the previously set ventilator rate by 2, 5, or 10. Tidal volume delivery, inspiratory time, and flow rate are determined by the main ventilator settings and are not influenced by the IMV rate control. Pause time (inspiratory hold) is not operative in the IMV mode. Because the volume compensation mechanism is inoperative in the IMV mode, the flow pattern should be set on square wave and the working pressure at a high value to avoid deceleration of flow and loss of volume delivery. CPAP may be accomplished by setting the ventilator at 0 in the IMV mode and using a PEEP valve on the exhalation orifice. Gas for spontaneous breaths in SIMV and CPAP modes is supplied on demand. Sensitivity is adjustable for SIMV, demand, and assisted breaths by adjusting the trigger level of the ventilator. This control must be adjusted to reference the sensitivity to an altered baseline when PEEP is added. A variety of PEEP valves may be added to the exhalation port to establish PEEP. A sigh setting provides for one sigh of double tidal volume every 100 breaths if chosen.

Alarms and displays: In addition to the traditional pressure manometer display, the 900B has a manometer display of minute ventilation, with adjustable audible and visible high and low alarms. As with the minute volume settings, these alarms and displays may be modified for use in infants.[13] An adjustable audible and visible high-pressure alarm that acts as a popoff is also included. An amber light indicates patient triggering of the ventilator.

Special features: Square-wave ventilation of infants is usually accomplished by using the inspiratory pause control of the Siemens. PEEP valve and blender normally provided

with this ventilator may not function well at the low volumes used for newborns and may need to be replaced with other models.[13] Humidifiers with constant water levels should be used to minimize compressible volume, as should minimally compliant ventilator tubing. The ventilator is readily adapted to the Siemens 930 CO_2 analyzer, which provides assessment of end-tidal CO_2, CO_2 minute production, and several other parameters and has been shown to measure accurately in the neonate. The ventilator can also be adapted to a monitor that provides tidal volume and minute volume monitoring on two different scales for adults and neonatal/pediatric patients and that displays peak, pause, and mean airway pressures, and to a lung mechanics calculator that displays peak pressure, pause pressure, inspiratory and expiratory resistance, compliance, and end-expiratory lung pressures.

Siemens–Elema Servo Ventilator 900C

Classification: The Siemens 900C (Fig. 13-7) is an assister–controller–guarantor with pressure support, SIMV, and CPAP, constant flow, nonconstant flow, or pressure generator, time cycled, with PEEP and inspiratory hold.

Operation: The 900C, like the 900B, is pneumatically powered and electronically controlled and is designed for use in all types of patients of all age groups. There are eight different modes of operation, some of which are combinations of others. In the volume-controlled ventilation mode, inspiratory time, optional inspiratory hold, and tidal volume (determined by rate and minute volume) are set. The patient is ventilated at the preset rate and volume. If the patient demands more ventilation, additional pressurized breaths of the same volume, time, and hold settings will be delivered, resulting in an increased minute volume. Inspiratory flow pattern is determined by the flow pattern setting, working pressure, and patient lung characteristics, as in the 900B. A second mode, volume-controlled ventilation plus sigh, allows for the addition of a double tidal volume (sigh) every 100th breath. In the pressure-controlled ventilation mode, a preset pressure will be maintained throughout the preset inspiratory time. This is analagous to the time-cycled, pressure-

limited capabilities of ventilators designed specifically for use in infants and produces a square-wave pressure pattern. The inspiratory pressure is adjustable up to 100 cm H_2O above PEEP but is limited to the maximum working pressure of the ventilator, which is 120 cm H_2O. Inspiratory pause is not used in this mode. In pressure-supported ventilation, the patient breathes spontaneously and gets a "boost" of pressure from the ventilator. This mode is useful in weaning patients and in reducing the work of spontaneous breathing. (It is described in more detail earlier in this chapter.) SIMV mode involves some pressurized machine breaths, which are delivered using the inspiratory time and volume settings of the ventilator, and some spontaneous breaths, gas for which is supplied on demand of the patient. Machine breaths are synchronized to patient breaths. A sixth mode involves a combination of SIMV and pressure-supported ventilation, in which spontaneous breaths are provided with an adjustable level of pressure support. The CPAP mode allows for spontaneous ventilation with varying levels of end-expiratory pressure adjusted by the overpressure valve. Finally, the mode setting may allow for manual ventilation through the ventilator.

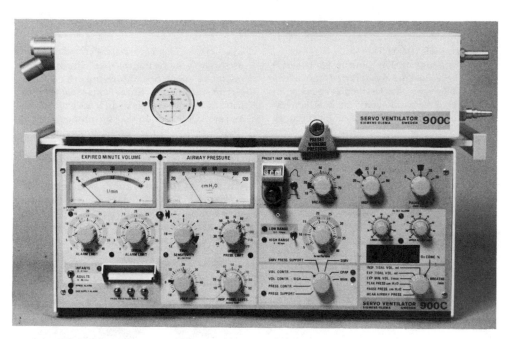

Fig. 13-7. The Siemens 900C Ventilator. (Courtesy of Siemens–Elema Corporation)

Unlike the 900B, the 900C does not use f/2, f/5, and f/10 settings to accomplish IMV rates. A separate rate control with a high rate panel (4–40 breaths/minute) and a low rate panel (0.4–4 breaths/minute) is used when SIMV modes are selected. The main rate control, used for volume and pressure control modes, is adjustable from 5 to 120 breaths/minute. Inspiratory time percentage is adjustable from 20% to 80%, allowing for a wide range of I:E ratios. Pause time is the same as that in the 900B. Trigger sensitivity and inspiratory pressure levels are automatically referenced to PEEP. The PEEP adjustment is built into this ventilator model and is adjustable to 50 cm H_2O.

Alarms and displays: The 900C incorporates an expired minute volume display that is similar to that of the 900B but which does not require modification for use in infants and children. This monitor and its associated high and low alarms (audible and visible) have two scales—0 to 4 liters and 0 to 40 liters—and a toggle switch that allows selection of the desired range. An apnea alarm with a 15-second time delay is also incorporated into the system. The high-pressure limit is adjustable up to 120 cm H_2O and provides audible and visual alarms, as well as cycling the machine to the expiratory phase to reduce pressure. An alarm for inadequate gas supply to the ventilator is also included. Digital displays of inspiratory and expiratory tidal volumes, expired minute volume, peak, pause, and mean airway pressures, frequency, and oxygen concentration may be selected by means of an eight-position switch on the front panel of the ventilator. High and low oxygen concentration alarms are also built in. Amber lights indicate selection of spontaneous breathing modes (pressure support, CPAP, and manual), selection of low IMV rate range and low minute volume range, oxygen alarm setting, and patient triggering.

Special features: Like the 900B, the 900C is readily adaptable to additional types of monitoring equipment.

VOLUME-CYCLED VENTILATORS

Bourns LS 104-150

Classification: The Bourns LS 104-150 (Fig. 13-8), commonly referred to as the "Volume Bourns," is classified as an assister–controller–guarantor, constant flow generator, volume cycled, with PEEP and inspiratory hold.

Operation: The Volume Bourns is electrically powered and must be supplied with a premixed, low-pressure gas supply. Figure 13-8 illustrates the Volume Bourns with the addition of the LS-145 oxygen blender, which supplies up to 20 liters per minute of gas flow. Other blending systems, including flowmeters attached to air and oxygen sources, may be

used. The Volume Bourns uses a linear-driven piston to displace volume into the patient circuit, producing a linear (square-wave) flow pattern. Mode settings include assist, control, and assist/control. In the assist mode, the patient determines the ventilator cycling rate. If the patient rate falls below 60% of the ventilator rate for 10 seconds, the ventilator will revert to the control mode and cycle for 5 seconds. At the same time, an apnea alarm will sound. This mode is unique to the Volume Bourns and was apparently designed to allow for the very common variation in respiratory rates seen in newborns, and also to

Fig. 13-8. The Bourns LS 104-150, shown with LS 145 Blender. (Courtesy of Bear Medical Systems)

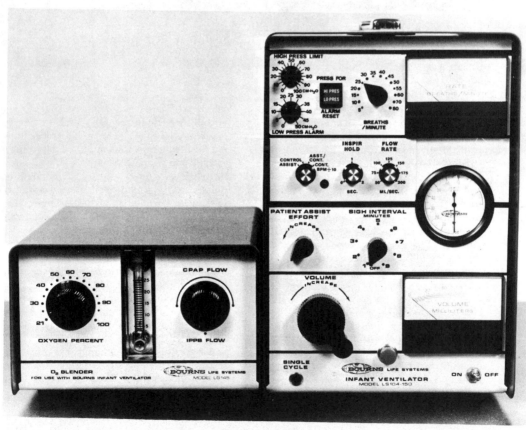

give an infant who is apneic a stimulus without completely taking over ventilation. The control mode locks out the patient from the ventilator and provides machine breaths at the preset rate. The ventilator can be adapted for IMV ventilation by supplying a continuous flow of gas with a reservoir bag through the ventilator and using the control mode to deliver volume-cycled breaths at a preset rate. Finally, assist/control mode allows for the infant to breathe above a preset rate but for the machine to take over if the infant's rate falls lower than this setting (guarantor).

The flow rate is adjustable from 50 to 200 ml/second, or from 25 to 200 ml/second in newer models. Tidal volume setting is adjustable from 5 to 150 ml and the rate, from 5 to 80 breaths/minute in 5-breath increments. A divide-by-10 switch on newer models allows lower rates. Tidal volume and flow settings determine inspiratory time. Rate determines total cycle time and, with tidal volume and flow, determines I:E ratio. Inspiratory hold is adjustable from 0 to 2 seconds. If inspiratory hold is used, it should be added to total inspiratory time before calculation of I:E ratio.

The Volume Bourns has a pressure popoff as well as a pressure limit, thus allowing both traditional volume ventilation with a safety pressure relief and "square-wave" pressure ventilation as commonly used in infants. The maximum pressure is limited to 100 cm H_2O. Prolonged inspiratory times require the setting of large tidal volumes and slow flow rates, which may result in excessive wear on the ventilator. Use of these settings in conjunction with the pressure limit provided on the rear of the ventilator, however, results in the desired effect of long inspiration with pressure plateau and may be useful if other ventilators are not available. A sensitivity adjustment (patient effort) allows patient triggering. An additional adjustment on the rear of the ventilator acts as a leak compensator and also increases machine sensitivity to patient demands. PEEP is adjustable to 18 cm H_2O. Sighs may be selected every 1 to 9 minutes, with a doubling of the set tidal volume.

Alarms and displays: The Volume Bourns has adjustable audible and visible high- and low-pressure alarms, as well as an apnea alarm previously described in the assist mode. Ventilator rate is displayed on a manometer. Spontaneous breaths are neither sensed nor displayed by this ventilator.

NEGATIVE-PRESSURE VENTILATORS

Air Shields Isolette Respirator

Classification: The Air Shields Respirator is a controller with IMV and CPAP, negative pressure generator, time cycled, with the equivalent of PEEP.

Operation: The infant's body is placed in the body compartment and separated from the head compartment by an iris collar, which forms a seal by pressing on the infant's shoulders. The head should be extended to maintain a patent airway. Care must be taken not to seal the collar tightly around the infant's neck to avoid interference with air movement and blood flow. Air is removed from the body compartment by a vacuum motor, creating negative pressure around the chest cage. This results in a reduction of intrathoracic pressure and a consequent flow of air into the lungs. The infant's head is placed in a chamber or bag containing warmed, humidified gas with the desired oxygen concentration. The length of time over which this negative pressure is applied is adjusted (inspiratory time), as is expiratory time, to determine rate and I:E ratio. A continuous negative pressure can be maintained during expiration, allowing for use of the negative pressure equivalent of PEEP (NEEP) and CPAP (CNP). Leaks reduce the effectiveness of this ventilator and also draw cool air into the body compartment, making it difficult to maintain infant body temperature. An assist mode with a thermistor (temperature sensor) at the nose to detect airflow is included but is not useful, since warmed gas must be provided around the infant's face. The respirator can cycle up to 80 breaths/minute and generate pressures of up to 60 cm H_2O.

Alarms and displays: None.

Clinical application of ventilators

Considerable controversy exists over the "best way" to ventilate newborns, and no convincing proof has been provided that one method is significantly superior to another. Advocates can be found for high or low rates, weaning oxygen or pressure first, and prolonging inspiratory time or not. The methods used to determine ventilator settings and subsequent monitoring and modification are thus variable depending on the individual physician or hospital protocol and, of course, on the underlying pathophysiology that has resulted in the need for ventilation. Some general principles can be helpful, however, in guiding the clinician when selecting ventilator parameters.

INDICATIONS FOR VENTILATION

The general indications for mechanical ventilation include the presence of complete apnea, or periods of apnea resulting in significant clinical deterioration that do not respond to other measures; acute hypercapnia (ventilatory failure); and acute hypoxemia not responsive to simpler therapeutic interventions. The level of hypercapnia that necessitates ventilation is controversial and depends on, to some degree, the rate of rise, underlying pathophysiology, gestational age, and birth weight of the infant. The level of hypoxemia that is allowed is also variable and dependent on similar factors. Reynolds has suggested that some infants, particularly those of more advanced gestational age, may tolerate lower P_{O_2}'s (less than 50 mm Hg) and higher P_{CO_2}'s (greater than 80 mm Hg) without adverse consequences, but this is by no means a widespread practice.[17] Some believe that a P_{O_2} that is unacceptable (less than 60 mm Hg) on high inspired oxygen (90% or greater, delivered by CPAP if appropriate to the underlying disorder) is a criterion for ventilation.[11] Others would argue that a P_{O_2} less than 50 mm Hg when inspired oxygen is above 40% requires ventilation, particularly if the infant is of low birth weight.[5] Other criteria that have been suggested for ventilation include symptoms of shock in any infant, regardless of perceived adequacy of gas exchange, and the presence of asphyxia or distress in any infant of less than 1000 g birth weight.[5]

TIME CONSTANTS

The concept of time constants is basic to the understanding of ventilator manipulations in the newborn. A time constant is a mathematical term, derived from the product of airway resistance and pulmonary compliance, and is measured in seconds. After a period of time equal to three time constants, more than 95% of the proximal airway pressure will be transmitted to the alveoli.[17] If the time constant is very short, airway and alveolar pressures equilibrate very quickly. This would be the case if airway resistance were fairly normal and lung compliance very low, as in hyaline membrane disease. It has been suggested that time constants may be as short as 0.5 seconds in infants with severe disease.[16] If the time constant were very long, it would take a longer period for equilibration. An example of a situation in which time constants would be increased is severe meconium aspiration, in which airway resistance is high and lung compliance is low or normal. During expiration, a low time constant produces a rapid expulsion of gas from the lungs, whereas a high time constant results in a long expiratory phase. Diseases that produce very short time constants lend themselves well to prolonged inspiratory and short expiratory phases, whereas the same settings in a disease with a long time constant would be disastrous. In the latter group of patients, expiratory time should be at least twice as long as inspiratory (I:E of 1:2 or less).

SETTING PARAMETERS FOR TIME-CYCLED VENTILATION

Most infant ventilators in common use are, as previously discussed, time cycled and pressure limited. The specific parameters that may be adjusted vary little among these ventilators, with the exception of the variability in the way that inspiratory time, expiratory time, I:E ratio, and respiratory rate may be determined (separate inspiratory and expiratory timers, inspiratory time and rate controls, or rate and I:E ratio controls). Other parameters that must be selected include pressure limit, flow, and PEEP. In addition, inspired oxygen concentration must be selected and is based on oxygen concentration and blood gas results obtained before initiation of ventilation. In some ventilators, depending on mode selection, it may also be necessary to adjust sensitivity and to choose demand or continuous flow for spontaneous breaths. In addition, pressure relief valves may be included in some ventilators.

Inspiratory time and I:E ratio

Because adjustment of inspiratory time is the primary method by which I:E ratio is altered, these two parameters will be discussed together. It is important to remember that adjustment of rate in some ventilators or expiratory time in others will also result in a change in I:E ratio and that subsequent adjustments in inspiratory time may also be necessary. The major consideration when adjusting inspiratory time and I:E ratio should be the specific type and severity of lung disorder for which mechanical ventilation is being used. In the early 1970s, Reynolds and others, in an attempt to find ways to ventilate infants at relatively low peak airway pressures and inspired oxygen concentrations, and thus to avoid the chronic sequelae often associated with mechanical ventilation of newborns, demonstrated that oxygenation in infants with hyaline membrane disease could be improved without increasing peak airway pressure by using a very long inspiratory phase, with a consequent reversal of the I:E ratio, such that inspiration was as long as or longer than expiration.[15] The rationale for this modification of ventilator parameters was based on the notion that, if alveoli could be held open for a larger part of each breathing cycle, gas exchange would be improved. The prolongation of inspiration and the shortening of expiration result in an increased period of positive pressure in the chest cage during each breathing cycle and thus increase the risk of side-effects of positive pressure (e.g., circulatory depression, barotrauma). In infants with very stiff lungs, pressure transmission to the circulatory system is minimal and risks may be small. In addition, short time constants in these infants allow expiration to occur over a very short time. If, however, prolonged inspiration is applied to an infant who does not have diffusely noncompliant lungs, side-effects may be pronounced. Thus application of this technique too early during the course of hyaline membrane disease or failure to alter the inspiratory time as the infant's condition improves, as well as application of this technique to infants with normal lungs or, even worse, to infants with prolonged time constants, will produce a high incidence of barotrauma and other side-effects and should be avoided. Even when the technique is properly applied, careful monitoring is essential and side-effects, particularly barotrauma, may still be expected. Many prefer to maintain a more normal I:E ratio, at least when ventilation is initiated, in an attempt to avoid possible adverse consequences.

Pressure limits and pressure popoffs

As previously discussed, pressure limits in an infant ventilator do not result in termination of the inspiratory phase but rather act to hold the pressure at the limit level for the remainder of the timed inspiratory phase, thus producing an inspiratory pressure plateau, commonly referred to as a square-wave pressure pattern. The time required for pressure to reach the preset pressure limit depends on a number of factors, including the characteristics of the patient's lungs and airways (compliance and resistance), the flow rate of gas set on the ventilator, and, in some cases, the waveform adjustment on the ventilator. Once the pressure limit has been met, the flow will decrease as needed to maintain the pressure at the preset level for the remainder of the preset inspiratory time. This means that flow is not constant throughout inspiration when the pressure limit is used, and volume thus cannot be calculated. The pressure limit setting is usually kept as low as possible because high peak airway pressure has been implicated as one of the possible causes of chronic lung disease (bronchopulmonary dysplasia) resulting from mechanical ventilation. An initial pressure setting of 20 to 25 cm H_2O has been suggested as an acceptable starting point in infants with hyaline membrane disease by Reynolds, who believes that if blood gas values are unacceptable on this setting, other parameters such as inspiratory time, ventilator rate, or PEEP should be adjusted first, in an attempt to avoid elevated airway pressures.[17] Finer and colleagues have suggested that increases in peak pressure and in PEEP are preferred before increasing inspiratory time or I:E ratio.[5] In ventilators without a pressure-limiting mechanism, inspiratory hold or pause may produce a similar pressure waveform and similar clinical results. Infants with normal lungs who require ventilation should require much lower peak pressures and are often ventilated in the constant volume mode.

It is possible to set the ventilator so that the pressure limit is not normally met during the set inspiratory time. This is done by setting inspiratory time and flow rate for a desired volume and by observing the pressure manometer. The pressure limit is then adjusted to a value greater than the required pressure shown on the manometer. This is sometimes referred to as *constant volume* ventilation. Because the flow remains constant throughout inspiration and the inspiratory time is preset, and because flow is a volume/time relationship, knowing time and flow, the operator can calculate the approximate tidal volume setting. The operator must also know or calculate ventilator and tubing system compliance so that an estimate of delivered tidal volume can be made (usually between 6 and 8 ml/kg). If, however, the clinical situation changes such that the pressure limit is met (increasing airway obstruction, decreasing compliance), volume calculation is no longer reliable. Many infants ventilated in this mode may have conditions in which meeting the pressure limit and providing a pressure hold with square-wave pressure ventilation may be detrimental. For instance, if an infant who has a tendency to develop frequent air leaks develops a pneumothorax, the pressure it takes to ventilate this infant will rise. The pressure limit may be met, and, if the ventilator has only a pressure limit, the infant will be placed on square-wave ventilation. This is certainly not the ideal way to treat a pneumothorax. A much better alternative would be for the ventilator to abort the inspiratory cycle in this instance or at least to cause a high-pressure alarm to sound and alert personnel. If a ventilator has a pressure popoff as well as a pressure limit, the popoff should be set for a value lower than the pressure limit in these infants, as well as in others who are prone to sudden changes in airway resistance and compliance (e.g., those with copious airway secretions who require frequent airway suctioning). If the ventilator does not have a popoff, a high-pressure alarm, either built into the ventilator or added to the ventilator, should be set to alarm at a value less than the pressure limit.

Ventilator frequency

Initial attempts to ventilate infants with hyaline membrane disease involved fast respiratory frequencies (60/minute or greater) in an attempt to mimic the spontaneous breathing rates of these sick infants. Reynolds and colleagues demonstrated that using rapid rates also required the use of high peak pressures and that the incidence of bronchopulmonary dysplasia in these infants was quite high.[14,18] Smith and colleagues subsequently demonstrated that oxygenation could be improved by decreasing the respiratory frequency, which was later confirmed by Reynolds.[15,19,20] Respiratory rate settings of about 30 to 40 breaths/minute are usually adequate for ventilation of these infants. Higher rates are generally reserved for infants who require mechanical hyperventilation to decrease carbon dioxide in an attempt to reverse pulmonary vasoconstriction and right-to-left shunting, a condition known as persistent pulmonary hypertension (see Chap. 9), but they have also been used in infants with pulmonary interstitial emphysema. Lower rates may be quite adequate for the infant who requires ventilation without significant underlying cardiopulmonary disorder (*e.g.*, the infant with apnea).

Flow rate

The ventilator flow rate is a major determinant of tidal volume delivery and, in many ventilators, also serves as the source of gas for spontaneous breaths in the IMV and CPAP modes. If the infant is breathing spontaneously most or all of the time, adequate flows to meet inspiratory demands must be provided. A "cushion" of flow is usually provided to allow for sudden changes in infant ventilation. Estimating the infant's minute ventilation (estimated tidal volume of 7 ml/kg times measured respiratory rate) and doubling this value is a helpful starting point. Careful observation of the pressure manometer will tell whether this flow rate is adequate; the infant who requires more flow will generate negative pressure swings that are noticeable and that generally are relieved by increasing the flow. If most or all of the infant's ventilation is from pressurized machine breaths, the flow rate should be set to achieve either the desired pressure limit or the desired tidal volume. When using pressure-limited ventilation, the flow rate is adjusted so that the pressure generated is slightly above the pressure limit, and the pressure limit control is then used to decrease this pressure to the desired value. When using volume-limited ventilation, the flow rate and the inspiratory time are adjusted to achieve the desired tidal volume. Increasing the flow rate will result in higher airway pressures, as well as potentially higher tidal volume delivery, in the volume-limited mode. In pressure-limited ventilation, increasing the flow rate will result in meeting the pressure limit sooner and increasing the length of the inspiratory pressure plateau; it will also potentially increase volume delivery to the infant. Increasing inspiratory time is the preferred method for achieving this prolongation of the square wave, rather than increasing flow, since high flow rates may provide excessive ventilation and may decrease air flow to the periphery due to the increased likelihood of turbulent flow patterns.

Positive end-expiratory pressure

The technique of PEEP is widely used in respiratory medicine. It is designed to keep alveoli from collapsing at the end of an expiration and may be used in conjunction with mechanical ventilation or with spontaneous ventilation (referred to as CPAP). This technique is very useful in the infant with diffusely noncompliant lungs and has become a mainstay of therapy for hyaline membrane disease. If alveoli can be kept from collapsing at the end of expiration, ventilating pressures for subsequent breaths can be reduced and oxygenation will be improved, since there is a longer period of time when air-filled alveoli and blood-filled capillaries are in contact with one another. Reynolds and colleagues have demonstrated that PEEP in conjunction with a prolonged inspiratory phase provides better oxygenation than either technique alone in the infant with severe respiratory distress syndrome.[9] PEEP is useful primarily for those patients in whom widespread alveolar dysfunction is a major cause of abnormal gas exchange. If PEEP is applied to patients who have normal lungs, localized restrictive disease, or airway obstruction, rather than diffuse alveolar disease, it is likely to cause alveolar overexpansion and to result in barotrauma, cardiovascular depression, and increased pulmonary vascular resistance. Overapplication of PEEP in infants for whom it is indicated may also result in these problems. Pulmonary vascular obstruction may be heralded by a rising Pa_{CO_2}, as ventilation/perfusion matching is worsened and increased areas of deadspace ventilation (ventilated but not perfused) develop. In general, a PEEP level of greater than 10 cm H_2O is not well tolerated in infants and will result in hypercapnia. When using prolonged inspiratory times, one may have to use lower PEEP levels than might otherwise be tolerated.

When adjusting PEEP, the clinician should remember that tidal volume delivery in a time-cycled, pressure-limited ventilator is influenced by the flow, the time, and the pressure gradient. If the baseline pressure (PEEP) is elevated without a concomitant change in peak pressure (PIP), the pressure differential will be narrowed, and the amount of volume delivered to the patient may decrease, thus affecting overall ventilation and carbon dioxide elimination.

Humidification

A variety of humidification systems have been developed for use with mechanical ventilators in the newborn. Ideally, the humidification system should have a system for maintaining a constant gas temperature and a constant water level. The latter avoids changes in compressible volume and consequent changes in delivered volume of gas. Compressible volume should be low, regardless of the system used. Both underhumidification and overhumidification are potential problems. Cool gas applied to the airway may result in significant heat loss through the respiratory tract, as well as drying and inspissation of respiratory tract secretions, with the usual consequence of an occluded endotracheal tube. Overhumidification may result in significant systemic fluid gain with consequent circulatory overload in the infant. A heated pass-over or wick-type humidifier is usually adequate to supply the humidification needs of the infant without great risk of overhydration, as long as adequate temperature control is maintained. One major problem associated with humidification of inspired gas has been accumulation of condensate in the ventilator tubing, which is quite narrow in most instances and very likely to become occluded or at least to interfere with gas flow to some degree. Recent introduction of heated ventilator circuits helps to alleviate this problem. Water traps placed in the ventilator circuit may also be useful.

Mean airway pressure

Several studies have suggested that mean airway pressure is the critical factor in determining gas exchange, particularly oxygenation.[2,3] Mean airway pressure is not a ventilator setting but rather the average pressure generated in the lungs over time. It is determined by several factors, including the pressure waveform, inspiratory time, expiratory time (which is influenced by rate settings), peak pressure, and PEEP. Manipulations of any of these settings may be useful in adjusting the mean airway pressure. Many infant ventilators and monitors now have the ability to continuously monitor and display mean airway pressure, allowing the clinician to see the effects of ventilator adjustments on this value. If oxygenation is adequate at a given mean airway pressure, altering ventilator settings (*e.g.*, prolonging inspiration and reducing peak pressure) without changing the mean airway pressure should maintain this oxygenation level. Thus monitoring of this parameter can be helpful in maintaining gas exchange while avoiding some of the harmful effects of mechanical ventilation.

HIGH-FREQUENCY VENTILATION

High-frequency ventilation has become increasingly popular in ventilation of the newborn over the past several years. Several techniques may be useful in administering high-frequency ventilation. High-frequency positive pressure ventilation (HFPPV) is defined as conventional positive pressure ventilation at ventilator rates higher than those normally used. In the newborn, rates in excess of 100 breaths/minute are generally considered high frequency. As previously discussed, this technique is useful primarily in creating respiratory alkalosis for the treatment of persistent pulmonary hypertension. Another technique, high-frequency jet ventilation (HFJV), has been shown in both adults and newborns to be useful in ventilating patients with pulmonary air leaks, as well as with other types of disease.[4,7,8,10,12] HFJV involves an entirely different type of ventilator from conventional positive pressure ventilation. These machines, referred to as jet ventilators, incorporate blended gas under high pressure with a time-cycling mechanism that allows control of inspiratory time or I:E ratio and a rate control. The high-pressure gas is passed through a very narrow tube ("jet") into the airway, using either a narrow-gauge catheter passed through an adapter directly into the endotracheal tube or a special endotracheal tube (Hi-Lo Jet Endotracheal Tube, NCC, Division of Mallinkrodt, Inc.) in which the narrow jet lumen is incorporated directly into the wall of the endotracheal tube. Airway pressure monitors are also provided when jet ventilation is used. The jet of gas will entrain surrounding gas, which is supplied either by a standard nebulizer with heated, humidified gas or by a standard infant ventilator. The entrained gas source, either from the nebulizer or the ventilator, also acts as a supply of gas for spontaneous breathing by the patient. A third system, high-frequency oscillation (HFO), which involves very rapid pulsation of the gas in the respiratory tree, without bulk gas flow, has also been used but is relatively uncommon.[1] The major advantage of high-frequency modes, particularly HFJV, is the ability to achieve adequate oxygenation and ventilation with reduced mean airway pressure, which is particularly useful when air leaks persist. The major disadvantage associated with all types of high-frequency modes has been tracheal damage. This damage has been attributed to a lack of adequate humidification, although its persistence despite various methods of humidification and its presence in patients ventilated with all types of high-frequency modes, including HFPPV, lead to the suspicion that high-ventilator rates may be causative, rather than humidification problems.[6,21]

COMPLICATIONS OF MECHANICAL VENTILATION

The major complications associated with any application of positive pressure to the airways are barotrauma (pneumothorax, pneumomediastinum, pulmonary interstitial emphysema) and cardiovascular depression (increased mean intrathoracic pressure, reduced venous return, reduced cardiac output). In addition, reduction of venous return from the head can result in increased risk of intracranial bleeding, particularly in very premature infants who are susceptible to intraventricular hemorrhage. Effects on the cardiovascular system are uncommon when ventilating infants with very stiff lungs, despite the use of prolonged inspiratory positive pressure combined with expiratory positive pressure. Barotrauma is most likely to result if the infant is very premature, if techniques that exaggerate the effects of positive pressure (e.g., reversed I:E ratio, PEEP) are applied too soon or to the wrong infants, and during the recovery phase from RDS, when careful attention must be given to the need to reduce pressures and inspiratory times as soon as gas exchange begins to improve (usually on the 3rd or 4th day).

A further complication that has been linked with positive pressure ventilation is the development of chronic lung disease (bronchopulmonary dysplasia). This disorder is discussed in detail in Chapter 8.

WEANING FROM MECHANICAL VENTILATION

Once an infant's condition has stabilized on the ventilator, weaning attempts can be begun. Some controversy exists over which parameters to wean first. Some believe that the primary consideration is lowering of peak pressures and PEEP and that inspired oxygen tensions may be left relatively high if necessary while reducing pressures, thus decreasing the likelihood of side-effects of positive pressure. It is important to recognize that prolonged inspiratory times must be shortened as the infant's condition improves, as previously discussed. Once the peak pressures, PEEP, and inspired oxygen tension have been lowered, the rate can be reduced gradually, allowing the infant to assume more and more spontaneous respiration as he progresses toward recovery. When respiratory rates are low, the infant generally can be placed on CPAP and observed before extubation. In some cases, infants may not tolerate rates of 0 on CPAP, probably because of high resistance of breathing through small endotracheal tubes. In these infants, rates of 5 to 10 breaths/minute may be necessary, proceeding directly to extubation if the infant tolerates these rates.[11] Another alternative in infants for whom narrow endotracheal tubes present a problem is the use of the pressure support mode, using just enough pressure to overcome the calculated tube resistance.

Manual ventilators

Manual ventilators are useful in the emergency setting, when the ventilator malfunctions, or when the infant requires special procedures such as suctioning or chest physical therapy. This technique may be applied with a mask to the nonintubated infant, as well as directly to the endotracheal or tracheostomy tube.

Two basic types of manual ventilators are used in the newborn: self-inflating and non-self-inflating (*e.g.*, Jackson–Reese, Mapleson bag). Examples of self-inflating bags that have been specifically designed for use in the infant and pediatric population include the Ambu Infant, Airbird Pediatric, Hope II Pediatric, Laerdal Infant, Laerdal Child, and Penlon manual resuscitators, with full bag volumes ranging from about 200 ml in the Laerdal Infant to 730 ml in the Hope II pediatric model. Non-self-inflating bags are often preferred because they may be more precisely adjusted to the needs of the infant and because they give a better "feel" for the condition of the infant's lungs during manual ventilation attempts. They can be difficult to use, however, unless the operator has frequent opportunity to practice. Several self-inflating models can provide similar advantages with proper modification and are much easier for the occasional operator to use safely and reliably.

Non-self-inflating bags are designed to be operated from either a blender, if control over inspired oxygen concentration is desired, or a pure oxygen source (primarily when used for emergencies, such as in the delivery room), using a calibrated flowmeter to adjust flow to the bag. The resuscitator unit usually consists of an anesthesia bag with a pressure relief valve and the patient's elbow attached. Adjustment of flow to the bag and adjustment of the pressure relief valve allow the operator fairly precise control over ventilation parameters. A pressure manometer is usually attached and monitored when the bag is used. Self-inflating bags may be used with reservoir attachments that allow blended gas or 100% oxygen to be accurately administered, and may also be adapted for continuous pressure monitoring. All non-self-inflating systems and most self-inflating systems allow the infant to breathe spontaneously while attached to the bag unit. Non-self-inflating units and some self-inflating units can be adapted to provide PEEP/CPAP. In summary, the most important aspects to be considered in selecting a manual resuscitator unit include ease of operation, range of delivered oxygen concentrations, availability of pressure monitoring, and availability of PEEP/CPAP.

Summary

Mechanical ventilation of the newborn is a controversial topic, with many variables to be considered. Undoubtedly, the most important variable is a staff that is able to evaluate the infant's condition and to operate and monitor knowledgeably and safely the ventilator and associated equipment used in treating these infants. Whether any specific protocol for ventilation will emerge as the "leader" remains to be seen.

Objectives

Having completed this chapter, the reader should be able to do the following:

1. Differentiate between positive and negative pressure ventilation.
2. List and describe all modes of ventilation, including CMV, augmented modes, CPAP, and pressure support.
3. Define I:E ratio, and explain the meaning of a reversed ratio.
4. Define the terms sensitivity, chattering, and self-cycling.
5. Define and state the purpose of PEEP.
6. Differentiate between continuous and demand flow.
7. Define and state an example of a servo-controlled function.
8. Differentiate between pressure limits and pressure popoffs in infant ventilation.
9. Describe the four phases of ventilator classification.
10. Define all terms used in classification of ventilators.

11. Differentiate between pressure and flow generators, and between constant and nonconstant flow generators.
12. Classify and describe the operation of all ventilators designed for or used for infant ventilation.
13. List and describe the indications for mechanical ventilation.
14. Discuss the meaning and significance of time constants in mechanical ventilation.
15. Describe the setting, including significance of alterations and rationale for use or adjustment, of each of the following ventilation parameters: inspiratory time, I:E ratio, pressure limit, pressure popoff, frequency, flow rate, PEEP, humidification, and mean airway pressure.
16. Describe the use of time-cycled ventilators for volume-limited ventilation in the newborn.
17. Describe and explain the rationale for use of high frequency ventilation in newborns.
18. Discuss the complications of mechanical ventilation.
19. Describe weaning from mechanical ventilation.
20. Describe the use of both self-inflating and non-self-inflating resuscitator bags in infants.

References

1. Bohn D, Tamura M, Bryan C: Respiratory failure in congenital diaphragmatic hernia: Ventilation by high-frequency oscillation. Pediatr Res 18:387A, 1984
2. Boros SJ: Variations in inspiratory:expiratory ratio and airway pressure wave form during mechanical ventilation: The significance of mean airway pressure. J Pediatr 94:114, 1979
3. Boros SJ, Metalon SV, Ewald R et al: The effect of independent variations in inspiratory:expiratory ratio and expiratory pressure during mechanical ventilation in hyaline membrane disease: The significance of mean airway pressure. J Pediatr 91:794, 1977
4. Boros SJ, Mammel MC, Coleman JM et al: Neonatal high frequency jet ventilation. Pediatrics 75:657, 1985
5. Finer NN, Kelly MA: Optimal ventilation for the neonate: II. Mechanical ventilation. Perinatology–Neonatology 7:63, 1983
6. Fox WW, Spitzer AR, Musci M et al: Tracheal secretion impaction during hyperventilation for persistent pul-

monary hypertension of the neonate. Pediatr Res 18: 323A, 1984

7. Harris TR, Christensen RD: High frequency jet ventilation treatment of pulmonary interstitial emphysema. Pediatr Res 18:326A, 1984

8. Harris TR, Christensen RD, Matlak ME et al: High frequency jet ventilation treatment of neonates with congenital left diaphragmatic hernia. Clin Res 32:123A, 1984

9. Herman S, Reynolds EOR: Methods for improving oxygenation in infants mechanically ventilated for severe hyaline membrane disease. Arch Dis Child 48:612, 1973

10. Karl SR, Ballantine TVN, Snider MT: High frequency ventilation at rates of 375 to 1800 cycles per minute in four neonates with congenital diaphragmatic hernia. J Pediatr Surg 18:822, 1983

11. Kisling JA, Schreiner RL, Liechty EA: Mechanical ventilation in the newborn. In Kisling JA, Schreiner RL (eds): Practical Neonatal Respiratory Care. New York, Raven Press, 1982

12. Pokora T, Bing D, Mammel M et al: Neonatal high frequency ventilation. Pediatrics 72:27, 1983

13. Rawlings DJ, McComb RC, Williams TA, Thompson TR: The Siemens-Elema Servo Ventilator 900B for the management of newborn infants with severe respiratory distress syndrome. Crit Care Med 8:307, 1980

14. Reynolds EOR: Indications for mechanical ventilation in infants with hyaline membrane disease. Pediatrics 46:193, 1970

15. Reynolds EOR: Effects of alterations in mechanical ventilator settings on pulmonary gas exchange in hyaline membrane disease. Arch Dis Child 46:152, 1971

16. Reynolds EOR: Pressure waveform and ventilator settings for mechanical ventilation in severe hyaline membrane disease. Int Anesthesiol Clin 12:259, 1974

17. Reynolds EOR: Ventilator therapy. In Thibeault D, Gregory G (eds): Neonatal Pulmonary Care. Menlo Park, California, Addison-Wesley Publishers, 1979

18. Reynolds EOR, Taghizadeh A: Improved prognosis of infants mechanically ventilated for hyaline membrane disease. Arch Dis Child 49:505, 1974

19. Smith PC, Daily WJR, Fletcher G et al: Mechanical ventilation of newborn infants: I. The effect of rate and pressure on arterial oxygenation of infants with respiratory distress syndrome. Pediatr Res 3:244, 1969

20. Smith PC, Schach E, Daily WJR: Mechanical ventilation of newborn infants: II. Effects of independent variation of rate and pressure on arterial oxygenation of infants with respiratory distress syndrome. Anesthesiology 37: 498, 1972
21. Tolkin J, Kirpalana H, Fitzhardinge P et al: Necrotizing tracheobronchitis: A new complication of neonatal mechanical ventilation. Pediatr Res 18:391A, 1984

Bibliography

Fox WW, Shutack JG: Positive pressure ventilation: Pressure- and time-cycled ventilators. In Goldsmith JP, Karotkin EH (eds): Assisted Ventilation of the Neonate. Philadelphia, WB Saunders, 1981

Hakanson DO: Positive pressure ventilation: Volume-cycled ventilators. In Goldsmith JP, Karotkin EH (eds): Assisted Ventilation of the Neonate. Philadelphia, WB Saunders, 1981

Kirby RR, Smith RA, Desautels DA: Mechanical ventilation. In Burton GG, Hodgkin JE (eds): Respiratory Care: A Guide to Clinical Practice, 2nd ed. Philadelphia, JB Lippincott, 1984

Kisling JA, Schreiner RL: Ventilators. In Schreiner RL, Kisling JA (eds): Practical Neonatal Respiratory Care. New York, Raven Press, 1982

McPherson, SP: Respiratory Therapy Equipment, 2nd ed. St. Louis, CV Mosby, 1981

Mushin WW, Rendell–Baker L, Thompson PW, Mapleson WW: Automatic Ventilation of the Lungs, 3rd ed. London, Blackwell Scientific Publications, 1980

14·
Bronchial
Hygiene
Therapy

Bronchial hygiene therapy refers to methods used to prevent the accumulation of secretions in the airways of the infant and to aid in the maintenance of airway patency. Specific measures used to accomplish these goals include various techniques of chest physical therapy (positioning or postural drainage, percussion of the chest wall, and vibration of the chest wall), administration of bland aerosol solutions to loosen secretions, and aministration of pharmacologic aerosols to either thin secretions or promote bronchodilation by relaxing bronchial smooth muscle. There is much controversy regarding the most effective and least harmful methods of chest physical therapy and the efficacy of various bland and pharmacologic aerosols. Specific procedures vary from region to region and even among institutions in proximity to one another, with little scientific rationale for any particular mode of therapy. Recent advances in the continuous monitoring of the infant's cardiopulmonary status using transcutaneous monitors and oximeters have helped to identify procedures that may be unduly stressful to the newborn. Identification of the efficacy of these procedures is more difficult to ascertain and remains uncertain.

Chest physical therapy

The techniques of chest physical therapy are designed to use positioning of the infant to drain various segments of the pulmonary system and to "shake" the infant's chest in an attempt to mobilize secretions into the major airways.

POSTURAL DRAINAGE

Positioning of the infant is referred to as postural drainage and relies on a thorough knowledge of the anatomy of the pulmonary system. Drainage positions for various lobes and segments are described in Table 14-1. Positioning of the infant should be performed on the basis of physical findings and the chest radiograph whenever possible. It is seldom necessary (or advisable) to use all drainage positions at one session because this is very stressful for the infant. Most infants have a localized problem, such as lobar atelectasis or pneumonia. If the

Table 14-1
Postural drainage positions for newborns

Lung segment	Drainage position
Posterior segments, upper lobes	Place infant on opposite side of involved area. Rotate infant forward slightly toward prone position. Elevate head of bed. Percuss and/or vibrate over upper back on involved side (Fig. 14-1).
	Alternative position: lean infant forward at a 30° angle from sitting and percuss/vibrate over upper back on involved side.
Anterior segments, upper lobes	Supine position. Percuss and/or vibrate over area between nipples and clavicles on involved side.
Apical segments, upper lobes	Supine position with head of bed elevated. Percuss and/or vibrate above clavicle on involved side.
	Alternative: Place infant in sitting position and percuss and/or vibrate above clavicles.
Right middle lobe and lingular segment of left upper lobe	Place infant on opposite side of involved area. Roll infant about one quarter turn toward supine position. Elevate infant's feet or hips. Percuss and/or vibrate over nipple area on involved side (Figs. 14-2, 14-3).
Lateral basal segments, lower lobes	Place infant on opposite side of involved area. Roll infant about one quarter turn toward prone position. Elevate infant's feet or hips. Percuss and/or vibrate over lower rib cage posteriorly on involved side (Fig. 14-4).
Superior segments, lower lobes	Place infant in prone position. Percuss and/or vibrate below scapula on involved side.
Posterior basal segments, lower lobes	Place infant in prone position. Elevate infant's feet or hips. Percuss and/or vibrate over lower ribs close to spine on involved side.
Anterior basal segments, lower lobes	Place infant on opposite side of involved area. Elevate feet or hips. Percuss and/or vibrate below axillary region on involved side.

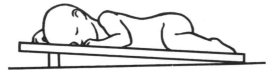

Fig. 14-1. Positioning of infant for drainage of posterior segment of upper lobe. Note position of infant on right side, with slight rotation towards the prone position, and elevation of head, for drainage of posterior segment of left upper lobe. Infant would be placed in same position on the left side for drainage of right upper lobe, posterior segment. (Blodgett D: Manual of Pediatric Respiratory Care Procedures. Philadelphia, JB Lippincott, 1982)

problem is generalized and the infant needs drainage of all areas of the lung, it is wise to alternate sides with each treatment. Use of continuous monitoring devices such as transcutaneous monitors or oximeters will help in evaluating the infant's tolerance of each procedure and position.

PERCUSSION

In addition to placing the infant in various drainage positions, some attempt is usually made to accelerate movement of secretions into the major airways, and thus to increase their rate of removal from the lungs through gravity drainage. The two techniques used to loosen secretions are referred to as percussion and vibration. Percussion involves striking the chest wall over the area to be drained with some device that will trap air between itself and the chest wall. This allows some force to be applied to the chest without directly striking the chest wall with a flat surface, which is very likely to cause

Fig. 14-2. Positioning of infant for drainage of right middle lobe. Note position of infant on left side, with rotation towards the supine position, and elevation of feet. (Blodgett D: Manual of Pediatric Respiratory Care Procedures, p 76. Philadelphia, JB Lippincott, 1982)

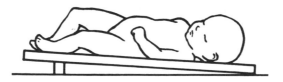

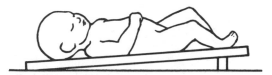

Fig. 14-3. Positioning of infant for drainage of lingular segment of left upper lobe. Note position of infant on right side, with rotation towards the supine position, and elevation of feet. (Blodgett D: Manual of Pediatric Respiratory Care Procedures, p 76. Philadelphia, JB Lippincott, 1982)

injury and discomfort. In pediatric and adult patients, the cupped hand is commonly used to apply percussion. In the infant, the chest cage is so small that this is usually impossible, and various devices have been developed to substitute for the cupped-hand technique. Many institutions have devised their own "percussors," such as medication cups with the rim padded, resuscitation masks with the bag connection occluded, bulb syringes cut in half and padded, and rubber feeding nipples. Mechanical percussors are also available, as are commercial variations of the "padded cup." One example of the commercial variety is the "Palm Cup" (DHD Medical Products, Canastota, NY), which is illustrated in Figure 14-5. These devices are available in various sizes, the smallest of which works quite well on the newborn chest.

Percussion should not be viewed as a routine or innocuous technique to be applied indiscriminately in the treatment of newborns with cardiorespiratory disorders. Infants who are critically ill and unstable will not usually tolerate this technique. Stabilization of the acute disease process should be the

Fig. 14-4. Positioning of infant for drainage of lateral basal segments of lower lobes. Note position of infant on right side, with rotation towards the prone position, and elevation of feet, for drainage of left lower lobe. The right lower lobe would be drained with the infant in the same position on the left side. (Blodgett D: Manual of Pediatric Respiratory Care Procedures, p 74. Philadelphia, JB Lippincott, 1982)

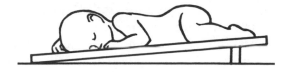

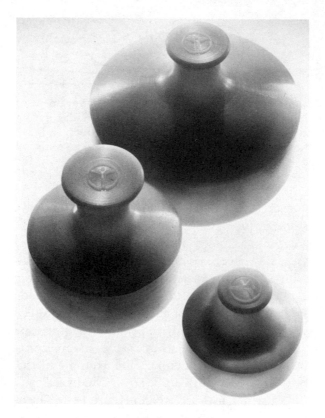

Fig. 14-5. Several sizes of "Palm Cup" percussors. The smallest size is suitable for use in the newborn. (Courtesy DHD Medical, Canastota, NY)

first priority in these infants. Once stabilization has been achieved, percussion may be very helpful in the treatment of atelectasis, pneumonia, or excessive secretions.

VIBRATION

Vibration refers to rapid movement of the chest wall rather than distinct clapping. Several techniques are useful in performing vibration, including placing the fingertips on the chest wall, tensing the muscles of the forearm, and rapidly "vibrating" the fingertips. Mechanical vibrators are available, and electric toothbrushes are a common substitute seen in many neonatal intensive care units. Vibration is usually applied only during the expiratory phase of each breath, so that movement of secretions may be enhanced by expiratory air flow. Although some investigators believe that vibration is less stressful to the infant than percussion, there is no general agreement on this subject.[1] Vibration may be harmful, especially to the unstable infant, and the same conditions should apply as for the use of percussion.

EFFECTS OF CHEST PHYSICAL THERAPY

The major desired effects of chest physical therapy techniques include increased removal of secretions, improved ventilation and oxygenation, and clearance of atelectasis and pneumonia. Chest physiotherapy does appear to increase the removal of secretions, when compared to suctioning, and percussion appears to be superior to postural drainage without percussion.[2-4] Oxygenation, as reflected by transcutaneous oxygen values, often decreases during the treatment, and it is not uncommon for infants to require an increased FI_{O_2} while chest physical therapy procedures are being performed. If the chest physical therapy is successful in relieving atelectasis and clearing airways, oxygenation should improve after the treatment, as was demonstrated by Raval and co-workers.[5] Auscultation of the chest before and after therapy as well as serial chest radiographs are also helpful in evaluating the effects of therapy.

Suctioning is usually performed after chest physical therapy to remove secretions. Suctioning procedures are described in Chapter 15.

Aerosols

Intermittent bland aerosol therapy finds little use in the treatment of the newborn. It is, of course, essential that adequate humidification of inspired gas be achieved, particularly if the infant is intubated. A heated humidifier, such as a cascade-type or wick humidifier, or a heated large-reservoir jet nebulizer may be used. Aerosols, particularly high-volume aerosols such as those produced by ultrasonic nebulizers, can provide a significant amount of fluid to the infant, and the risk of fluid overload with these devices is appreciable. Adequate humidification of inspired gas should alleviate the need for bland aerosol therapy to facilitate secretion removal.

PHARMACOLOGIC AEROSOLS

Pharmacologic aerosols include three types of drugs: bronchodilators, vasoconstrictors, and mucolytics. Vasoconstrictors are used primarily to treat postextubation edema of the upper airway and will be discussed in Chapter 15. For bronchial hygiene, both bronchodilators and mucolytics may be used. Aerosolized bronchodilators are usually adrenergic (sympathomimetic) drugs such as isoetharine (Bronkosol) and isoproterenol (Isuprel). The usual newborn dosage of these drugs is 0.25 ml in 3 ml or more of diluent, usually normal saline. Racemic epinephrine (Vaponefrin) is also an adrenergic bronchodilator but is more commonly administered for its alpha-adrenergic (vasoconstrictor) effects. Metaproterenol (Alupent), another adrenergic bronchodilator, is not recommended for infants and small children.

The adrenergic bronchodilators mimic the action of the sympathetic branch of the autonomic nervous system by stimulating receptors called beta-two receptors in bronchial smooth muscle. Stimulation of these receptors results in relaxation of bronchial smooth muscle and thus in bronchodilation. These drugs are usually not effective in the newborn, who has relatively little smooth muscle in his airways. In the older infant with chronic lung disease, such as bronchopulmonary dysplasia, bronchoconstriction and consequent wheezing may play a significant role, and these patients may find good relief with the administration of aerosolized bronchodilators. The major side-effect associated with these drugs is cardiac stimulation, caused by their effects on beta-one receptors in cardiac muscle.

Mucolytics are also not widely used in the management of the newborn. The major agent administered for its mucolytic properties is acetylcysteine (Mucomyst), which acts by rupturing the bonds in mucus, thus making the mucus more liquid and more easily mobilized. There are few diseases in the newborn period that result in the retention of thick, viscid secretions, and thus few patients who benefit from the administration of acetylcysteine. Occasionally, infants with bronchopulmonary dysplasia will have significant problems with secretion clearance and may benefit from aerosolized mucolytic therapy. The major adverse side-effect associated with the administration of acetylcysteine is the precipitation of bronchospasm. Acetylcysteine is often administered either with or after one of the adrenergic bronchodilators.

EQUIPMENT AND ADMINISTRATION

All aerosolized drugs are administered with small-volume jet nebulizers, which are powered from a flowmeter that may be attached to any 50 psig gas source. They may also be powered from a small compressor. Whenever possible, they should be attached to a blender for precise control of inspired oxygen. Using oxygen as a nebulization source may result in the administration of excessive oxygen concentration, which has been shown to have toxic effects even for short periods of time in premature infants. Using air as a power source may result in hypoxemia during the treatment. Aerosolization of the drugs should occur within 5 to 10 minutes. Liquid output of these nebulizers is low, and intermittent use should not result in significant addition of fluid to the infant.

Objectives

Having completed this chapter, the reader should be able to do the following:

1. List the procedures that are included in bronchial hygiene for the newborn.
2. Describe the rationale for use of postural drainage.
3. State the correct drainage position for each area of the lungs.
4. Explain the monitoring of the patient during drainage.
5. Describe the rationale for use of percussion and vibration.
6. List the various types of devices that may be used for percussion and vibration in the newborn.
7. Describe the proper procedure for percussion and vibration in the newborn, including monitoring of the patient.
8. State the desired effects of chest physical therapy procedures, and explain how these effects may be assessed.

9. Discuss the use of bland and pharmacologic aerosols in the newborn with cardiorespiratory disease.
10. Describe the procedures used to administer pharmacologic aerosols to the newborn.

References

1. Curran C, Kachoyeanos M: The effects on neonates of two methods of chest physical therapy. MCN 4:309, 1979
2. Etches PC, Scott B: Chest physiotherapy in the newborn: Effect on secretions removed. Pediatrics 62:713, 1978
3. Finer NN, Boyd J: Chest physiotherapy in the neonate: A controlled study. Pediatrics 61:282, 1978
4. Finer NN, Grace MG, Boyd J: Chest physiotherapy in the neonate with respiratory distress. Pediatr Res 11:570, 1977
5. Raval D, Mora A, Yeh TF, Pildes RS: Changes in TcPO$_2$ during tracheobronchial hygiene in neonates. J Pediatr 96: 1118, 1980

15·
Airway
Care

Establishment and maintenance of a patent airway are important considerations in the newborn patient, as in other age groups. Several factors, however, including the relatively small size of the infant's airway and the flexibility of the infant's neck, make clinical airway obstruction more likely to occur. Careful attention to the status of the airway is thus of paramount importance.

Pharyngeal suctioning

In an infant who does not have an artificial airway in place, secretions must be removed from the upper airway by suctioning of the pharynx, either nasally or orally. This procedure may be necessary at any time but is most commonly performed after chest physical therapy procedures.

TYPES OF SUCTION EQUIPMENT

Several techniques or types of equipment may be used for the suctioning procedure. A suction catheter may be attached to a mechanical vacuum source, such as a wall suction unit or a portable suction machine. Alternatively, the catheter may be attached to a DeLee trap, which is operated by suction from the operator's mouth. The safest method of pharyngeal suctioning is the use of a bulb syringe, although this method does not allow for deeper suctioning if it becomes necessary.

AVOIDING COMPLICATIONS

The procedure used for suctioning the infant should be systematic, both to assure maximum effectiveness and to avoid possible complications. Table 15-1 outlines the steps to be taken in suctioning an infant. Careful attention to aseptic technique is necessary to avoid introducing pathogens into the infant's airway. Minimal monitoring of the infant should include a heart monitor, although a transcutaneous oxygen monitor or oximeter is preferred for rapid detection of hypoxemia during the suction attempt. Before suctioning, the infant should be well oxygenated and ventilated because the suction procedure may remove both volume and oxygen from the infant's airway. This hazard increases in likelihood when the infant is intubated but may still exist during pharyngeal suctioning; thus, providing bag breaths with enriched oxygen is recommended. The infant should also be ventilated and oxygenated during and after each suction attempt. The oxygen concentration used should be the same as the concentration

Table 15-1
Suctioning procedure

1. Prepare equipment
   a. Select appropriate-sized catheter
   b. Determine catheter insertion distance, if possible
   c. Adjust vacuum pressure to 50 to 80 mm Hg with main suction line occluded
   d. Use sterile glove on dominant hand
   e. Maintain sterility of catheter
2. Prepare patient
   a. Oxygenate and ventilate infant with manual resuscitator, using transcutaneous monitor or oximeter as a guide, if possible
   b. Instill through endotracheal tube with normal saline or sodium bicarbonate solution when necessary
   c. Observe baseline heart rate and oxygenation
3. Perform suction procedure: pharyngeal suctioning
   a. Insert catheter into oral cavity without suction
   b. Remove catheter while applying intermittent suction
   c. Observe monitors for bradycardia/hypoxemia
   d. Oxygenate and ventilate patient between suction attempts
   e. Limit suction time to 10 seconds or less
   f. Insert catheter into nostril, moving catheter straight back and applying gentle pressure
   g. Remove catheter while applying intermittent suction
   h. Limit suction time to 10 seconds or less
4. Perform suction procedure: nasotracheal or orotracheal
   a. Insert catheter without suction during inspiration while applying gentle pressure over the larynx
   b. Remove catheter while applying intermittent suction
   c. Observe monitors for bradycardia/hypoxemia
   d. Oxygenate and ventilate infant between suction attempts
   e. Limit suction time to 10 seconds or less
5. Perform suction procedure: endotracheal tube
   a. Insert catheter without suction the predetermined length, or insert catheter without suction until resistance is met and pull catheter back 1 cm
   b. Remove catheter while applying intermittent suction, or remove catheter while applying constant suction and twirling catheter between thumb and forefinger
   c. Observe monitors for bradycardia/hypoxemia
   d. Oxygenate and ventilate infant between suction attempts
   e. Limit suction time to 10 seconds or less

that the infant is generally receiving, although some infants may require a slight increase in inspired oxygen to avoid hypoxemia. The common practice of using 100% oxygen during suctioning should be discouraged because even short-term administration of high oxygen concentrations may have undesirable effects on retinal vessels and effects on alveolar stability through denitrogenation. This procedure is most efficient when the transcutaneous monitor or oximeter is used to guide the amount and frequency of ventilation and oxygenation needed to avoid desaturation.

Because bag and mask ventilation requires two hands, this procedure is much easier with two operators: one to provide oxygenation and ventilation, and the other to suction. If two operators are not available, the infant should still be oxygenated and ventilated before the suction procedure is started. Oxygenation alone may be used between suction attempts, followed by reaeration and oxygenation when the suction procedure has been completed.

Before attaching the suction catheter to the suction source, the line should be occluded so that the maximum suction pressure can be observed and adjusted as necessary. In general, suction pressures of 50 to 80 mm Hg are considered safe and effective for the newborn, although some authors recommend suction pressures as high as 100 mm Hg.[2,12] The hand that will guide the catheter should be covered with a sterile glove. The suction catheter should be removed from its sterile packaging without contamination and attached to the suction line. A size-5 French suction catheter is preferred for oropharyngeal or nasopharyngeal suctioning.

INSERTION AND MONITORING

After the infant has been preoxygenated and ventilated, the catheter should be inserted into the oropharynx to clear secretions from this region and to prevent their subsequent aspiration during nasopharyngeal suctioning.[5] Care should be taken to avoid trauma to the oral mucosa by gently moving the catheter and by applying suction with the thumb on the control vent intermittently. The cardiac monitor should be observed for bradycardia caused by vagal stimulation, and the oximeter or transcutaneous monitor for signs of hypoxemia or desaturation. If either occurs, the suction procedure should be aborted immediately and the infant hand-ventilated until the heart rate or oxygen reading returns to an acceptable level. In addition, suction should not be applied for more than 10 seconds before the infant is reoxygenated.

NASOPHARYNGEAL SUCTIONING

After removal of oropharyngeal secretions, the nasopharynx may be suctioned. If nasal suctioning is performed first, the stimulation of the catheter in the nose may result in aspiration of pharyngeal secretions into the airway. The same considerations apply for oxygenation, ventilation, and careful attention to technique. The catheter should be gently directed straight back from the nostril along the septum and should never be forced. Suction should be applied intermittently during removal of the catheter. The entire procedure should be limited to 10 seconds or less. Suction applied too vigorously or for an extended period is likely to result in bradycardia, apnea, and significant trauma to the nasal passages.[4] It is well to remember that the newborn infant is an obligate nose breather and that the nose produces about half of the airway resistance of the newborn.[7] Trauma to the nasal mucosa causing inflammation and swelling may result in increased airway resistance, and thus in increased work of breathing for the infant. In addition, severe swelling may obstruct the nasal passages and result in apnea and the need to establish an artificial airway with its attendant problems. While the nasal passages must be kept clear of secretions for these reasons, vigorous and repeated suctioning may exacerbate the problem rather than relieve it. A bulb syringe is usually safe and sufficient for removal of nasopharyngeal secretions.

Nasotracheal or orotracheal suctioning

In some instances, it may be necessary to attempt to pass the suction catheter below the vocal cords into the trachea itself. This may be accomplished either through the nasal or oral passageway. The initial procedures for preparation for suctioning and for catheter insertion are the same as those for nasopharyngeal or oropharyngeal suctioning. The operator then attempts to insert the catheter into the airway during inspiration. Pressure applied externally over the cricothyroid area may be helpful in these attempts. This technique greatly increases the risk of trauma, atelectasis, hypoxemia, bradycardia, and apnea. Many institutions do not attempt it for these reasons. If the infant has a large volume of secretions that he cannot raise into the upper airway, suctioning under direct visualization with a laryngoscope or insertion of an artificial airway will probably be necessary.

Suctioning through a tube

The general procedure for suctioning and the hazardous consequences of this technique are not different when suctioning through a tube, although several additional considerations are necessary. Choosing an appropriate catheter size and determining the length of catheter to be inserted are critical to the avoidance of serious side-effects of suctioning. Catheters should not occlude more than two thirds of the internal diameter of the endotracheal or tracheostomy tube; exceeding this ratio results in occlusion of the airway with the possible consequences of severe hypoxemia, lung collapse, and development of pulmonary air leaks.[10] Catheters that are inserted too far may occlude a major branch of the airway. Additionally, the endotracheal or tracheostomy tube provides a direct route for introducing pathogenic microorganisms into the airway. Sterile, disposable catheters should always be used and handled with a sterile gloved hand.

SELECTING A CATHETER

Endotracheal tube sizes are usually expressed in millimeters, whereas suction catheters are expressed in French units. Dividing the French size by three will give an approximate estimate of the diameter of the suction catheter (*e.g.*, a size-5 French suction catheter has an external diameter of about 1.67 mm, which is approximately two thirds of the inner diameter of a size-2.5 endotracheal tube). Table 15-2 provides helpful guidelines for selecting an appropriate catheter size.

INSERTION AND WITHDRAWAL PROCEDURES

There are several ways in which the depth of insertion of the catheter can be determined. Ideally, the catheter should not be inserted past the end of the endotracheal tube because it can easily occlude a main airway, particularly those leading to the right middle and upper lobes, and lead to lobar collapse. Catheters with external markings of length are now available that allow the operator to determine the precise depth of insertion. Alternatively, the catheter may be inserted until resistance is met and then withdrawn about 1 cm before suction is applied. This does not assure that the catheter will not be inserted too deeply but does help to prevent the tip of the catheter from being lodged in a bronchus or wedged against mucosal tissue when suction is initially applied.

Once the catheter has been inserted, it should be withdrawn while suction is applied and while gently twirling the catheter between thumb and forefinger. Alternatively, suction may be applied intermittently as the catheter is removed. The entire procedure for insertion and removal should last no longer than 10 seconds. Of course, the infant should be oxygenated and ventilated as outlined above before, during, and after the suction procedure and monitored carefully to detect side-effects. Turning the head to each side may facilitate entrance of the catheter into the opposite main stem bronchus,

Table 15-2
Catheter and tube sizes

Endotracheal tube (mm)	Catheter (French units)
2.5	5
3.0	6½
3.5	6½
4.0	8

although it is questionable whether this procedure is successful in increasing the probability of the catheter's entering the left main stem bronchus.

INSTILLATION

Instillation of either normal saline or sodium bicarbonate solution into the endotracheal tube may be necessary. A few drops of sterile saline are routinely instilled into the endotracheal tube before suctioning in many hospitals. Unit-dose preparations of sterile saline designed for use in aerosol devices are easily available and convenient for this purpose. Unused portions of an opened vial should be discarded at the end of each shift. After instillation, several breaths with a manual ventilator will help to distribute the saline. If the infant has very thick, tenacious secretions, instillation of sodium bicarbonate solution (1:4 dilution with normal saline), administered for its mucolytic properties, may be helpful.

Endotracheal intubation

The major reasons for insertion of an artificial airway in the newborn are essentially the same as those in older patients: for connection to mechanical ventilation or other form of positive airway pressure (*e.g.,* CPAP); to bypass upper airway obstruction (*e.g.,* in choanal atresia); to protect the airway from aspiration (*e.g.,* with the presence of tracheoesophageal fistula); and to facilitate removal of secretions or other material from the tracheobronchial tree (*e.g.,* at delivery when meconium has been aspirated).

SELECTION OF EQUIPMENT

Before beginning the intubation procedure, all equipment needed should be assembled and checked for operation. A size "0" Miller laryngoscope blade is adequate for almost all newborns and may be attached to either a regular adult-sized laryngoscope handle or to a pediatric handle. An appropriately sized tube should be ready, as well as a tube one size larger and one size smaller, if possible. A 2.5 mm ID endotracheal tube is used for very small newborns (under 1000 g), and a size 4.0 for infants above 3500 g. Infants between 1000 and 3500 g will need a 3.0 or 3.5 mm tube. In the past, Cole tubes were commonly used. These tubes have a larger diameter than does a normal endotracheal tube (Murphy tube) except for the distal end, which is narrow. This creates a "shoulder" at the end of the tube, which naturally rests on the larynx, thus preventing intubation of a main stem bronchus. The Cole tube is also stiffer and thus does not require an obturator for insertion. These tubes are more likely to become occluded, however, and the incidence of damage to the larynx is greater, particularly if used with long-term ventilation. At present, Cole tubes are not commonly used except for emergency orotracheal intubation, particularly in the delivery room.[11]

In addition to the laryngoscope blade and handle and a selection of endotracheal tubes, equipment for suctioning, ventilating, and securing the tube after insertion should be available. A stylet is usually used to maintain rigidity of the tube during insertion of orotracheal tubes. A stethoscope for postintubation auscultation should be ready and the infant kept under a warmer during the intubation procedure.

OROTRACHEAL INTUBATION

The procedure for intubation of the newborn is very similar to that for older patients. An endotracheal tube may be inserted either orally or nasally. The choice of route depends largely on the preference of the intubator. Oral intubation is preferred in an emergency because it is faster and easier to accomplish. For prolonged ventilation, nasal intubation is preferred because the tube is easier to stabilize. Nasal intubation is often limited in the newborn by the size of the nasal passages. For oral intubation, the infant is placed supine with the head in the "sniffing" position (Fig. 15-1). Care must be taken to avoid hyperextension of the neck because the infant's neck is very flexible and extreme hyperextension with subsequent occlusion of the airway is possible. The laryngoscope handle is held in the left hand, between the thumb and index finger, and introduced into the right side of the mouth. As the blade is advanced, it is moved to midline to move the tongue out of the field of vision. The third and fourth fingers may be

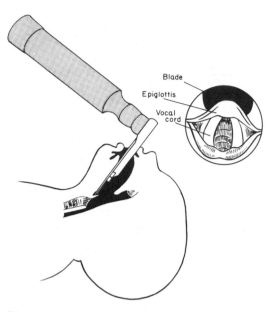

Fig. 15-1. Orotracheal intubation. Note the position of the infant's head, and the insertion of the tip of the blade into the vallecula. The cords should be visualized below the blade and epiglottis to ensure proper tube placement. (Avery GB: Neonatology: Pathophysiology and Management of the Newborn, 2nd ed, p 415. Philadelphia, JB Lippincott, 1981)

used to elevate the chin and maintain the "sniffing position," and the fifth finger may be used to apply pressure to the larynx to bring it in line for better visualization. The tip of the blade is then advanced into the vallecula, which is a space between the base of the tongue and the epiglottis. The entire laryngoscope is then lifted upward to elevate the epiglottis and expose the glottis. The gingiva of the infant should not be used as a fulcrum for the laryngoscope blade because this may cause permanent damage to the underlying teeth. Suctioning may be necessary at this point. Once the glottis is exposed, the endotracheal tube should be inserted along the right side of the mouth and passed through the glottis under direct visualization, with the tip of the tube about 2 cm past the glottis. The approximate insertion distance can be estimated by using the "rule of 7-8-9" proposed by Tochen: the 7 cm mark should be at the lip line for a 1 kg infant, the 8 cm mark for a 2 kg infant, and the 9 cm mark for a 3 kg infant.[14] The infant larynx is narrowest at the cricoid cartilage rather than at the glottis, and it is not uncommon to pass a tube easily through the glottis but find its forward passage blocked below this level. The tube should not be forced if this happens because it will result in significant trauma to the airway.[1]

During the intubation procedure, heart rate and rhythm should be monitored. If bradycardia (heart rate less than 100/min) occurs, the intubation procedure should be aborted and immediate bag/mask ventilation with elevated oxygen concentration performed until the heart rate returns to normal. If the infant is not attached to a cardiac monitor, an assistant should listen to the apical heart beat with a stethoscope or feel the umbilical pulse during the intubation attempt.

NASOTRACHEAL INTUBATION

If the tube is to be inserted nasotracheally, it should be lubricated with a water-soluble lubricant to facilitate passage through the nares. Petroleum-based lubricants should be avoided because they cause a chemical pneumonitis when inhaled. The laryngoscope is placed as for oral insertion and the glottis visualized. The tube is passed through the nostril into the nasopharynx. Magill forceps may be used to grasp the tube and guide it through the glottis, although an experienced intubator may not need this instrument. Insertion distance may be ascertained using charts that compare body weight, head circumference, and crown–heel length to the distance from naris to cords and naris to carina.[3] Alternatively, 1 cm may be added to the "7-8-9" rule proposed by Tochen.[9]

TUBE POSITION

After insertion, tube position should be checked by auscultating for equal breath sounds bilaterally in the axillary regions and by observing symmetrical movement of the chest cage. If the movement or breath sounds are diminished on one side, it is likely that one of the main stem bronchi has been intubated, and the tube should be slowly withdrawn until equal breath sounds are heard; however, breath sounds are often "referred" from an aerated area to an unaerated area in the newborn chest, and a follow-up chest x-ray is needed to confirm proper placement. The tip of the tube should be approximately midway between the cords and the carina with the infant's head neither flexed nor extended. The mark on the tube at the lip line should then be noted, and often is marked with adhesive tape, so that movement of the tube can be identified and corrected.

SECURING THE TUBE

Once correct position of the tube has been assured, the tube must be secured so that movement of the infant or traction from attached equipment does not cause the tube to become displaced or dislodged. Several systems have been proposed, including placement of Elastoplast on the upper lip following application of benzoin to the skin, with suturing or taping of the tube, or both, to the Elastoplast.[6] Alternatively, a roll of one-half inch adhesive can be prepared, with one end wrapped around the endotracheal tube, the roll then passed under the infant's neck, and the other end again wrapped around the tube. Benzoin is used to prepare the skin as before.

COMPLICATIONS

Most of the problems associated with endotracheal intubation of the newborn are related to the intubation process itself, including intubation of the esophagus, intubation of a main stem bronchus, and trauma to the upper airway. Prolonged intubation may result in damage to the larynx, trachea, and vocal cords, although most heal spontaneously and few result in long-term sequelae.

EXTUBATION

Intubation is no longer needed when the original conditions that required it are no longer present. In most cases, the tube was placed to provide better access to the airway for mechanical ventilation and CPAP. When the infant is breathing spontaneously and requires low inspired oxygen and CPAP levels over several hours, extubation should be considered. The infant should be suctioned thoroughly before extubation and the stomach emptied, if possible. After inflation with a manual resuscitator, the tube is removed. Some prefer to apply suction to the endotracheal tube during removal to facilitate removal of any mucous plugs that may be attached to the tube or tracheal wall. After extubation, the infant should be observed for signs of respiratory distress while receiving warmed, humidified oxygen. In some nurseries, routine aerosol treatments with 0.25 ml of racemic epinephrine are given after extubation to prevent the development of clinically significant laryngeal edema. Chest physiotherapy may also be indicated because many infants develop right upper lobe or right middle lobe collapse.[8,13]

Objectives

Having completed this chapter, the reader should be able to do the following:

1. List the types of equipment that can be used to suction the infant's airway, and describe the operation of a DeLee suction trap.
2. Describe the major complications of suctioning, and discuss the procedures that can be used to prevent complications.
3. State suction pressure ranges for the newborn.
4. Describe the procedure for insertion of the catheter and monitoring of the infant with nasopharyngeal and oropharyngeal suctioning.
5. Discuss the procedure for orotracheal and nasotracheal suctioning, and explain why this procedure is not performed in some hospitals.
6. Describe the procedure for determining appropriate catheter size and insertion distance when suctioning through an endotracheal tube.
7. Discuss the consequences of using catheters that are too large and of inserting catheters too far into the airway.
8. Describe the procedures for insertion and withdrawal of suction catheters when suctioning through an endotracheal tube.
9. Describe the instillation process, and state two solutions that can be instilled.
10. List the reasons for endotracheal intubation.
11. Describe the equipment needed for intubation of the newborn.

12. Compare Cole tubes to Murphy tubes.
13. Describe the procedure used for orotracheal and for nasotracheal intubation of the newborn.
14. List the major reasons for choosing the oral or nasal route.
15. Discuss the "rule of 7-8-9."
16. Explain how the anatomy of the infant's airway differs from that of the adult.
17. Discuss the monitoring of the infant during the intubation procedure.
18. Describe the ways in which tube position is monitored after intubation.
19. Describe methods used to secure endotracheal tubes.
20. Discuss the complications associated with intubation.
21. Describe the indications and procedure for extubation.

References

1. Applebaum EL, Bruce DL: Tracheal Intubation. Philadelphia, WB Saunders, 1976
2. Blodgett D: Manual of Pediatric Respiratory Care Procedures. Philadelphia, JB Lippincott, 1982
3. Coldiran JS: Estimation of nasotracheal tube length in neonates. Pediatrics 41:823, 1968
4. Cordero L, Hon EH: Neonatal bradycardia following nasopharyngeal stimulation. J Pediatr 78:441, 1971
5. Fletcher MA: Respiratory distress syndrome and other respiratory diseases in neonates. In Burton GC, Hodgkin JE (eds): Respiratory Care: A Guide to Clinical Practice, 2nd ed. Philadelphia, JB Lippincott, 1984
6. Gregory GA: Respiratory care of newborn infants. Pediatr Clin North Am 19:311, 1972
7. Hodson WA, Truog WE: Special techniques in managing respiratory problems. In Avery GB (ed): Neonatology: Pathophysiology and Management of the Newborn, 2nd ed. Philadelphia, JB Lippincott, 1981
8. Levine MI, Mascia AV: Pulmonary Diseases and Anomalies of Infancy and Childhood: Their Diagnosis and Treatment. New York, Harper & Row, 1966
9. Nugent J, Hanks H, Goldsmith JP: Pulmonary care. In Goldsmith JP, Karotkin EH (eds): Assisted Ventilation of the Neonate. Philadelphia, WB Saunders, 1981
10. Rosen M, Hillard EK: The effects of negative pressure during endotracheal suction. Anesth Analg 41:50, 1962

11. Schreiner RL, Stevens DC, Lemons JA, Greshman EL: Resuscitation. In Schreiner RL, Kisling JA (eds): Practical Neonatal Respiratory Care. New York, Raven Press, 1982
12. Slonim NB, Schneider S, Weng T, Fields L: Pediatric Respiratory Therapy: An Introductory Text. New York, Glenn Educational Medical Service, 1974
13. Smith RM: Anesthesia for Infants and Children, 3rd ed. St Louis, CV Mosby, 1968
14. Tochen ML: Orotrachael intubation in the newborn infant: A method for determining depth of tube insertion. J Pediatr 95:1050, 1979

16·
Resuscitation of the Newborn

Kathleen M. Beney

Persons experienced in resuscitation of the newborn should be present in the delivery room for all high-risk births and be readily available for situations that suddenly and unexpectedly become high risk. These persons, including physicians, nurses, and respiratory therapists, should be knowledgeable in perinatal physiology, skilled in resuscitation techniques, and familiar with all delivery room equipment and techniques. This chapter will review the integral parts of providing effective resuscitation for the newborn, including anticipation of the need for infant resuscitation, recognition and management of the infant in distress, stabilization, and follow-up care.

Anticipation of need

HIGH-RISK DELIVERIES

Many situations involving infant resuscitation are predictable based on knowledge (or *lack* of knowledge) involving various maternal factors, fetal problems during pregnancy, and complications that present during labor and delivery (see Chap. 3). When these situations are identified, skilled personnel should be notified, be given the opportunity to review the specific problems that may be encountered, and be present at the time of delivery in order to respond to any resuscitative efforts that may be necessary. The resuscitation of a severely depressed infant requires the skills of at least two, and preferably three, persons to coordinate ventilation and airway management, insertion and monitoring of intravascular catheters, administration of drugs and fluids, and performance of chest compression.

EQUIPMENT AND SUPPLIES

All necessary equipment and supplies must be present and operating properly, and *all* personnel having any contact with the newborn infant in the delivery room must know how to locate and operate each piece of equipment. An area within each delivery room should be set up for infant care within a few feet of the delivery site, complete with oxygen supply, suction apparatus, radiant warmer, a table that allows access to the infant from at least three sides, and storage space for all infant resuscitation equipment, supplies, and drugs.

Recommendations for equipment, supplies, drugs, and fluids for the storage area or cart are listed in Table 16-1.

Before the delivery, equipment should be prepared in advance whenever possible. The radiant warmer and transport incubator should be turned on; all suction and oxygen apparatus set up and functional; and estimated sizes of laryngoscope blades, endotracheal (ET) tubes, catheters, and other equipment set up and available. The resuscitation bag should be readied and set up with the appropriate flow of oxygen.

All equipment, supplies, and medications should be reviewed in a check-off type procedure performed on a routine basis (daily or weekly, depending on how often the delivery suite is used), and before and after each resuscitation effort. This is necessary to ensure that all equipment is functioning properly, all supplies are present and easily located, and outdated medications are replaced.

Recognition of the infant in distress

IMMEDIATE EVALUATION AND MANAGEMENT

Although various and progressive methods of evaluation of oxygenation and perfusion of the infant usually begin before the actual delivery occurs, at birth rapid, thorough, and continuous assessment begins immediately. Resuscitation is necessary for any infant who, for any reason, cannot establish adequate ventilation for effective gas exchange or maintain adequate circulation to perfuse major organ systems within the first few minutes after delivery.

Fortunately, about 90% of all infants are delivered without these complications and require only nasal and oral suctioning, drying of the skin, and maintenance of body temperature.[4] These infants generally have Apgar scores between 8 and 10. The Apgar scoring system, devised by Dr. Virginia Apgar, provides a means to assess rapidly the need for, and success of, resuscitation and has been reviewed in detail in Chapter 4.

As the infant's head is delivered, the mouth is cleared first to prevent aspiration of pharyngeal contents with the first breath, and the nose is then suctioned, both with a bulb syringe. If meconium is present, more aggressive suctioning

Table 16-1
Supply list for emergency resuscitation in the delivery room

Equipment and supplies	Medications and fluids
Radiant warmer	Atropine 0.5 mg/ml
Transport incubator	Sodium bicarbonate 8.4%
Oxygen source with flowmeter	(1 mEq/ml)
Bubble humidifier with connecting tubing	Calcium chloride 10%
Suction devices with manometers (2)	Dextrose in water 10% and 50%
Suction catheters (5, 6, 8, 10F)	Epinephrine 1:10,000
Bulb suction and DeLee trap	Albumisol 5%
Cardiotachometer with ECG oscilloscope	Naloxone 0.02 mg/ml
"Clothespin" ECG leads	Sterile water
Neonatal resuscitator bag with pressure manometer	Normal saline
Face masks (sizes 0–4)	Heparin
Oral airways (sizes 0–000)	
Endotracheal tubes (sizes 2.5–4.0 mm)	
Laryngoscope	
Laryngoscope blades, straight (sizes 00–1)	
Extra bulbs and batteries for laryngoscope	
Stethoscope	
½" tape	
Rolled diaper	
Tincture of benzoin	
Umbilical catheters (sizes 3.5 and 4.0F)	
Sterile umbilical artery catheterization tray	
Sterile scissors	
Sterile cord clamp	
Three-way stopcocks	
Y-connector	
Infant feeding tubes for gastric decompression (sizes 5 and 8F)	
Syringes (sizes 3, 5, and 10 ml)	
Several sizes of needles	
Alcohol wipes	
Iodophore solution	
Gauze sponges	
Dextrostix	
Hematocrit tubes	
Laboratory tubes	
Blood gas syringes	
Dry, warmed blankets	

should be performed (see Chap. 8). When fully delivered, the infant should be held at the level of vaginal delivery (introitus) while being dried off with warmed towels. Drying will help to maintain the infant's body temperature and at the same time stimulate the initiation of ventilation. Holding the infant at the level of the introitus will optimize blood flow between placental and infant circulations while the umbilicus is still intact. When the infant has begun to breathe and pulsations in the umbilical cord have subsided, the cord may be clamped and cut.[4] At this time, the infant should be placed on a radiantly heated bed with the head tilted slightly downward and lying on his side. The airway may be further cleared with gentle suctioning of the nose and mouth with the bulb syringe. After the 5-minute Apgar score has been obtained, and assuming that all vital signs are stable, a suction catheter may be inserted through each nostril into the hypopharynx to rule out choanal atresia, and then through the mouth into the esophagus and stomach. If difficulty or resistance is encountered, the possibility of esophageal atresia should be investigated. Once in the stomach, if more than 25 ml of fluid is removed, the presence of a small bowel obstruction should be suspected.[4] When this procedure has been completed and the infant is stable, he may be wrapped in a warm blanket and given to his parents.

Skill in identifying the depressed infant is essential for the appropriate initiation of resuscitation efforts.[1] Although it is relatively easy to differentiate between the infant who appears healthy and responsive and the infant who is severely compromised, intermediate situations may be less obvious. The 10% of infants who require more aggressive intervention and resuscitative efforts may present with varying degrees of asphyxia. Although the Apgar score can be helpful in indicating the extent of asphyxia, and will be used here to describe progessive stages of asphyxia, it is important to realize its limitations.

Most importantly, resuscitation should be started immediately when required, and not delayed for the assessment of the score at 1 minute. Additionally, the evaluation of need for, or response to, resuscitation may be assessed more accurately by evaluating heart rate, respiratory activity, and neuromuscular tone than by the total score.[3] It is also significant to note that even when the 1-minute score reflects stability, the infant should be carefully re-evaluated at 5 minutes of age. Some infants who appear fine at birth deteriorate rapidly.

MILD ASPHYXIA

Infants with an Apgar score of 5 to 7 may have experienced a mild asphyxia just before birth, usually during the birth process. Generally, they require only stimulation by gently slapping the feet or rubbing the back, and oxygenation provided by a simple face mask with a continuous flow of oxygen. If they are slow to respond, they may be ventilated with a high concentration of oxygen by bag and mask.

MODERATE ASPHYXIA

An Apgar score of 3 or 4 usually reflects moderate asphyxia. These depressed infants appear cyanotic and have very little respiratory effort. If *some* breathing is present, they can be assisted with bag-mask ventilation and will usually "pink up" with continued support. If, however, they have not made an inspiratory effort or begun to breathe, bag-mask ventilation will be difficult without an ET tube in place because of the increased airway resistance, and may result in preferential flow of gas to the esophagus. Intubation should be performed if the infant does not respond quickly to bag-mask ventilation.[4]

SEVERE ASPHYXIA

Infants with an Apgar score of 2 or less are severely asphyxiated and require immediate and vigorous resuscitation. These infants will appear flaccid, pale, limp, and cyanotic as they are delivered. As a result of the immediate and necessary response to this situation (clamping of the cord to begin resuscitation measures), the infant may also be hypovolemic.

Management of the infant in distress

The principles of newborn cardiopulmonary resuscitation (CPR) are the same as those used for an adult. Initially, the personnel involved with the resuscitation attempt should concern themselves with the "ABC's of CPR": *a*ssessment and *a*irway management; *b*reathing; and *c*irculatory support. Once this has been accomplished, steps can be taken involving the "D's": drug therapy, dysrhythmia recognition, defibrillation, diagnosis, and decisions for treatment. The only additional measure that needs to be included in the newborn is immediate attention to the importance of maintaining body temperature by drying the infant and carrying out resuscitative measures on a radiant heated bed.

TEMPERATURE REGULATION

There is a substantial difference in temperature between being in a controlled intrauterine environment and the temperature of the normal delivery room. Therefore, care must be taken to provide all newborns with a warm environment immediatcly at birth. Supplying extrinsic heat by completely drying the infant with towels and immediately placing him under a radiant heating device will minimize the need for intrinsic heat production by the infant.

It is especially crucial to minimize the need for intrinsic heat production in infants who have undergone a prolonged, difficult delivery or who have been born with any degree of asphyxia. These infants have varying degress of acidosis, compromised oxygen reserves, and unstable thermoregulatory mechanisms, all of which will be compromised further if they must increase oxygen consumption while attempting to produce heat. If unable to produce enough heat, they will develop hypothermia, which will further delay recovery from acidosis. For these reasons, it is essential that all resuscitation efforts take place under conditions in which the infant is kept warm.

AIRWAY MANAGEMENT

Assessing responsiveness and ventilation, establishing a patent airway, and preventing aspiration are of primary and immediate concern. Apnea is the most common type of respiratory disorder in the newborn. If spontaneous breathing is not present after suctioning the mouth and nose with a bulb syringe and drying the infant with warmed towels, the infant should immediately be placed under a radiant warmer in a slight

Trendelenberg position and the following steps taken: [1] check apical or femoral pulse; [2] gently suction with a catheter, once through each nare; [3] establish an optimal anatomic airway by holding the chin forward to ensure that the tongue is not obstructing the posterior pharynx; [4] stimulate infant by rubbing his soles; and [5] consider naloxone administration.

If there is no response to these additional stimuli, begin bag-mask ventilation immediately. Inserting a nasogastric tube at this time will aid gastric decompression, preventing distention and consequent compromise to ventilation.

Initially, a ventilatory rate of 30 to 40 breaths per minute at a pressure of 30 to 40 cm H_2O should provide adequate ventilation for most infants. This can be further assessed by evaluating bilateral chest expansion both visually and by auscultation, and by noting an increase in heart rate and an improvement in color of the infant.

Inability to deliver adequate ventilation with bag-mask ventilation indicates the need for the immediate intubation of the trachea. Size of the ET tube may be ascertained by matching the diameter of the infant's little finger to the diameter of the tube or by correlation with birth weight (Table 16-2). Because the incidence of apnea in newborns is often

Table 16-2
Selecting appropriate sizes of equipment
for resuscitation of the newborn

	Weight in grams				
	<1000	1000–1250	1250–2500	2500–3000	>3000
Oral airway	000	000	00	0	0
Endotracheal tube (mm)	2.5–3.0*	3.0	3.0	3.0–3.5	3.5–4.0
Suction catheter (French)	5	5 or 6	6	6 or 8	8
Mask for bag-mask resuscitation	0	0	0–1	1	1–4
Laryngoscope blade	00–0	0–1	0–1	0–1	1

* A 2.5 mm ET tube should not be used unless absolutely necessary, as it is difficult to suction and frequently occludes.

secondary to some type of airway obstruction, laryngoscopy should be performed with the laryngoscope in one hand and a suction catheter in the other. *It is crucial that suction apparatus be ready at the time of initial laryngoscopy,* in order to allow for immediate clearance of the airway to visualize the vocal cords. Failure to follow this procedure will often necessitate additional laryngoscopy, which becomes more difficult with each subsequent attempt because of resultant trauma and edema inherent to the procedure.

Apnea is not the only indication for bag-mask ventilatory assistance. Any time that ventilation is not adequate to maintain a heart rate of at least 100 per minute, bag-mask ventilation should be initiated. Critical determinants of adequate bag-mask ventilation include use of the proper mask size, correct application of the mask with an adequate seal, use of an in-line pressure manometer, ability to deliver 100% oxygen, familiarity with the bag-mask setup in use, and adequate flow if a non-self-inflating bag is in use.

The two types of resuscitation bags used in infant ventilation are self-inflating and non-self-inflating (anesthesia) bags. Each has advantages and disadvantages and requires practice in order to learn how to use it effectively. *It is essential that individuals responsible for using these devices receive adequate training and frequent practice in their use.* This will ensure optimal results when the procedure is necessary. Only when resuscitation bags or adjunctive equipment is missing or malfunctioning should mouth-to-mouth breathing be initiated. If this circumstance arises, the mouth and nose of the infant should be covered and sealed with the rescuer's mouth, and small "puffs" of air adequate to cause the chest to rise should be delivered once every 2 to 3 seconds.

ENDOTRACHEAL INTUBATION

Intubation of the trachea in the delivery room is necessary under certain circumstances. The first indication occurs after an infant has been delivered through thick or particulate meconium or has aspirated blood.[3] In this situation, intubation and thorough suctioning should be done *before* any other measures of resuscitation, especially bag-mask ventilation, in order to prevent further aspiration of these substances. A second indication is if an obstruction appears to be preventing adequate bag-mask ventilation. In this situation, the ET tube will usually by-pass the obstruction and allow for adequate ventilation. Intubation may also be indicated if the infant being ventilated with a bag-mask system has not shown significant improvement in heart rate and color, or demonstrated a return of spontaneous breathing after a few minutes of assisted ventilation or when cardiac compressions become necessary.

Endotracheal intubation is much more likely to be successful on the first attempt if the following steps are taken before the initial laryngoscopy:

1. Select proper size and prepare ET tube, carefully inserting stylet. In addition to size selected, have one size larger and one size smaller at hand. A stylet provides rigidity and appropriate curvature to the ET tube to facilitate rapid intubation, but it is important that the tip not project beyond the distal tip of the tube. In the absence of a stylet, the tube may be placed "on ice" to facilitate rigidity.
2. Choose laryngoscope blade and handle, lock in place, and check that the light is bright enough and that the bulb is screwed tightly in place.
3. Make sure that suctioning equipment is set up, functioning properly, and that a sterile suction catheter is attached and ready for use. Suction pressures generally should not exceed −80 mm Hg.
4. Properly position infant's head in the "sniff position" to obtain a straight line axis of the pharynx and trachea. Slight elevation of the occipital skull will facilitate this. Gentle pressure exerted over the larynx may also help the operator to visualize the opening to the airway.
5. Adequately hyperinflate and hyperoxygenate the infant for *at least* 10 seconds before attempting intubation.

The procedure to be used for insertion of an oral ET tube is described in Chapter 15. Throughout the procedure, one must be sure that the infant receives adequate oxygen, and after 30 seconds (or sooner if bradycardia occurs) the intubation attempt must be stopped so that the infant may be reventilated with 100% oxygen by bag-mask system.

Once the tube is in proper position and secured, ventilations should be delivered with a volume just large enough to allow for adequate chest movement and should be delivered once every 2 to 3 seconds, for an overall rate of 20 to 30 breaths per minute. Ventilating with more volume than necessary may result in gastric distention and possible aspiration and may also lead to pneumothorax.

There are several ways in which effectiveness of ventilation can be evaluated. In addition to evaluation of breath sounds (auscultation), one should look for the return of normal skin color, a rapid rise in heart rate to at least 120 beats per minute, and progressive return of spontaneous breathing and movement. If these changes do not occur, steps should be taken to rule out airway obstruction, inadequate seal of the mask, misplacement of the ET tube, pneumothorax, or circulatory failure.

CIRCULATORY SUPPORT

Whenever the heart rate of the newborn drops to less than 80 to 100 beats per minute and does not immediately respond to effective ventilation, cardiac compression should begin.[2,4] In newborns, the two-handed chest encircling method of chest compression (Fig. 16-1) is generally preferred whenever sufficient personnel are present, rather than the technique that requires compression of the sternum with two fingers (Fig. 16-2). The hands should encircle the chest, both thumbs side-by-side just below the nipple line on the midportion of the sternum. The fingers should be wrapped around and supporting the chest cage, without compressing the rib cage. Care should be taken to avoid limitation of movement of the thorax with encircled hands, which is especially likely to occur if the infant is large or the rescuer's hands are small and may result in changes in intrathoracic pressure, compromised circulation, and compromised ventilation. In this case, the two-finger method would be preferred. In a very small infant, the thumbs may have to be superimposed.

The sternum should then be compressed about one half to three fourths of an inch, at a rate of 5 compressions within 2 to 3 seconds, resulting in an overall compression rate of 100

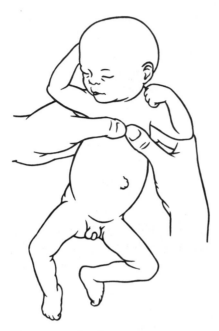

Fig. 16-1. Cardiac compression in the newborn, using two-handed chest encircling method. (Blodgett D: Manual of Pediatric Respiratory Care Procedures, p 119. Philadelphia, JB Lippincott, 1982)

Fig. 16-2. Cardiac compression in the newborn, using two-finger compression of sternum. (Blodgett D: Manual of Pediatric Respiratory Care Procedures, p 116. Philadelphia, JB Lippincott, 1982)

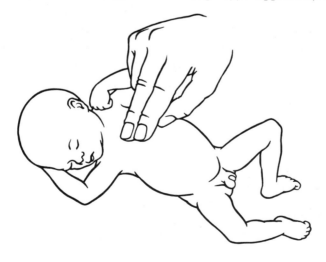

to 150 per minute. Each compression should generate a systolic pressure of at least 80 mm Hg. This, plus a heart rate of about 120 per minute, should maintain diastolic pressure at 15 to 20 mm Hg, which is probably adequate for coronary perfusion. Care should be taken to avoid compressing the lower portion of the sternum because of the high potential for damage to underlying organs from contact with the xiphoid process.

After every fifth compression, a breath should be given as the pressure on the sternum is released. If for any reason the ventilation appears inadequate, time should be taken to deliver a second breath before restarting compressions. When there is inadequate or no response to ventilation and compression, drug therapy should be initiated.

DRUG THERAPY AND FLUID ADMINISTRATION

Infants who do not respond rapidly to stimulation, ventilation, intubation, and cardiac compression need to receive fluids and drugs through a central line placed as quickly as possible. The preferred placement of a central line is into the umbilical artery and secondly, into the umbilical vein. Although umbilical artery catheterization may be more difficult to perform, it offers several advantages: It allows for direct and continuous measurement of blood pressure; arterial blood samples may be easily obtained; and it may be left in place for several days to allow for continued monitoring and fluid/drug infusion in the postresuscitation management period. An umbilical venous catheter is usually removed immediately after resuscitation to prevent possible infection and clotting of the portal vein.

Initial drug therapy and fluid administration are directed toward correcting acidosis, hypoglycemia, hypovolemia, and hypotension.

Acidosis

Because the presence of acidosis decreases the effectiveness of other resuscitation drugs, the pH should be raised above 7.2 as soon as possible. Respiratory acidosis is caused by accumulation of carbon dioxide that results from lack of adequate ventilation, and is corrected by assisting ventilation with a manual resuscitator attached to either a mask or ET tube. *The importance of achieving and maintaining effective ventilatory support cannot be overemphasized.*

Metabolic acidosis is caused by inadequate tissue oxygenation leading to anaerobic metabolism and subsequent lactate production and accumulation. Inadequate tissue oxygenation is usually the result of inadequate perfusion during cardiopulmonary arrest and is corrected by administering sodium bicarbonate, by expanding blood volume, and by cardiac compression; however, great care must be taken to minimize the potential complications of sodium bicarbonate administration in this situation. These complications include hypertension, too rapid expansion of intravascular volume, and a significant increase in Pa_{CO_2}. A substantial increase in Pa_{CO_2} may result and will worsen the acidosis, possibly causing death; it may also dilate the cerebral vessels, increasing the risk of intracranial hemorrhage.

Because of these risks, mild to moderate metabolic acidosis usually does not require sodium bicarbonate administration. If the *pH* can be maintained above 7.15 with ventilation, compression, and volume expansion, bicarbonate therapy should be delayed. If acidosis progresses beyond this point, sodium bicarbonate should be diluted 1:1 with sterile water and infused at a rate of 1 to 2 mEq/kg/min, aiming to correct one fourth of the base deficit. If blood gases and *pH* are not available, 1 mEq/kg should be given by slow push (30–60 seconds) every 10 minutes during the resuscitation attempt.[2,4] Whenever possible, the overall dosage of sodium bicarbonate given over 24 hours should not exceed 8 mEq/kg. Amounts exceeding this dosage may be associated with increased risk of intracranial hemorrhage.[1]

Hypoglycemia

Hypoglycemia is defined as a blood glucose level of less than 30 mg/dl in the full-term infant and less than 20 mg/dl in the infant weighing less than 2500 g. These abnormally low blood glucose levels occur frequently in asphyxiated newborns because their glycogen stores are easily depleted under stress. Untreated, hypoglycemia may rapidly cause death secondary to cardiac failure or hypotension. Signs of hypoglycemia include apnea, irritability, lethargy, tremors, hypotonicity, and seizures; however, before any of these signs have the opportunity to appear, immediate bedside glucose levels should be measured from blood sampled at the heel. Serum analysis can then be performed by the laboratory for confirmation. Hypoglycemia should be treated by providing glucose to supplement glycogen stores. A rapid infusion of glucose should be administered as an intravenous bolus of 1 ml/kg of 50% dextrose, followed by a continuous infusion of 10% dextrose at 4 ml/kg/h. Recognizing that a rapid infusion of dextrose will correct even undiagnosed hypoglycemia and simultaneously replace depleted glycogen, it is currently recommended that documentation of blood glucose levels should not delay dextrose administration.[2]

Hypovolemia

It is not unusual for asphyxiated infants to be hypovolemic at birth. This may be related to the fact that their umbilical cords are clamped early in order to proceed with resuscitation measures. Hypovolemia should be considered in these infants, as well as in those who have undergone delivery complicated by partial umbilical cord occlusion, accidental placental transection during C-section, placental abruption, or any maternal bleeding before or during delivery.

At physical examination, these infants may appear gray, pale, or mottled and usually have poor perfusion and capillary filling pressures manifested by cold, cyanotic extremities and weak or absent peripheral pulses. Hypovolemia should be suspected if mean arterial pressures are low, if systolic pressure decreases more than 5 mm Hg with inspiration, or if the central venous pressure is less than 4 cm H_2O.

Hypovolemia is treated by intravascular volume expansion with albumin, crystalloid, or blood (15 ml/kg infused over 5 to 10 minutes). Care should be taken not to overexpand the intravascular volume because this may result in hypertension and subsequent intracranial hemorrhage. The presence of central venous and arterial lines greatly facilitates optimal fluid management in these infants.

Hypotension

Hypotension in newborns is frequently secondary to hypovolemia, and therefore is corrected as fluids are given to correct the volume deficit. Other possible causes may include intrapulmonary gas leaks that interfere with venous return to the heart, hypoglycemia, hypocalcemia, hypomagnesemia, severe anemia, and alcohol or magnesium intoxication. Mean arterial pressures consistent with hypotension vary with birth weight (less than 50 mm Hg for 3000 g; less than 40 mm Hg for 2000 g; and less than 35 mm Hg for 1000 to 2000 g); regardless of weight, however, systolic pressure should be maintained above 40 mm Hg.

Treatments other than volume expansion may include epinephrine or atropine. Epinephrine is administered in an initial dose of 0.1 ml/kg of 1:10,000 solution, to be repeated every 5 minutes. Its use results in an increased heart rate, increased force of myocardial contraction, and increased vascular resistance. Atropine is indicated if the major problem is persistent bradycardia (less than 100 beats/min) and is administered in a dose of 0.03 mg/kg, which may be repeated twice.[2] Both drugs should be used following attempts to restore adequate cardiopulmonary function with ventilation and external compressions and may be administered intravenously or by instillation.

Maternal narcotic use

If it is suspected that respiratory depression is secondary to maternal narcotic administration during labor and delivery, naloxone hydrochloride (Narcan) may be administered at a dosage of 0.01 mg/kg every 2 to 3 minutes until the effects of the narcotic analgesic no longer interfere with the ability to ventilate. Naloxone hydrochloride should not, however, be given to infants of mothers who are chronically addicted to narcotic drugs because it may precipitate narcotic withdrawal in these infants, leading to further complications.

Stabilization and follow-up care

PREPARATION FOR TRANSPORT

As the infant in distress is being resuscitated, contact should be established immediately with the nearest neonatal special care facility and arrangements made for transport. Stabilization of the infant while awaiting the arrival of the transport team is crucial and involves the management of hypothermia, hypotension, hypoglycemia, and altered acid–base status, as well as gas exchange.[6]

MANAGEMENT AND FOLLOW-UP CARE

Initial management will be similar whether the infant is being transferred to another facility or to the newborn nursery in the hospital where delivered. Care should be taken to correct hypothermia by placing the infant in an isolette with temperature set to maintain a neutral thermal environment (see Chap. 7). All oxygen delivered should be warmed and humidified. Vital signs including blood pressure should be monitored every 15 minutes for the first hour, and systolic pressure should remain above 40 mm Hg regardless of birth weight. When necessary, blood products (fresh frozen plasma, whole blood, or packed red blood cells, if available) or lactated Ringer's solution should be infused at 10 to 20 ml/kg over 5 to 10 minutes to maintain blood pressure.

Bedside screening for hypoglycemia (*e.g.,* Dextrostix) is particularly important in infants who have had problems at delivery, because glycogen stores are easily depleted in these infants. Glucose levels should be monitored carefully at the bedside with blood samples obtained from heelsticks. It may be necessary to infuse a dextrose solution in infants whose glucose levels fall below 20 to 30 mg/dl, depending on body weight.

To monitor acid–base and oxygenation/ventilation status, it is always preferable to obtain arterial blood samples when possible. This is greatly facilitated when an umbilical arterial line is in place. Arterial values and trends should be evaluated carefully at frequent intervals and appropriate adjustments made to assure optimal oxygenation, ventilation, and the correction of both metabolic and respiratory acidosis. Nonin-vasive monitors such as transcutaneous monitors and oximeters may be helpful in early detection of derangements in some of these parameters. Early recognition of the need for positive pressure ventilation may minimize the progression of severely altered acid–base status.

Other tests that should be obtained as soon as possible after stabilization of the infant include a chest radiograph and complete blood count.

Summary

Resuscitation efforts in the delivery room are intended to facilitate the necessary physiologic changes that must occur in the transition from fetal to neonatal life. When these respiratory and circulatory changes require assistance, only immediate and correct action will prevent injury and possible death. Resuscitation efforts are much more likely to be successful when the medical team is knowledgeable, skilled, and familiar with all aspects of complications in the newborn and with delivery room equipment and procedures.

Objectives

Having completed this chapter, the reader should be able to do the following:

1. Discuss the equipment and supplies that should be available in the delivery room for resuscitation of the asphyxiated infant.
2. Describe the immediate evaluation and management of the newborn infant in the delivery room.
3. Discuss the use of the Apgar score in evaluating asphyxia in the newborn.
4. Differentiate between mild, moderate, and severe asphyxia, in terms of recognition and treatment.
5. Discuss the importance of temperature regulation in the newborn.
6. Describe the initial steps to be taken if a newborn infant does not begin to breathe.
7. Explain how adequacy of ventilation during resuscitation may be evaluated in the newborn.
8. Discuss the use of laryngoscopy during resuscitation.
9. State the indications for the use of bag-mask ventilation.

10. List the factors that influence the adequacy of bag-mask ventilation.
11. Describe the circumstances under which mouth-to-mouth ventilation would be used in the delivery room, and explain how it is performed in the newborn infant.
12. Discuss the indications for endotracheal intubation in the newborn who requires resuscitation.
13. List and describe steps that should be taken before inserting an ET tube.
14. State the proper breathing rate and breath intervals for resuscitation of the newborn.
15. Discuss the ways in which the effectiveness of ventilation can be evaluated.
16. State the circumstances under which cardiac compression should be initiated.
17. Describe the two methods used for cardiac compression in the newborn, and compare their advantages/disadvantages.
18. State the proper compression rate and depth for resuscitation of the newborn.
19. Discuss the integration of ventilations and compressions when performing CPR in the newborn.
20. List the four major deficits that drug and fluid administration is used to correct.
21. Differentiate between respiratory and metabolic acidosis, and discuss the treatment of each.
22. Discuss the problems associated with the use of sodium bicarbonate in treating acidosis in the newborn.
23. Discuss the treatment of hypoglycemia in the newborn.
24. List the infants who are likely to be hypovolemic immediately after birth, and describe their usual appearance.
25. Discuss the treatment of hypovolemia and hypotension.
26. Explain the rationale for using epinephrine, atropine, and naloxone in newborn resuscitation.
27. Describe the procedures to be followed for stabilization and follow-up care in the newborn who has been resuscitated.

References

1. Boere RC Jr: Resuscitation of the Newborn. Ann Arbor, Michigan Perinatal Education Project, University of Michigan, 1977

2. Chameides D, Melker R, Rave JR et al: Resuscitation of the newborn. In McIntyre KM, Lewis AJ: Textbook of Advanced Cardiac Life Support. Dallas, American Heart Association, 1981
3. Fletcher MA: Respiratory distress syndrome and other respiratory diseases in neonates. In Burton G, Hodgkin J (eds): Respiratory Care. A Guide to Clinical Practice, 2nd ed. Philadelphia, JB Lippincott, 1984
4. Gregory GA: Resuscitation of the newborn. In Shoemaker WC, Thompson WL, Holbrook PR: Textbook of Critical Care Medicine. Philadelphia, WB Saunders, 1984
5. Jastremski MS, Cantor RM, Olson CM, Smith RW, Tyndall GJ: The Whole Emergency Medicine Catalog. Philadelphia, WB Saunders, 1985
6. Tadres ID, Rogers MC: Methods of external cardiac massage in the newborn infant. J Pediatr 86:781, 1975

17·
Home
Health
Care
of the
Newborn

Michael Boroch

Treating pediatric respiratory therapy patients in the home is not a new phenomenon, but the intensity and the scope of care are changing dramatically. Although several factors are responsible for this change, the most significant is that children with chronic, stable disease are leaving the hospital and going home.

Respiratory therapy has played a role in the transition from hospital to home and is a significant factor in home care. Advances in the area of pediatric respiratory home health care, which improve the quality of life for both the child and the parents, are tied directly to the driving forces in the health care industry. With the improvement of pediatric home health care technology, chronic disease can often be treated outside an institution without sacrificing the quality of care.

As with many dynamic topics, descriptions vary and change with time. The Discursive Dictionary of Health Care, a document prepared for the Subcommittee on Health and Environment of the U.S. House of Representatives, describes home health care as "the provision of health services rendered to an individual as needed in his/her home environment. Services are provided to aged, disabled, or sick or convalescent individuals who do not need institutional care." The American Medical Association's definition—"provision (under medical supervision) of needed health care and supportive services to a sick or disabled person in his/her home surroundings"— stresses the human factor, whereas the guidelines of the Department of Health and Human Services, formerly the Department of Health, Education, and Welfare, focus on the technical aspects: "A wide range of services from the highly skilled to maintenance care, personal care and related services in various combinations."

All of these definitions agree on the setting (at home), the care (a wide range of services), and the providers (skilled), the last two under the general directions and orders of a physician. Yet none mention the potential financial savings of home health care, the benefits of familial emotional support, and the resulting normalcy of the home environment on childhood development.

A major financial motive in support of home health care arose when it was discovered that Medicare and Medicaid would be financially insolvent between 1988 and 1992 unless significant expenditure reductions or increased revenues into the system, or both, occurred.[8] Because the federal government is the single largest payer of health care costs, proposals for less costly treatments were developed (prospective payment). Traditionally, most of the Medicare dollars are spent on in-hospital care; therefore, changes or restraints were developed and passed by Congress to create incentives for alternative (*i.e.*, less expensive) health care delivery systems. One of the alternatives considered is home health care. Other alternatives include nursing homes and "half way" or rehabilitation centers.

Pediatric home health care is often a difficult task to manage because of the complexity and diversity of individual cases. A total, multi-disciplinary team approach is recommended. Maintaining the quality of care can usually be achieved, and savings are often significant. Many who have private insurance may quickly reach the maximum levels of reimbursement in a few years. At costs of $30,000 to $50,000 per month for care, reaching a million dollar cap does not take long. Because home care can reduce the costs of hospitalization, it extends the length of time of insurance benefits, which is particularly significant with young children who may require health care services for many years. Home health care is continuing to gain acceptance as a preferred option for many children with chronic respiratory related problems. The major issues are quality of life for the patient and family, cost of care, normal child development, and family participation in the care of the child.

This chapter will cover the major therapies and related monitoring for pediatric respiratory care patients, including oxygen therapy, aerosol therapy, apnea monitoring, and home mechanical ventilation. Specifically reviewed will be developing the care plan, problems and safety measures, discharge planning, physician ordering information, and monitoring.

Oxygen therapy

INDICATIONS

Oxygen therapy is indicated when hypoxemia exists. In 1984, the American College of Chest Physicians and the National

Heart Lung and Blood Institute (ACCP–NHLBI) held a National Conference on Oxygen Therapy. The conference developed institutional guidelines for long-term oxygen therapy, such as would occur in home health care. Although the study did not specifically address the pediatric patient, the guidelines are generally applicable.

The study indicated that long-term oxygen therapy should be considered only for those patients who have been on an optional regimen for 30 days or more.[4] The generally recommended Pa_{O_2} for adult patients was 55 mm Hg or less to document the need for oxygen therapy. Although the exact values were not applied to pediatric patients, if persistent hypoxemia exists after all other treatment modalities have been attempted (*i.e.* bronchial hygiene, treatment of bronchospasm, and cardiac stabilization), oxygen therapy is indicated.

The ACCP–NHLBI conference also referred to oxygen needs when [1] oxygen therapy significantly improved exercise or activity duration and performance or capacity; [2] patients exhibit nocturnal hypoxemia; and [3] patients have evidence of hypoxic organ dysfunction.

Because oxygen therapy can have beneficial effects, such as decreasing the work of breathing, reducing pulmonary vascular resistance, and decreasing stress on the heart, it should be considered when it is indicated. The ACCP–NHLBI suggests that the following four conditions be met before initiating oxygen therapy.

1. An accurate, current diagnosis must have been established.
2. An optional medical regimen prescribed by a physician knowledgeable in chest diseases must be in effect.
3. The patient should have recovered from any exacerbation of his disease and should have been in a stable state for about 1 month. (It is important to note that the need for stability before long-term oxygen therapy is begun does not preclude short-term [1–30 days] oxygen therapy, especially if the latter oxygen therapy allows the patient to be safely discharged from the hospital sooner.)
4. Oxygen therapy has been shown, or can reasonably be predicted, to improve the hypoxemia or evidence of tissue hypoxia and to provide overall clinical benefit.

Oxygen therapy is indicated to maintain an adequate resting and activity blood P_{O_2} level. Patients with chronic pulmonary disease may not have the same oxygen requirements as do those without pulmonary disease. A situation may exist in which the amount of oxygen required to achieve a desired P_{O_2} and the apparatus needed to deliver the oxygen are not always safe and practical in the home setting. Thus, accepting lower but physiologic Pa_{O_2} levels may be an appropriate alternative. Determining the exact oxygen requirements varies from patient to patient, and these requirements should be established through evaluation during the hospital stay. This determination in the hospital is essential. No one formula exists for determining the exact amount and duration of oxygen therapy, but the severity of the patient's disease and resultant secondary abnormalities should determine the longevity of oxygen use.[7]

HOME OXYGEN PRESCRIPTION

Oxygen therapy is indicated in home use to relieve hypoxemia, just as it is in the hospital. Specific information must be provided to obtain the necessary equipment and to ensure that it is covered by medical benefits. First, a prescription is essential to acquire this drug. The prescription should include the following:

Patient's name, age, and address

Diagnosis, including current ABG or saturation, PFTs, and other related laboratory data or complications

Oxygen required in liters per minute

Delivery device (*e.g.*, mask, cannula, tent)

System required (*e.g.*, liquid, concentrator, or compressed gas)

Expected use/dosage (*e.g.*, % concentration or liters/min)

Expected number of days, weeks, months, or years needed (projected use)

Special concerns (*e.g.*, ability to comply with Rx, family support, electrical and telephone service, mental status)

Reimbursement information (*e.g.*, Medicare, Medicaid, and other insurance information)

Obtaining sufficient detailed information and providing the correct therapy with the right oxygen delivery system will help ensure appropriate therapy. It will also minimize time, reduce confusion, prevent changes because of inadequate information, and improve the probability for reimbursement of the therapy provided.

HOME OXYGEN EQUIPMENT AND DELIVERY SYSTEMS

Oxygen therapy for pediatric patients is usually delivered by means of face masks, tracheostomy masks, nasal cannulas, nasal catheters, oxygen hoods, and, occasionally, in conjunction with mist tents. The device that most easily provides the needed oxygen in an appropriate fashion should be chosen. This is rarely a problem because the apparatus used in the hospital usually is appropriate for the home setting. The decision in oxygen therapy has traditionally involved the distinction of the three major systems of delivery: cylinders of compressed gas, liquid oxygen systems, and oxygen concentrators. It should be noted that reimbursement changes and oxygen-saving devices are changing the decision process regarding the selection of oxygen systems. Continual monitoring of changes in technology and reimbursement is essential.

Oxygen Cylinders

The most common oxygen cylinders used in the home are the H(K) and the D and E cylinders. The D or E cylinders are usually used for ambulation outside the home or as a backup for a concentrator or a large cylinder. The H(K) cylinders are for long-term use in the home. If an H or K cylinder is being used at 2 liters per minute (lpm), it will last about 57 hours, or almost 2½ days. The D or E cylinder at 2 lpm will last 3.5 to 5 hours, respectively (see Table 17-1). Because these pressurized cylinders can be hazardous, precautions must be taken. No alarm system exists to indicate low contents in these systems; however, some battery-powered external devices are being developed that attach to the pressure gauge to alarm at preset pressures. Some are concerned about the safety of high-pressure relief valves when these cylinders are used. A humidifier may provide this desired safety feature.

Table 17-1
Oxygen cylinder duration examples

Oxygen cylinder size	Usage/lpm	Longevity
H or K	2 lpm continuously	57 hours/2½ days
D or E	2 lpm continuously	3.5 to 5 hours respectively

Liquid Oxygen

Thermos-type reservoirs containing liquid oxygen stored at $-297°F$ can be used in the home and are advantageous when patient portability is possible. Many of the present units weigh between 60 and 90 pounds and contain 20 to 30 liters of liquid oxygen (1 liquid liter of oxygen = 860 liters of gaseous oxygen). A 30-liter container holds 25,800 liters of gaseous oxygen. At 2 liters/minute, the tank will last about 215 hours, or 8.9 days. Liquid reservoirs and portable systems vent gaseous oxygen into the surrounding air at about 1 lb/day. The evaporation/venting varies with different units based on manufacturer specifications so that one must include this fact when calculating how long a reservoir will last (see Table 17-2). Higher temperatures will increase the venting rate. Because of the venting, neither the portable unit nor the reservoir should be stored in a small space, such as a closet. The liquid systems are valuable for patients who are ambulatory, that is, wheel chair or carriage. Portable units are filled from the main reservoir, and most hold 6½ to 11 pounds. At 2 liters/minute they will last 4 to 8 hours. Lighter and larger volume portable units are becoming available to extend the time of use.

Most liquid systems have a metering device or a weighing scale to indicate the amount of oxygen in the cylinder or in the portable unit; therefore, calculations for usage and refill time can easily be ascertained. One should refer to each manufacturer's instructions on individual units for functioning and safety guidelines.

Oxygen Concentrator

An oxygen concentrator is an electrically powered device that provides a constant source of oxygen from ambient air. A molecular sieve bed in the concentrator separates oxygen from nitrogen, trace gases, and water. Oxygen concentrations vary from 80% to 95% depending on the liter flow, the unit's capability to separate gases, and the cleanliness of the sieve bed and filters. As liter flows to the patient are increased, the delivered oxygen concentration decreases. This decrease is rarely a clinical problem because the concentration varies only a small amount with the prescribed oxygen flow rates.

Occasionally an oxygen concentrator is used as a "bleed-in" for an air-compressor-powered nebulizer to provide low oxygen concentrations during humidity therapy. As the flow is increased, the oxygen concentration may fall below the required level. Turning the flow rates down on both the concentrator and the compressor in an effort to increase F_{IO_2} may not provide adequate total flow rates to meet patient needs. Additionally, the oxygen concentrator does not generate enough pressure to power nebulizers or Venturi masks.

Although oxygen concentrators have somewhat revolutionized the available choices for oxygen therapy, they must be well maintained to function properly. Periodic analysis of the F_{IO_2} delivered and a check on the accuracy of flow rate readings are important. Electrical power failures can occur, and backup oxygen systems (i.e., a cylinder) are necessary.

These concentrators usually are on wheels and are portable from room to room; as a rule, however, they are stationary. Often up to 30 feet of oxygen tubing is provided to

Table 17-2
Liquid oxygen duration example

Liquid container size	Gaseous equivalent	Usage/lpm	Longevity
30 liquid liters	25,800 liters	2 lpm continuously	215 hours or 8.9 days

Evaporation/venting and portable usage need to be considered when determining longevity.

the patient to allow some mobility from room to room; therefore a pressure compensated flowmeter is needed. Also, the ACCP–NHLBI study indicates that there is no subjective or objective evidence that routine humidification of oxygen is necessary at flow rates of 1 to 4 liters/minute when environmental humidity is adequate.[4]

Another oxygen system called an "enricher" uses a polymeric membrane that is permeable to oxygen and water vapor. These polymeric membrane enrichers deliver 30% to 40% oxygen from 1 to 10 liters/minute. These enrichers often are adjusted by the manufacturer to deliver flow rates three times the setting in an effort to equal oxygen delivery by a system that provides 100% oxygen. Some patients have exhibited "air hunger" when treated with lower flows at 100% after becoming accustomed to the higher flows from membrane enrichers.

The following should be considered when making decisions about the best choice of the oxygen device for a particular patient and environment: cost, geography, mobility of patient, safety, travel requirements, and the patient's clinical needs. If, for example, a patient lives a long distance from the delivery site, it might be more cost effective to provide a concentrator even though cylinders would technically meet the patient's needs. A liquid system or cylinders may be considered in an area where considerable electrical power failures make a concentrator unsafe. Also, patients without electricity or with poor wiring might require liquid or cylinders instead of a concentrator.

Costs to the patient will vary from state to state and from vendor to vendor. From a cost-effective standpoint, the quantity of oxygen used has been the determining factor in choosing a system. For example, cylinders are the least expensive when their usage rates are low. For very high usage rates (*i.e.*, greater than 6 liters/minute), they can be the most expensive oxygen source.

Concentrators are most cost-effective in mid-to-high usage rates because the cost of a concentrator remains the same regardless of use. But if a patient needs mobility, the liquid system is more appropriate. Liquid system costs, however, vary with usage. Thus for a patient who is only occasionally mobile, as

during a trip to the doctor's office, the concentrator and a backup E cylinder may be the most economical form of therapy. Oxygen concentrators also increase electrical use and, therefore, cost to the patient. The average concentrator will have a power consumption ranging from 265 to 420 watts, and the cost of electricity may be $30/month or more, which is not reimbursable. Obviously, each case must be evaluated to meet the patient's needs.

Because cost is an increasing concern, additional methods are being evaluated to provide less expensive oxygen therapy. A recently available nasal cannula, for example, has a reservoir that holds about 18 ml of oxygen. When the patient inspires, he receives a "bolus" of oxygen when the flap valves open. During exhalation, these flaps (or valves) close and the reservoir fills. In theory, the oxygen liter flow requirements are less because less oxygen is wasted. Liquid oxygen systems are now available that have a demand valve attached to the unit that opens only on inspiration. Again oxygen use is minimized. These items are relatively new, but great savings are being realized.

Another approach to conserving oxygen is the use of transtracheal oxygen. Here, oxygen is delivered by means of a Teflon catheter placed percutaneously into the trachea between the second and third tracheal rings. This system was devised by Henry Heimlich in an effort to reduce oxygen use from 2 to 4 liters/minute to ¼ to 1½ liters/minute, and studies thus far have been positive. Many of these devices are being used on adults, but their success may provide new developments and cost savings for pediatric patients as well.

Efforts to halt spiraling health care costs have impacted the reimbursement for home oxygen therapy. In most parts of the United States, Medicare now reimburses for oxygen therapy by cubic foot usage per month. This change is known as the PATROL initiative and was instituted to provide the patient with the lowest cost alternative for home oxygen therapy. New regulations have been proposed that call for a monthly rental for the oxygen-saving devices or for a capitation amount for oxygen therapy. As technology and reimbursement change, those who refer to home health care agencies, as well as to home care providers, will need to evaluate options on the basis of cost as well as the adequacy of meeting consumption and mobility needs on an individual, case-by-case basis.

In addition to cost considerations, patients and families may want to resume activities that might include travel over several days. This can be safely accomplished with detailed planning. The following are suggested tips for persons traveling with oxygen:

1. Be sure to have available the written prescription for oxygen from your physician.

2. Identify the location of oxygen suppliers and their hours of service.
3. Calculate how much oxygen will be needed each day.
4. Plan travel around oxygen refill stops.
5. Be aware of and avoid the possible hazards of oxygen use.

The technology in this area continues to improve. Some manufacturers are developing lightweight, portable, battery-packed oxygen concentrators. These innovations will continue to make home administration of oxygen to patients easier, cheaper, and better.

HOME ASSESSMENT

Home assessment of the safe use of oxygen is performed by many respiratory therapy home care companies. For most patients on oxygen therapy, however, this assessment is made only when equipment is delivered to the home and the ordering physician is notified that the environment is unsafe. Before this type of notification occurs, all available options should be considered. Although the home environment is often not as clean and safe as that in the hospital, it is usually acceptable.

The home assessment often consists of the following:

1. Electrical checks (for concentrators) to note sufficient numbers of safe outlets, as three-prong grounded outlets are recommended. Also, 15 amp circuit breakers are preferred over fuses. The electrical outlet used by the oxygen concentrator should not have any other heavy-current-utilizing devices on the same breaker (*e.g.*, air conditioners, heaters, stoves). One should ask the family about the occurrence and frequency of power outages.

2. A quick observation of the support structure of the home. Many children have bedrooms on the second story, and adding oxygen cylinders, concentrators, or liquid systems may be too heavy for the floor to support. Heaters and other potential fire hazards should be checked and removed. General cleanliness should be noted and the family encouraged to remove sources of flammable materials.

An experienced individual can assess a home for oxygen therapy in minutes. This review should be documented and necessary changes noted. Some families may want to have some additional electrical work performed, such as adding a dedicated electrical circuit to the patient's room. Although most third-party payers will not cover this renovation, it is sometimes allowable as a tax-deductible expense because the medical bill usually exceeds the IRS minimal medical requirements. The family should be encouraged to contact the local IRS to be sure that their tax deductions are acceptable. The therapist or the durable medical equipment (DME) technician can and should make recommendations concerning rearrangement of household items to create ease and safety of treatment. One must be helpful, creative, and supportive of the family during these difficult times.

MONITORING

A major difference between monitoring the patient at home and in the hospital is that the patient is seen much less frequently by the health care provider; therefore, good clinical assessment skills, thorough progress notes, and adequate patient and family instructions are important. Some of these chronically ill children normally look quite sick, and understanding this should prevent unnecessary calls to the physician, especially when a new health care provider makes a home visit.

Communication between care providers is essential. The therapist may be the only source of information for the physician and may be asked questions related to other medications or treatment by the family. Appropriate transmission of these inquiries to the physician is necessary. Telephone communication with the patients and their families can make the transition to the home favorable and minimize problems.

From a clinical standpoint, monitoring of oxygen can be performed on pediatric patients using clinical assessment, transcutaneous monitoring, arterial blood gas determinations, or noninvasive oxygen saturation measurement by means of an ear/pulse oximeter. Some of these tests are rarely needed, but arrangements should be made in the event that they are indicated. The noninvasive devices such as transcutaneous monitoring and oximetry are becoming easier to use, lighter, more accurate, and less expensive. Oxygen saturation monitoring is now a popular monitoring technique and enables superior monitoring capabilities of arterial oxygen saturation. Reimbursement systems are leaning toward periodic documentation of oxygen needs. Therefore, the trend for monitoring the clinical use of oxygen therapy in the home will also increase.

PROBLEMS AND SAFETY

Problem and safety concerns often arise in the home health care setting. Listed below are some of these potential concerns that one might be faced with while treating a pediatric patient receiving oxygen:

> Overuse of the oxygen, (*i.e.*, not following the prescribed dose).
> Running out of oxygen (coordinating oxygen deliveries).
> Electrical failure with oxygen concentrators.
> Smoking near the oxygen and resultant fire.
> Travel problems with portable oxygen systems.
> Third-party reimbursement.
> Family not coping with the home situation.
> Increased electrical costs.
> The need for hospital readmission.
> Transferring of oxygen and related hazards.

Prudent planning, detailed education, and communication with follow-up can minimize these problems and make the environment safer. If several of these problems are present in the home environment, it may be advisable not to send the child home. Notification of these problems and corrective action directed by the physician are appropriate. Often the physician's support can alleviate concerns and help the family create a more efficient environment. Documentation in the home care chart of the physician's suggestions is important protection against malpractice.

PHYSICIAN ORDERS AND COMMUNICATION

As mentioned earlier, adequate therapy and equipment ordering information are important in patient care, liability, saving time, and reimbursement. Written progress notes, changes in physician's orders, and telephone communication are also important. Often the respiratory therapist is the only health care provider who sees the patient. In this setting, the physician has to rely heavily on the therapist's assessment for continuation or change of the care plan. Third-party reimbursement and liability again can be affected by this documentation. Physicians are in a difficult position because they are the case manager of a patient whom they rarely see, and they may also have several patients in this situation. The physician, therefore, has increased liability, is busier, and is paid less. Because the physician will be expecting a great deal from the respiratory therapist, communication should be accurate and concise. The exact amount of communication depends on the patient's needs and conditions, as well as third-party reimburser's requirements. These details should be worked out with the physician.

In summary, oxygen therapy to pediatric patients is safe and effective in the proper situations as described above. More patients who are stable but require oxygen therapy will be going home, and the current technology and the social/psychological assistance make this treatment more available and less expensive. A well-organized, caring clinical therapist can become the catalyst for successful home oxygen therapy for the pediatric patient.

Aerosol and humidity therapy

The administration and the equipment used for aerosol therapy in the home generally are similar to those used in the hospital setting. As in other home health care modalities, documentation, appropriate prescription information, and monitoring are very important components of this therapy.

Aerosol therapy uses a nebulizer to generate a mist or suspension of medication and can be classified into three components: intermittent bland aerosol therapy, continuous bland aerosol therapy, and intermittent medication (pharmacologic) aerosol therapy.

Intermittent bland aerosol therapy nebulizes sterile water or a saline solution that is delivered to the respiratory tract to liquify secretions, promote and induce a productive cough, and decrease laryngeal edema. Continuous bland aerosol has similar functions and is also used to reduce humidity deficit during long-term oxygen therapy.

Intermittent medication aerosol therapy involves nebulizing pharmacologic agents to reduce or reverse bronchoconstriction, to reduce laryngeal and airway edema, to control and prevent bronchial asthma symptoms and attacks, to loosen viscid or purulent secretions, and occasionally to deposit antibiotics in the airways.

For specific pharmacologic agents, actions, dosages, indications, and hazards, see Table 17-3.

The following represents a complete physician's order for bland aerosol therapy:

Type of therapy—intermittent or continuous therapy.
Frequency and duration of intermittent treatments.
Solution to be nebulized.
Cool or heated mist.
Type of aerosol generator to be used.
Device or appliance to deliver aerosol to patient.
Related monitoring.
Oxygen percentage if appropriate.

An intermittent medication aerosol order should include the following data:

Type and amount of medication to be used.
Frequency of use.
Device or appliance to be used.
Duration of treatments.
Whether powered by oxygen or air.
Related monitoring.

Again, the orders need to be specific, particularly in terms of the equipment, as this will assist third-party reimbursement. The hospital respiratory therapy department and the home health agency can be very helpful to the physician in this area. Figure 17-1 is an example of a patient-admitting form that is used as a guide for gathering necessary information.

METHODS AND DELIVERY SYSTEMS

Intermittent and continuous bland aerosol therapy uses large-bore tubing attached to an aerosol generator. The patient de-

Table 17-3
Drugs for aerosol therapy

Generic name	Trade name	Dosage	Indications	Common side-effects/hazards
Bronchodilators				
Isoetharine	Bronkosol (solution)	¼ to ½ ml in 3 ml saline q4h	Relieve bronchospasm in asthma, emphysema, chronic bronchitis	Tachycardia, palpitations, tremor, headache, BP changes
	Bronkometer (metered dose)	56 mg/delivery Adults: 2 to 3 inhalations	Relieve bronchospasm in asthma, emphysema, chronic bronchitis	Tachycardia, palpitations, tremor, headache, BP changes
Isoproterenol	Isuprel (solution 1:200 or 1:100)	1:200 strength 0.5 ml in 3 ml saline (adults); 0.25 ml in 3 ml saline (children)	Relieve bronchospasm in asthma, emphysema, chronic bronchitis	Tachycardia, nervousness, palpitations
	Isuprel Mistometer (metered dose) Medihaler-ISO	Adults and children: 125 µg/delivery 2 to 3 inhalations up to 5 times daily	Relieve bronchospasm in asthma, emphysema, chronic bronchitis	Tachycardia, nervousness, palpitations
Metaproterenol	Alupent (solution) Metaprel (metered dose)	Not recommended for children under 12 Adult dose 0.65 mg/delivery 2 to 3 inhalations q4h. No more than 12 inhalations in 24 hours.	Relieves bronchospasm	Tachycardia, hypertension, palpitations
	Alupent (solution)	Not recommended for children under 12 0.3 ml in 3 ml saline q4 to 6h	Relieves bronchospasm	Tachycardia, hypertension, palpitations
Bronchodilator/vasoconstrictor				
Racemic epinephrine	Micronephrine (solution)	0.2 to 0.4 ml in 3 to 5 ml sterile H_2O	Croup—postextubation	Tachycardia, nervousness
	Vaponefrin (solution)	0.5 ml in 3.5 sterile H_2O	COPD—reduction in airway edema Decrease in bronchospasm	
Vasoconstrictor				
Phenylephrine	Neo-synephrine (solution)	0.2 ml in 4 ml to 0.5 ml in 4 ml	Local vasoconstriction Shrinkage of bronchial mucosa	Local irritation

Table 17-3
(continued)

Generic name	Trade name	Dosage	Indications	Common side-effects/hazards
(continued)				
Steroids				
Beclometha-sone dipro-pionate	Vanceril (me-tered dose)	Children (6–12) 1 to 2 inhalations 3 to 4 daily; max, 10 inhal/day Adults 2 to 3 in-halations 3 to 4 daily; max, 10/day	Control of bronchial asthma symptoms	Adrenal insufficiency Local mouth infection with *Candida albicans, Aspergillus niger* Throat irritation
Dexametha-sone phosphate	Respihaler (Decadron) (Metered dose)	Adults 3 inhala-tions 3 to 4 daily; max, 12 inhal/day Children 2 inhala-tions, 3 to 4 daily; max, 8 inhal/day	Control of bronchial asthma symptoms	Adrenal insufficiency Throat irritation
Mucolytics				
Acetylcysteine	Mucomyst (so-lution 10% or 20%)	Aerosol Adults and chil-dren—3 to 5 ml of 20% or 6 to 10 ml of 10% 3 to 4 times a day Instillation 1 to 2 ml of 10% to 20% directly into trachea Also comes as 10% acetyl-cysteine and 0.05% isopro-terenol	Thick, viscid inspis-sated mucus Use to decrease chance of bronchospasm	Nausea Rhinorrhea Bronchospasm (espe-cially in asthmatics)
Antibiotics				
Kanamycin	Kantrex	250 mg with 3 ml N/S 2 to 4 times/day	Gram-negative bacteria	Bronchospasm Hypersensitivity
Neomycin		50 to 400 mg with saline 2 to 4 times/day	Gram-negative bacteria	Bronchospasm Hypersensitivity
Streptomycin		Children 4 to 10 40 mg/kg q6h Adults 2 to 4 g/day	Gram-negative bacteria	Bronchospasm Hypersensitivity

(continued)

Table 17-3
(continued)

Generic name	Trade name	Dosage	Indications	Common side-effects/hazards
Miscellaneous				
Cromolyn sodium	Arane Intal	One capsule 3 to 4/day	Prevention of asthma attacks	Local irritation Pneumonitis Bronchospasm
Ethyl alcohol	Ethanol	20% to 50%	Pulmonary edema	Bronchospasm Irritation of lung tissue
Pancreatic dornase	Dornavac	100,000 units in saline 2 to 3 times/day	Purulent secretions	Bronchospasm

(Blodgett D: Manual of Pediatric Respiratory Care Procedures. Philadelphia, JB Lippincott, 1982)

livery devices include aerosol face mask, tracheostomy mask, face tent, or t-tube (Briggs adaptor). Heated aerosol systems are usually used for tracheostomy patients.

Intermittent medication aerosol devices generate aerosol by means of a medication nebulizer powered by air or oxygen and deliver the mist through aerosol face masks, tracheostomy masks, t-tubes, or mouthpieces.

The aerosol devices used in the hospital are usually the same as those used in the home. The compressors that power them are simple and easy to use and maintain if specific manufacturer instructions are followed.

MONITORING

Pediatric monitoring is important because clinical conditions can change rapidly. As mentioned above, parents may become the primary care providers. They must be properly instructed in the delivery of treatments and the safe monitoring of both the patient and the equipment.

Monitoring oxygen with aerosol patients is mentioned above. This includes examining the safety of the system and the actual clinical response to therapy. Clinical monitoring includes clinical assessment, ascertaining arterial blood gas values, transcutaneous oxygen monitoring, and ear/pulse ox-

Financial class _____

Call taken by: _____ Date/time _____

Caller name/title: _____ Caller phone: _____

Patient name: _____ Phone: _____

Address: _____ County: _____

City/state: _____ DOB/age: _____

Dx: _____

Hospital: _____ Physician: _____

Discharge date: _____

Oxygen
_____ concentrator, _____ liquid & stroller
_____ liquid, _____ cylinder- _____ size
_____ liters per minute, _____ hours/day
_____ nasal cannula, _____ Venti-mask,
_____ percentage O_2, _____ other
_____ therapeutic objective(s)

Chest physiotherapy
what lobes
frequency _____ /day
precautions (SOB, osteoporosis, clotting
time)

Medication nebulizer (aerosol)
medications
frequency of treatments _____ /day
therapeutic objective(s)

Suction equipment
_____ size of catheters
_____ frequency
pressure _____ cm/H_2O
_____ O_2 cylinder must accompany suction

IPPB
medications
frequency _____ /day
pressure _____ cm/H_2O
therapeutic objective(s)

Bland aerosol (high volume nebulizer)
_____ frequency
_____ mode-mask
_____ mouthpiece
_____ trach collar
_____ heated, _____ cool
_____ NaCl, _____ sterile H_2O

Estimate of need: _____ Months

SSN/Medicare/Medicaid # _____

Name of insured _____

Employer _____

Insurance co. _____

Is patient covered?   Yes _____   No _____

Billing address:

_____

_____

_____

Policy no. _____

SSN of insured _____

Fig. 17-1. Patient referral information/insurance worksheet.

imetry when indicated and ordered by the physician. Equipment monitoring might include the monitoring of temperatures, as with heated nebulizers.

The clinical effects of the aerosol are monitored in several ways. The viscosity of secretions is one sign of adequate treatment. Also, sputum should be evaluated in terms of volume, consistency, color, and odor. Because overhydration is a concern with continuous humidity therapy, weighing the child and observing for peripheral edema are two procedures helpful in allaying these concerns. One should be familiar with volume output of nebulizers so that adjustments can be made if patient needs are not met or are exceeded. Ausculation and percussion are important assessment functions of the health care provider during visits. One should note wheezing and findings consistent with fluid buildup, consolidation, or atelectasis. In addition, the pulse rate should be documented during a medication nebulizer treatment. Obviously some pediatric patients will have tracheostomies, and as the child grows the tracheostomy tube may become too small and need replacement. Continual evaluation of tube size and airway patency is essential.

PROBLEMS AND SAFETY

By taking proper steps to provide education and monitoring, many potential problems can be minimized. Issues that the hospital and the home respiratory care providers should be aware of to effect a smooth, safe transition to the home include the following:

Fire hazards with oxygen used with an aerosol. Avoid smoking and heaters (especially kerosene).

Compressors can overheat. Clean filters and check for adequate ventilation.

Overmedication—improper family instruction.

Infection—poor cleaning of equipment, not changing equipment as ordered, poor suctioning technique. Instruct to dispose of water each time nebulizer is filled and not to drain hoses back into nebulizer).

Increased cost of electricity, particularly with continuously running compressors.

Overheating of nebulizer heaters.

Noise of compressor.

Heat of compressor.

Underhydration—faulty nebulizer jet, failure to fill neb-
ulizer, particularly at night.
Overhydration.
Overmobilization of secretions.
Decrease in air flow or FI_{O_2} when water fills up tubing.
Child growing and requiring larger tracheostomy tube.
Children's bed clothing recommended to be 100% cotton
because of combustion in presence of oxygen.

The family is often the primary care provider and, therefore, has a great deal of responsibility. Proper planning and
education are important for the patient's comfort, care, and
for everyone's safety.

Apnea monitoring

Apnea is a pause in breathing common among infants, children, and adults. When it is present for longer than 20 seconds,
it is considered abnormal and seems to occur primarily in infants younger than 1 year of age. In the newborn, it is thought
to be a symptom of delayed maturation of the part of the brain
that controls breathing. A prolonged apneic episode may be
accompanied by bradycardia and eventually death.[6]

Weinstein and Steinschneider[9] have classified major types
of infantile apneas as prolonged sleep apnea, feeding-induced
apnea, gastroesophageal reflux-induced apnea, and seizure-
associated apnea. Appropriate diagnostic tests are indicated
to differentiate these types of apnea.

Guilleminault[5] categorized apnea as central, obstructive,
and mixed. Central or diaphragmatic apnea existed when no
thoracic or abdominal impedance was recorded and, simultaneously, no respirations were recorded by nasal thermistor.
Obstructive apnea was noted when impedance strain gauges
exhibited continuous deflections of chest movement but no
air exchange was recorded by nasal thermistor. Progressive
increases of pressure with diaphragmatic movements occurred
during obstructive apnea. Mixed apnea was defined when a
central apnea was followed by an upper airway apnea during
one cessation of air exchange. The type of apnea should be
accurately determined to rule out underlying disease that may
be the cause of prolonged infant apnea.

Infants exhibiting apnea may be at risk for developing sudden infant death syndrome (SIDS). Although a great deal has been learned about SIDS over the past few years, much still remains a mystery. In 1971, 10,000 children in the United States died of SIDS. On April 23, 1974, the government passed legislation providing funds for the study of SIDS and aiding the bereaved families. SIDS is by far the leading cause of death of infants between 1 month and 1 year of age, with an estimated incidence of 2 to 3:1000. A relationship exists between SIDS and apnea although they are not synonymous terms, and thus home apnea monitoring has gained popularity.

The psychological and emotional impact on the family is profound.

DISCHARGE PLANNING FOR INFANT APNEA

Preparation of the family before discharge is one of the most important aspects of the entire process of home infant apnea monitoring. The proper discharge planning activities not only will review all points of discharge preparation, but also may raise other legitimate concerns that dictate the need to extend the in-hospital teaching segment. Listed below are major areas that should be part of the discharge planning process:

Psychosocial assessment (*e.g.,* does the family understand, and can they cope with the responsibility?).

Review of the costs and reimbursement issues.

Parent teaching, to include definition of apnea, feeding precautions, community resources, psychosocial needs/resources, assessment skills to identify life-threatening situations, infant CPR, apnea monitoring options.

Preparation of the home and a child's room.

Community support such as parent groups, the local physician, baby sitters, public health nurses, social services.

Home electrical assessment.

Assurance of a working telephone.

Identification of language problem with parents or babysitters.

Often equipment-related problems are not due to equipment malfunction or faulty equipment but to the parents' lack of understanding of the equipment. As one can easily see, a great deal of education is required. In addition to instruction and demonstration to the parent, written instructions should be provided.

HOME SUPPORT FOR THE FAMILY

At home, a follow-up support team helps the family cope with the situation in general and deal with specific problems that arise. A typical full-service program includes the following elements:

Daily telephone calls the first week.

Weekly telephone calls after the first week; additional social services and psychology calls as needed.

Twenty-four-hour call.

Visit to home by home health care company providing monitoring equipment 1 week after initial setup.

Monthly evaluation at pediatric outpatient clinic.

Monthly pneumogram. (A pneumogram is usually a 12-hour recording of the infant's respiratory pattern and heart rate.)

Local psychosocial support systems identified in the national SIDS group, infant apnea support groups, local social service agency, community health nursing service.

Notification of police, local rescue service, telephone company, and power company of the infant apnea monitor.

Encouragement of parents to treat baby as normally as possible, hold baby, and so forth.

Most mothers take time to do household chores while the baby is asleep. These activities can be arranged to ensure that the monitor alarm can be heard within 10 seconds. Before discharge, some hospitals actually simulate the home environment in a private room for 1 or 2 days. This allows the parent(s) to become more comfortable with the monitor and have immediate help if necessary. Literature containing stories of families who have monitored a child at home also helps to build parents' confidence and can be made available at this time. Health professionals provide that first step of family preparation for home apnea monitoring. This is a challenging task that can be accomplished with detailed planning, appropriate knowledge, proper teaching, and caring.

Unfortunately, despite proper discharge planning and home support, the infant may die. The home health care provider is often the first to know and to make contact with the family after a SIDS death. This is obviously a critical time, and sensitivity can make a significant difference for the family. Some parents will be hysterical; others will be calm or in a state of shock. Most parents are young and have not dealt with the death of a child. A misinformed health professional may aggravate the situation rather than alleviate guilt and other emotional problems.

CRITERIA FOR DISCONTINUATION OF MONITORING

Most infant monitoring is discontinued when the following criteria exist:

> The infant is free of events requiring vigorous stimulation or resuscitation for at least 3 months, or 2 months if no critical problems have existed since the presenting episode.
>
> No monitor alarm for at least 2 months on an apnea setting of 20 seconds or a heart rate below 60 beats/minute.
>
> During the asymptomatic period, the infant must have experienced the stress of nasopharyngitis or DPT immunization without a recurrence of symptoms.
>
> A normal pneumogram exists indicating no persistent cardiorespiratory abnormalities.

To discontinue home apnea monitoring, a physician's order and a discussion with the parents are needed. Social services' support is helpful for those who have difficulty with discontinuance. Usually, 1-month and 6-month telephone follow-up calls are appropriate.

In summary, home apnea monitoring requires a knowledgeable, dedicated, and sensitive person to provide the needed services. Obviously, apnea monitoring is not a cure for any situation or disease but a means of helping the baby through an at-risk point of development. To be part of this caring team, one must realize that a great deal of specific knowledge is necessary, such as risk factors related to medications and respiratory fatigue. This requires that one keep abreast of current literature, techniques, and technology. With the many new apnea monitors becoming available, some people believe that monitor manufacturing for infants should be regulated more stringently to assure proper clinical testing. At present, the FDA places infant monitors in the Class II category; some would prefer that it be elevated to Class III, as drugs are regulated at this classification. Concern also exists in two other areas: First, some infants are being monitored without adequate evaluation of need; and second, inadequate family education may exist (families may believe that the monitor can prevent SIDS).

Mechanical ventilation

Many major clinical studies have recently been published that describe the potential benefits of home mechanical ventilation. The benefits described range from improving quality of life for the patient and family to cost savings for the patient, the hospital, and the insurer. The Medicare/Medicaid insolvency issue is a driving force behind sending patients home on ventilatory support. Most agree that when a patient meets the appropriate discharge criteria, the option of going home should be available. One major concern is that the potential profits to be made by home care companies might cause some to accept patients without having the resources to render the needed services safely. It is much safer to wait or decide against home ventilation than to provide services inadequately and have an avoidable emergency or readmission occur. On the other hand, some home care companies have developed very comprehensive and thorough programs to handle complex patient problems in the home. It should be mentioned that health care providers effective in the hospital setting may not be as efficient in the home.

A look at patients on mechanical ventilator support at home in the past shows that most of these patients were older than 50 years of age and had polio or spinal cord injury. An increasing number of pediatric patients, however, are going home, for two major reasons: One, more experience in the process of home ventilator care now exists, making the process easier and safer; and two, the technology of neonatal respiratory care has improved dramatically over the past 2 decades. Infants who previously would not have lived are now surviving. The Surgeon General's conference on ventilator-dependent patients concluded that "ventilator dependence" is not a diagnosis but rather a condition. This new attitude is creating hope for these complex situations.

PATIENT SELECTION/DISCHARGE CRITERIA

Success with home ventilation depends critically on the proper selection of the patient. The following criteria should be considered to identify candidates for home ventilation:

1. *Medical stability.* The patient should not have acute cardiopulmonary dysfunction, significant oxygen disorders, or other major system problems. This patient should have had no major therapeutic or diagnostic intervention during the month preceding ventilation. Formerly, patients could go home on a ventilator if they had not been weaned from oxygen. Each patient's situation must be dealt with individually; for example, infants 6 months old have been sent home on ventilators requiring 60% oxygen with 5 cm H_2O PEEP. One particular patient had severe bronchopulmonary dysplasia (BPD). This infant had been on the ventilator almost since birth and was relatively stable. The pediatric pulmonologist provided a realistic but poor prognosis for this infant. The mother wanted to take her child home because she was tired of spending the night in the hospital. After extensive discussions and evaluations by both the hospital personnel and a comprehensive home health care team, planning began for discharging the infant, which included 24-hour pediatric nursing at home and respiratory therapy visits at home. This was a very unusual situation but shows the need for individualization of selection criteria.

2. *Family evaluation.* The family must genuinely want their child at home. The child's illness and therapy will demand most of their time, energy, and resources; thus they must try to balance these duties with some semblance of nor-

malcy. The sick child cannot dominate their entire existence. The family must also show motivation and be capable of gaining the skills and knowledge necessary to care for their child. Support systems such as an extended family, the clergy, and friends are important. In addition, the financial effects should not overburden the family.

3. *Selection of home health care company.* One should be selected that has proper equipment and a 24-hour call by qualified and knowledgeable personnel. In addition, they should [1] provide personnel, equipment, and supplies within a reasonable geographic location; [2] have experience in home ventilator care; [3] supply all needs efficiently and economically; and [4] be versed in reimbursement to assist in financial matters.

These selection criteria help determine whether a patient is a reasonable risk for home ventilation. At this point the important details of home assessment and discharge planning can begin.

DISCHARGE PLANNING FOR MECHANICAL VENTILATION PATIENTS

Discharge planning or discharge management is the process of preparing the patient, the family, and the home for the patient's transport and care at home. A review of these important components to discharge planning follows:

1. *Care plan.* The first step is to develop a clinical plan covering all areas of patient care. A common approach is to detail the patient's needs and then determine the personnel, equipment, and supplies required for adequate and safe treatment. This is developed by the hospital and home health care teams and submitted to the attending physician for approval.

2. *Reimbursement.* The care plan indicates the necessary equipment, supplies, medications, and professional care providers. Before a patient goes home, payment for the services must be considered or arranged. If the care plan is incomplete, it will be difficult, if not impossible, to secure more funds once a patient is home. Detailed planning is important because many supply items not individually charged in the hospital

can easily be missed. Again, the increase in costs incurred in electrical use should be noted because it is not reimbursable. The family must have a clear picture of the financial burden before discharge. Even though the patient meets the clinical and home assessment criteria, his home care may not be affordable.

3. *Parent teaching.* Teaching the parents, who will become the primary care providers, is a process that will take several days, even weeks. The parents probably will have become familiar with much of the care while the child is still in the hospital. One must now define the roles and schedule of the tasks at hand. Developing a problem review list with goals is often a good approach. This is accomplished by the hospital and the home care company. The following are examples of goals:

> Maintain adequate respiratory status
> Prevent respiratory infection
> Increase the child's weight
> Increase muscle strength
> Work on cognitive and motor development skills
> Administer medications safely
> Relieve parent from duty with a qualified sitter (private time for parents)

Specific teaching might include the following concepts:

> Disease process related to the patient's diagnosis
> Tracheostomy care
> Changing tracheostomy tube
> Suctioning
> Infant CPR
> Medication delivery and monitoring
> Cardiac monitoring
> Postural drainage and chest percussion
> Medication nebulizer therapy
> Mechanical ventilator operation, circuit change, troubleshooting, alarms, and humidifier functions (routine checks)
> Equipment cleaning
> Nutrition
> Physical therapy/range of motion exercises

Oral care
Emergency care

A great deal of knowledge must be gained by the family. Demonstrations by hospital personnel and by parents are important, and handouts of educational materials are helpful. It is important to be flexible, because some days will be more productive than others. Evaluation of the parents' level of education and coping skills is also important.

4. *Home assessment.* The home assessment is a very important aspect of discharge planning and could in itself prevent discharge. The home must be thoroughly inspected for safety. The first step is to work with the family to determine which room in the house will be the safest and most efficient for all the equipment needed. Oxygen will probably be part of the equipment, and related safety measures must be exhausted. Because several pieces of heavy equipment may be used, the child's bedroom on the second floor may not have the necessary structural support. From an electrical standpoint, the room will require several three-pronged (grounded) outlets. These outlets must be checked for general safety, current leakage, and grounding. A circuit breaker is preferred over fuses, and specific identification of the circuits is essential. Because a great deal of equipment will be used, the total wattage consumption needs to be calculated to be sure the present system is sufficient. Remember, this may include an air conditioner, clocks, radios, and lights on that circuit as well. Additional electrical work may be required and often is not covered by insurance. It is suggested that the parents contact the IRS to see whether these improvements are tax deductible.

5. *Preparation of the home.* Preparation includes notification of police, ambulance service, lifeline, apartment management, and electric, gas, and telephone companies that life support systems are in place and that priority status for services should be granted. This notification should be made by telephone and in writing and double checked by the home care company. Developing adequate storage space for supplies can be worked out with the parents. Both delivering and testing all the ordered equipment before discharge are essential.

6. *Transportation home.* The proper equipment, personnel, and coordination of care are imperative. This is an anxious

time for the family, and every effort should be made for the move to be timely and efficient.

The discharge planning process is important to create a smooth transition to home and a mood conducive to a successful home stay. This, in turn, builds confidence for the family and their ability to handle the situation adequately. It is also necessary for the family to decide which medical institution they will use in an emergency situation. Will the discharging hospital and the reimburser agree to readmit the patient if home ventilator care is no longer possible or unsuccessful? Checking these details can prevent many potential problems.

METHODS AND EQUIPMENT

Home ventilation usually requires many pieces of equipment. Here is a list of some of the equipment and supplies often used:

Ventilator with backup
Air compressor
Oxygen system with backup
Oxygen analyzer
Suction machine with backup
Resuscitation bag
Hydrogen peroxide
Thermometer
Nebulizers
Percussor
Oxygen and aerosol tubing
Gloves
Syringes
Nebulizer heater
Incontinence pads
Blood gas kits
Tape
Scale

Ventilator circuits and humidifiers
Tracheostomy tube taped on bed
Suction catheters and tubing
Sterile water
Normal saline
Medication nebulizer
Water-soluble lubricant
Tracheostomy dressing and supplies
Hospital crib/bed
Medications
External ventilator battery
Remote battery cable
Spirometer
Apnea monitor
Oxygen bleed-in adapters

Resuscitation bag   Disinfectant solution
                                        and containers
                                     Sphygmomanometer
                                     Ventilator filters

Simple written descriptions of assembly, function, and cleaning are important references for the family. Also, cleaning of filters, circuits, and humidifiers and maintenance of the equipment should be of prime concern. Two additional points should be considered: first, as previously mentioned, the cost of electricity will increase, and this is usually not reimbursable; and second, calculation of the oxygen use for many pneumatic ventilators requires not only the calculation of oxygen required to meet the flow rates and FI_{O_2} needs, but also the needs to operate the machine and the PEEP valves. This may exceed 10 liters/minute; therefore the oxygen system requirements and costs will vary according to the specific setup.

MONITORING

Monitoring of patients on mechanical ventilatory support in the home depends on the needs of the patient and the capabilities of the family/care providers. Clinical monitoring of the patient and the equipment is essential.

In terms of the patient, clinical monitoring performed by the home care company and primary care providers should include at least the following signs and symptoms:

1. Physical signs such as color, mental alertness, secretions, and respiratory patterns should be noted.
2. The weight of the child can give information relative to fluid balance and nutrition.
3. Vital signs such as heart rate, blood pressure, and respiratory rate must be checked.
4. Oxygenation may be checked periodically with an oxygen saturation monitor, transcutaneous monitor, or arterial blood gas determinations.
5. Chest excursion/ventilation is an observation taught to the family. The health care providers should assess the chest during visits.

Detailed review of this clinical monitoring is taught to the family.

Equipment monitoring performed by the home care company and the primary care providers includes the following points:

1. Leaks in circuit should be checked after emptying the tubing.
2. Overall function of the ventilator and accessory alarms must be checked to see that they are functioning properly.
3. Backup systems (as in the ventilator and suction systems) should function properly and be at the same settings as the primary system. The backup oxygen should also be checked.
4. Oxygen concentration with an oxygen analyzer can be checked on a predetermined basis.
5. Review of the cleaning/disinfection procedure is important.

These general areas must be methodically reviewed with the parents. Immediate, 24-hour/day service must be available from qualified professionals should an emergency arise. The home health care companies should also provide proper equipment maintenance and have backup equipment available.

It is important to remember that infants change significantly during the first year of life. The average infant in the first 12 months of life, for example, has a fourfold lung volume increase, and the number of alveoli increases by 500%.[2] When these changes occur, the equipment and supplies may require adjustment to meet new needs. As development occurs in older babies and children, similar changes must be made in the equipment and care plan.

Proper selection criteria, planned family education, and proper monitoring can provide high probability for success in home ventilation. This technique can achieve the goals once thought to be impractical to provide a safe, cost-effective alternative to hospitalization to the stabilized patient needing mechanical ventilation. The U.S. Surgeon General's interest and commitment, along with that of health care professionals, will continue to create new advances in this area of home care.

Summary

The significant advances in pediatric and neonatal home health care have resulted in favorable outcomes. The home environment creates a quality of life for the infant and the family that is lost when hospitalization occurs, and normal development of the child seems more likely in this setting. In many situations the cost savings are significant and sometimes extend the number of years of an insurance policy coverage.

With all of these significant advantages, one must not forget that this is far from an easy process. The family may not be willing or capable of handling the situation. To assure the chances of success, a methodical approach, hard work, appropriate knowledge, and caring are essential.

This chapter has touched on many issues. The professional education of care providers on changes in the technology and approach to alternative care sites is essential to meet the needs and achieve an improved life for these pediatric patients. An increased awareness of this approach, emphasizing the psychological aspects of the family and child, is needed. Technology is improving and expanding to assist these children. The funding issue is improving but is often still inadequate. Family involvement and follow-up must be part of the care. Effective discharge assessment and planning should include an assessment of mental/psychosocial status, medical needs, technological support, financial status, and logistics planning. Evaluation and selection of home care providers are important aspects. Those families who are incapable or unwilling to provide care in their home may be presented with other alternative discharge sites. The liability aspect of home care should be taken into account even though little litigation has occurred to date. Detailed and adequate discharge planning/management is important and should consist of the care plan, reimbursement consideration, parent teaching, home assessment, actual preparation, and transportation to the home. Proper monitoring and safety measures will improve the chances of successful home treatment. The details of planning and monitoring will vary depending on the patient, family, and environmental needs. Finally, public policy and ethical issues, which are not covered but are upcoming concerns, will need collective efforts to continue these positive steps and further enhance the lives and families of these chronically ill children.

Objectives

Having completed this chapter, the reader should be able to do the following:

1. Discuss the various definitions of home health care.
2. Discuss the financial implications of home health care.
3. Describe the indications for home oxygen therapy.
4. Explain the components of an adequate prescription for home oxygen therapy.
5. Compare and contrast the various types of home oxygen equipment and delivery systems available.
6. Describe the home assessment to be performed before oxygen therapy in the home is begun.
7. Discuss the ways in which infants receiving home oxygen therapy should be monitored.
8. Describe the problems and safety measures associated with the use of oxygen in the home setting.
9. Discuss the importance of physician orders and communication in relation to home oxygen therapy.
10. Describe the uses of aerosol and humidity therapy in the home.
11. Describe the methods and delivery systems used for home aerosol and humidity therapy.
12. Discuss the monitoring of the patient on aerosol/humidity therapy at home.
13. Describe the problems and safety measures associated with the use of aerosols and humidity at home.
14. Discuss the various types of infant apnea that may require monitoring in the home.
15. Explain the process of discharge planning for infant apnea.
16. Describe a typical home support system for the family.
17. State the criteria for discontinuation of home monitoring.
18. Discuss patient selection and discharge criteria for mechanical ventilation in the home.
19. Describe the steps in discharge planning for home mechanical ventilation patients.
20. Discuss the monitoring of home ventilator patients.

References

1. American Association for Respiratory Therapy: Proceedings of the Surgeon General's Regional Workshop on Home Care AARTimes, 8:4, 1984

2. Anton B: Pediatric respiratory therapy beyond the neonatal ICU. Resp Ther 8:19, 1984
3. Blodgett D: Manual of Pediatric Respiratory Care Procedures. Philadelphia, JB Lippincott, 1982
4. Fulmer JD, Snider GL et al: ACCP–NHLBI National Conference on Oxygen Therapy. Chest 86:2, 1984
5. Guilleminault C: Apnea during sleep in infants: Possible relationship with sudden infant death syndrome. Science 190:677, 1975
6. Guilleminault C: Sleep apnea syndromes, impact of sleep and sleep states. Sleep 3(314):277, 1980
7. O'Ryan J, Burns DG: Pulmonary Rehabilitation: From Hospital to Home. Chicago, Year Book Medical, 1984
8. US Government Health Care Financing Administration, Medicare and Medicaid Expenditures, 1983
9. Weinstein S, Steinschneider A: Prolonged infantile apnea: Diagnosis and therapeutic dilemma. J Respir Dis 1(8):76, 1980

Bibliography

Bach J, Alba A et al: Long-term rehabilitation in advanced stages of childhood onset, rapidly progressive muscular dystrophy. Arch Phy Med Rehabil 62:7, 1981

Banaszak EF, Travers H, Frazier M, Vinz T: Home ventilator care. Respir Care 26:1262, 1981

Bell CW, Blodgett D, Goike CA et al: Home Care and Rehabilitation in Respiratory Medicine. Philadelphia, JB Lippincott, 1984

————: Commentaries: Home monitoring and its role in the sudden infant death syndrome. Pediatrics 73:7, 1983

Fisher BA, MacIntyre M: The ethics and responsibilities of home monitoring. Pulm Med Tech 1:4, 1984

Fisher BA, Prentice WS: Feasibility of home care for certain respirator-dependent restrictive and obstructive lung disease patients. Chest 82:739, 1982

Giovannoni R: Chronic ventilator care from hospital to home. Rx Home Care 7:51, 1985

Goldberg AI: Home care for a better life for ventilator-dependent people. Chest 84:4, 1983

Kahn L: Ventilator-dependent children heading home. Hospitals 58:54, 1984

LaMontagne M et al: Home apnea monitoring: Preparing the family. Coordinator 3:30, 1984

Lawrence P: Home care for ventilator-dependent children: Avoiding a chance to live a normal life. Dimens Crit Care Nurs 3:42, 1984

————: Nocturnal oxygen therapy trials: Continuous or nocturnal oxygen therapy in hypoxemic chronic lung disease. Ann Intern Med 93:391, 1980

Purcell JH: Home apnea monitoring: Around-the-clock support. Rx Home Care 6:61, 1984

Waring WW, Jeansonne LO: Practical Manual of Pediatrics, 2nd ed. St. Louis, CV Mosby, 1982

Wasserman AL: A prospective study of the impact of home monitoring on the family. Pediatrics 74:323, 1984

Index

The letter *f* following a page number indicates a figure; the letter *t* following a page number indicates a table.